Milestones in Drug Therapy
MDT

Series Editors
Prof. Dr. Michael J. Parnham
PLIVA
Research Institute
Prilaz baruna Filipovica 25
10000 Zagreb
Croatia

Prof. Dr. J. Bruinvels
INFARM
Sweelincklaan 75
NL-3723 JC Bilthoven
The Netherlands

Modern Immunosuppressives

Edited by H.-J. Schuurman, G. Feutren and J.-F. Bach

Springer Basel AG

Editors

Dr. Henk-Jan Schuurman
Novartis Pharma AG
present address:
Immerge BioTherapeutics
Building 75
3rd Avenue, Charlestown Navy Yard
Charlestown, MA 02129, USA

Dr. Gilles Feutren
Novartis Pharma AG
4002 Basel
Switzerland

Prof. Dr. Jean-François Bach
Immunologie Clinique
Hôpital Necker
161 Rue de Sèvres
Paris Cedex 15
France

Library of Congress Cataloging-in-Publication Data
Modern immunosuppressives / edited by H.-J. Schuurman, G. Feutren, and J.-F. Bach.
    p. ; cm. — (Milestones in drug therapy)
    Includes bibliographical references and index.

    1. Immunosuppressive agents. I. Schuurman, H.-J. (Henk-Jan), 1950- II. Feutren, G. (Gilles) III.
Bach, Jean-François. IV. Series.
    [DNLM: 1. Immunosuppressive Agents—therapeutic use, 2. Autoimmune Diseases—therapy.
3. Biological Products—therapeutic use, 4. Immunosuppression. 5. Transplantation Immunology.
QW 920 M689 2001]
RM373 .M63 2001
615'.37—dc21

2001020346

Deutsche Bibliothek Cataloging-in-Publication Data
Modern Immunosuppressives / ed. by H.-J. Schuurman .... - Basel ; Boston ; Berlin : Birkhäuser, 2001
    (Milestones in drug therapy)

© 2001 Springer Basel AG
Originally published by Birkhäuser Verlag, Basel, Switzerland in 2001

Printed on acid-free paper produced from chlorine-free pulp. TFC ∞
Cover illustration: Mechanism of action of RAPA (see p. 45)

9 8 7 6 5 4 3 2 1

Table of contents

Perspectives

Abbreviations

AAV	adeno-associated virus
ADA	adenosine deaminase
ADCC	antibody-dependent cellular cytotoxicity
ALG	anti-lymphocyte globulin
AMP	adenosine monophosphate
ASC	ascomycin
ATG	anti-thymocyte globulin
AUC	area under the curve
CDC	complement-dependent cytotoxicity
CDR	complementarity-determining region
CI	combination index
C_{max}	maximum blood concentration
$C_{min}0$	pre-dose (trough) level
CMV	cytomegalovirus
CNS	central nervous system
CsA	cyclosporine A
CTL	cytotoxic T-lymphocyte
CYP	cytochrome P
D	dose
Dexa	dexamethasone
Dm	median-effect dose
DRI	dose-reduction index
DSG	15-deoxypergualin
DT	diphtheria toxin
ED	effective dose
ED_{50}	median-effect dose
EDTA	ethylene diamine tetraacetic acid
Ep	enisoprost
ER	estrogen receptor
FasL	Fas ligand
FGF	fibroblast growth factor
FK506	tacrolimus
FKBP	FK-binding proteins
GMP	guanosine monophosphate
GVHD	graft-*versus*-host disease
HAMA	human anti-mouse antibody
HPLC	high performance liquid chromatography
HSP70	heat-shock protein 70
HSV	herpes simplex virus
IC_{50}	median-effect concentration
IFN	interferon
Ig	immunoglobulin

IL-2	interleukin 2
IL-2R	interleukin-2 receptor
IL-10	interleukin 10
IMP	inosine monophosphate
IMPDH	IMP dehydrogenase
IT	immunotoxin
m	exponential coefficient signifying the sigmoidicity of the dose-effect curve
6-MP	6-mercaptopurine
MHC	major histocompatibility complex
MLR	mixed lymphocyte reaction
MMF	mycophenolate mofetil
MMP	matrix metalloprotein
MoLV	Moloney leukemia virus
MPA	mycophenolic acid
MPAG	mycophenolic acic glucuronide
Mtor	mammalian target of RAPA
NIMA	non-inherited maternal antigen
NIPA	non-inherited paternal antigen
PAH	p-aminohippurate
PD	pharmacodynamics
PDGF	platelet-derived growth factor
PEA	*Pseudomonas* exotoxin A
PK	pharmacokinetics
PRPP	phosphoribosyl-1-pyrophosphate
PTDM	post-transplant diabetes mellitus
PTK	protein tyrosine kinase
PUVA	psoralen ultraviolet A
r	linear regression coefficient of the median-effect plot
RAPA	rapamycin
RCMV	rat cytomegalovirus
RSV	Rous sarcoma virus
SA	sulfonamide
SST	somatostatin
SSTR	somatostatin receptor
SV40	simian virus 40
TCR	T-cell antigen receptor
TDM	therapeutic drug monitoring
TGF	transforming growth factor
Th1/2	T-helper type 1/2
TLI	total lymphoid irradiation
t_{max}	time when highest drug levels were measured
TMP	trimethoprim
TNF	tumor necrosis factor
TRL	tacrolimus

List of contributors

Einari Aavik, Transplantation Laboratory and Rational Drug Design Program, Biomedicum, University of Helsinki and Helsinki University Central Hospital, P.O. Box 21, (Haartmaninkatu 3), FIN-00014 Helsinki, Finland; e-mail: einari.aavik@helsinki.fi

Jean-François Bach, INSERM U25, Hôpital Necker, 161 Rue de Sèvres, F-75015 Paris, France; e-mail: bach@necker.fr

Thomas Bühler, Novartis Pharma AG, Transplantation Research, WSJ-386/906, P.O. Box, CH-4002 Basel, Switzerland; e-mail: thomas.buehler@pharma.novartis.com

Suphamai Bunnapradist, Kidney Transplant Program, Cedars-Sinai Medical Center, 8635 W. 3rd Street, Suite 590 W, Los Angeles, CA 90048, USA; e-mail: Mike.Bunnapradist@cshs.org

Roy Calne, Cambridge University, UK (emeritus professor of surgery)

Lucienne Chatenoud, INSERM U25, Hôpital Necker, 161 Rue de Sèvres, F-75015 Paris, France; e-mail: chatenoud@necker.fr

Ting-Chao Chou, Molecular Pharmacology and Therapeutics Program, Memorial Sloan-Kettering Cancer Center, 1275 York Avenue, New York, NY 1002, USA; e-mail: chout@mskcc.org

Gabriel Danovitch, UCLA Medical Center, Renal Transplantation Unit, Department of Nephrology, 10833 LaConte Avenue, Los Angeles, CA 90024, USA; e-mail: gdanovitch@mednet.ucla.edu

Reto A. Gadient, Novartis Pharma AG, Transplantation Research, WSJ-386/906, P.O. Box, CH-4002 Basel, Switzerland

Majed M. Hamawy, University of Wisconsin Medical School, Department of Surgery, 600 Highland Av., Madison, WI 53792-7375, USA; e-mail: hamawy@surgery.wisc.edu

Pekka Häyry, Transplantation Laboratory and Rational Drug Design Program, Biomedicum, University of Helsinki and Helsinki University Central Hospital, P.O. Box 21, (Haartmaninkatu 3), FIN-00014 Helsinki, Finland; e-mail: pekka.hayry@helsinki.fi

Johnny C. Hong, Division of Organ Transplantation, Department of Surgery, The University of Texas Medical School at Houston, 6431 Fannin Street, Suite 6.240, Houston, Texas 77030, USA; e-mail: Johnhong@pol.net

Barry D. Kahan, Division of Organ Transplantation, Department of Surgery, The University of Texas Medical School at Houston, 6431 Fannin St., Suite 6.240, Houston, Texas 77030, USA; e-mail: Barry.D.Kahan@uth.tmc.edu

Paul A. Keown, Vancouver General Hospital, 855 West 12th Ave., Vancouver, BC V5Z 1M9, Canada

Stuart J. Knechtle, University of Wisconsin Medical School, Department of Surgery, 600 Highland Av., Madison, WI 53792-7375, USA; e-mail: stuart@tx.surgery.wisc.edu

Christophe Legendre, Service de Néphrologie, Hôpital Saint Louis, 1, Avenue C. Vellefaux, F-75010 Paris, France; e-mail: christophe.legendre@sls.ap-hop-paris.fr

Gary A. Levy, Multi Organ Transplant Program, Toronto General Hospital, University Health Network, 621 University Avenue, NU-10-116, Toronto, ON, Canada M5G 2C4; e-mail: fgl2@msn.com

Marcel Luyten, Novartis Pharma AG, Transplantation Research, WSJ-386/906, P.O. Box, CH-4002 Basel, Switzerland; e-mail: marcel.luyten@pharma.novartis.com

N. Rao Movva, Novartis Pharma AG, Transplantation Research, WSJ-386/906, P.O. Box, CH-4002 Basel, Switzerland; e-mail: rao.movva@pharma.novartis.com

Gerard F. Murphy, Novartis Pharmaceuticals Canada, 385 Boul. Bouchard, Dorval, PQ, Canada H9S 1A9

Hanna Savolainen, Transplantation Laboratory and Rational Drug Design Program, Biomedicum, University of Helsinki and Helsinki University Central Hospital, P.O. Box 21, (Haartmaninkatu 3), FIN-00014 Helsinki, Finland; e-mail: hanna.savolainen@helsinki.fi

Terry B. Strom, Department of Medicine, Harvard Medical School, Division of Immunology, Beth Israel Deaconess Medical Center, Research North, Room 380, P.O. Box 15707, Boston, MA 02215, USA

Eric Thervet, Service de Néphrologie, Hôpital Saint Louis, 1, Avenue C. Vellefaux, F-75010 Paris, France

David J.G. White, Robarts Research Institute, University of Western Ontario, Siebens Drake Building, 1400 Western Road, London, Ontario, Canada N6G 2V4; e-mail: david.white@rri.on.ca

Serdar Yilmaz, Transplantation Laboratory and Rational Drug Design Program, Biomedicum, University of Helsinki and Helsinki University Central Hospital, P.O. Box 21, (Haartmaninkatu 3), FIN-00014 Helsinki, Finland; e-mail: serdar.yilmaz@crha-health.ab.ca

Preface

Clinical immunosuppression has made substantial advancements during the last decade. This is first evident by the introduction of new immunosuppressives on the market. Hallmarks of the 1980s were the introduction of cyclosporine, which boosted an expansion in clinical transplantation, and subsequently, the introduction of OKT3 monoclonal antibody for induction/rejection treatment, that being the first monoclonal antibody approved for therapeutic use. The 1990s witnessed the introduction of more immunosuppressives, including tacrolimus, mycophenolate mofetil, leflunomide and most recently sirolimus, as well as new monoclonal antibodies including anti-CD52 and anti-CD25 antibodies or anti-TNF α, antibody or fusion-receptor protein. Although most of these new therapeutics have been introduced for clinical transplantation, some of these have been launched for other indications, like anti-TNF α, antibody or leflunomide for rheumatoid arthritis and the anti-CD52 antibody for lymphomas. The anti-CD25 antibodies basiliximab and daclizumab are the first antibodies in clinical medicine that have been genetically engineered, i.e., a chimeric antibody or hyperchimeric or humanized antibody, respectively. Thanks to the larger number of immunosuppressives available, clinicians can design individualized treatment protocols and search for optimal balance between immunosuppression and side-effects in individual patients. Although transplantation forms the major indication of immunosuppressives today, other indications have been established and validated in clinical trials, including for autoimmune diseases like rheumatoid arthritis and psoriasis.

The second boost in clinical immunosuppression has come from a better understanding of the immune system and the host response that need to be suppressed in order to prevent or avoid pathology. To give an example, the interplay between various T-helper subsets (Th1 and Th2) cells and their cytokine products can be mentioned which play different roles in the intitiation of graft rejection and autoimmune diseases. Accompanying this increase in knowledge, phenomena like immune tolerance (in the transplant setting operationally defined as the maintenance of a functioning graft without the need of continuous immunosuppression) are gradually becoming better understood. However, there is a certain imbalance between progress in understanding the immune system and modalities (drugs) presently available to interfere in specific pathways of the immune response. Most immunosuppressive drugs (bio-

---

[1] www.phrma.org/pdf/charts/biotech2.pdf

logicals excluded) have a broad spectrum of interference in immune reactions, which evidently is related to their mechanism of action.

As editors of *Modern Immunosuppressives* we welcomed the opportunity to review present knowledge on immunosuppressive drugs, and to offer this work in the series *Milestones in Drug Therapy*. Although the basis of this monograph focuses on new drugs and advanced clinical development of new modalities, the editors have also chosen to highlight some new avenues in immunosuppression. We are pleased that a number of experts in the field have contributed to this work which comprises three main parts: current immunosuppressives, immunosuppressive biologicals and emerging new therapies for immunosuppression. The latter addresses two major issues that have yet to be resolved, namely chronic graft vasculopathy and immune tolerance, and also reviews the status of gene therapy in organ transplantation. The final section has two chapters dealing with perspectives in immunosuppression. T.-C. Chou and B.D. Kahan present their long experience in dealing with drugs given in combination treatments aimed to achieve synergy in immunosuppression. As synergy is often not used correctly, the mathematical approach outlined is particularly recommended for obtaining proper conclusions on synergy in clinical studies and preclinical models dealing with drug combinations. Finally, J.-F. Bach contributed an overview on the use of cyclosporine in treatment of autoimmune disease. This experience not only addresses the potential use of the immunosuppressive for this indication, but also the incidence of adverse effects which apparently differ from those observed in clinical transplantation. This last chapter clearly illustrates that not only do immunosuppressive drugs developed for the indication transplantation have potential for other indications, but also that experience gained from other indications has value in the transplantation settting. Although the way in which immunosuppressives are applied in various indications might differ, the experience presented shows in a more general sense how clinicans and their patients can benefit from the experience with drugs in other indications.

We determined to compile this monograph of use to clinicians working with immunosuppressives in daily patient care, and for researchers in preclinical and clinical studies. We hope that this volume will give the reader an overview of this fast developing field in biomedicine.

Henk-Jan Schuurman
Gilles Feutren
Jean-François Bach

Modern Immunosuppressives
ed. by H.-J Schuurman, G. Feutren and J.-F. Bach
© 2001 Birkhäuser Verlag/Switzerland

Introduction, global perspectives and history of immunosuppression

Roy Calne[1] and David J.G. White[2]

[1] *Emeritus Professor of Surgery, Cambridge University, and* [2] *Imutran Ltd (A Novartis Pharma AG Company), P.O. Box 399, Cambridge CB2 2YP, UK*

Introduction

For the first 20 years of clinical organ grafting, from the mid-1960s to the mid-1980s, azathioprine and corticosteroids were the lynchpins of immunosuppression. There were some preparations of polyclonal antilymphocyte sera that had proven efficacy although batch variation was a worry to clinicians. Following the introduction of cyclosporine A (CsA) in the early 1980s the results of organ transplantation improved to such a degree that this drug served as a watershed, changing transplantation from a speculative, dangerous and often unsuccessful enterprise, into a form of therapy that was widely used. Clinical transplantation units were established world-wide for transplanting not only kidneys but also hearts, liver, lung, pancreas and multiple organ transplants. Recently this spectrum has been further extended by the early success in transplantation of the hand. The results achieved with CsA stimulated the development of new potent immunosuppressive agents broadly divided into drugs, all of which have side-effects, and biologicals like antibodies.

Related to their mechanism of action, i.e., interference in cellular pathways that are ubiquitous in all celll types, most drugs have serious side-effects. Most immunosuppressive drugs have generalised but some have a more selective immunosuppressive activity. Biologicals like anti-lymphocyte agents present another approach to retaining selectivity of immunosuppressive activity while limiting side-effects. Powerful polyclonal agents have been available since the mid-1960s (anti-thymocyte globulin, ATG; anti-lymphocyte globulin, ALG), of which the use is limited to induction immunosuppression and anti-rejection therapy. Anti-lymphocyte antibodies are not general poisons in the same sense as other drugs but the target molecules against which they react may be present in cells and tissues which are not part of the immune system and therefore undesired effects can still be produced. Monoclonal antibodies are today more attractive as these are directed against a specific (well-defined) molecular target, and quality control is easy and excellent. The anti-T-cell CD3 monoclonal antibody was the first antibody to receive registration approval in the mid-1980s.

Drugs and antibodies together now provide extremely powerful immuno-suppressive cocktails: with the burst of new agents appearing during recent years, the clinician is faced with difficulty in optimal use of the available agents. One special dilemma is that excessive immunosuppression may not only predispose the patient to infection and malignancy but also prevent the natural active control mechanisms that prevent immune reactions from contin-uing in an aggressive manner. Thus excess immunosuppression may prevent the objective of immunological tolerance from being achieved.

The immune system and transplantation

In the 1950s the biological barrier to grafting of tissues within a species was defined and shown to be part of the protective immune system. During embry-onic life the developing immune system is programmed to "live in peace" with its own antigenic profile and can be persuaded to accept as self extraneous for-eign material artificially or accidentally introduced during this formative embryonic state [1].

Once the repertoire "self" products have been established foreign antigen is treated as an invading organism and powerful imunological mechanisms are set in motion to recognise and destroy these "non-self" products, which include bacteria, fungi, viruses, potentially malignant cells, and unfortunately organs and tissues transplants from other individuals. The potential value of organ grafting was first demonstrated clinically by successful kidney grafting between identical twins, where there was no immunological barrier to be over-come. The immune response to grafted tissue is complex and still only par-tially understood but there are two categories: the more primitive non-specific reaction to an invader by neutrophils, macrophages and "natural killer" cells, and acquired specific immunity of lymphocytes. This specific immunity is pri-marily driven by T-cells which can directly destroy the transplant. T-cells can also interact with B-cells to produce antibodies specifically directed towards the transplanted tissue.

The immune system is vital for survival of the individual. Fortunately if one part is destroyed other components can compensate for the defect, i.e., there are alternative resources available. Total destruction of the immune system is only compatible with survival if an alternative new immune system is provid-ed, as in bone marrow transplantation, but the conditioning required for this was found to be too traumatic for sick recipients of organ grafts. Tissue-match-ing for major histocompatibility complex (MHC) antigens between donor and recipient must be close to prevent graft-*versus*-host disease, thereby limiting its application as a method of preventing organ transplant rejection. Although rejection cannot occur before grafting, a patient may be already sensitized by previous blood transfusion, pregnancies or failed grafts. The closer the MHC tissue match between donor and recipient, the better are the results. However, for graft survival other factors like damage to the organ from ischaemia during the operative procedure are also important and so is the innate immune responsiveness of the recipient.

Rejection can occur anytime after grafting: the response varies from immediate hyperacute haemorrhagic destruction of the organ, to (acute) cellular rejection mediated by sensitized T-effector cells, and finally to chronic destruction with arteriole obliteration after years, which currently is still almost irreversible. The common occurrence of acute cellular rejection usually 7–21 days after grafting can in most cases be reversed by pulses of high-dose corticosteroids for a few days or a short course of powerful cytotoxic poly- or mono-clonal anti-lymphocyte antibodies.

Immunosuppressive drugs

In 1959, Schwartz and Darnashek [2] suggested that drug treatment might return the immune system to its receptive embryonic state for a short period during which foreign protein could be injected and would be accepted as "self", even in an adult individual. Rabbits given 14 days treatment with the anti-leukaemia drug 6-mercaptopurine failed to produce antibodies against human serum albumin even after the drug treatment was stopped. 6-Mercaptopurine also prolonged renal allograft survival in dogs [3, 4].

A derivative of 6- mercaptopurine, azathioprine, when used in combination with anti-inflammatory corticosteroids, was the start of effective immunosuppression for clinical renal allograft recipients. However, the results were variable, providing spectacular therapy for some patients, but failure and graft loss in nearly half the cases within a year [5].

The idea that immunological techniques could be used to produce immunosuppressive agents is very old but it was not until the 1960s that effective polyclonal anti-lymphocyte antibodies were available, produced by injecting human lymphocytes in animals [6, 7]. These agents had many specificities and batches varied in efficacy and toxicity. However they proved a useful adjunct to azathioprine and steroid therapy.

In the early 1980s the discovery of the immunosuppressive properties of a fungal metabolite, cyclosporine A (CsA), changed organ transplantation from a risky, unpredictable endeavour to a respectable and much desired form of therapy for many previously untreatable conditions [8]. The development of monoclonal anti-lymphocyte antibodies, each with a single molecular target, was a significant advance on the old polyclonal ALGs or ATGs especially when foreign species protein was removed by genetic egineering techniques to form "humanised" or "chimeric" monoclonal antibodies [9].

In the past decade many new immunosuppressive agents have been studied, some are registered and in clinical use, others are nearly through their clinical trials. The clinician is embarrassed with riches, but there is a danger of adding agents to produce excessive immunosuppression with the risks of infection, malignancy and inhibition of the normal "switch-off' mechanisms that are probably necessary for achieving the goal of tolerance, i.e., maintenance of long-term good graft function without the need of continuous immunosuppression. How can the clinician find a way through the maze of immunological data and theories, much of it derived from studies of animals where species differences in response to drugs in both efficacy and toxicity vary greatly?

The agents available now or to be registered in the near future fall into four categories which are considered by their site of action in relation to the immune response (Tab. 1) [10]:
• Calcineurin inhibitors inhibiting expression of early T-cell activation genes, for instance the expression of interleukin-2 (IL-2) receptors (CsA, FK-506)
• Rapamycins inhibiting growth factor-induced cell proliferation, i.e., the response to IL-2 (Rapamycin, RAD)
• Inhibitors of purine/pyrimidine biosynthesis, i.e., cell proliferation: azathioprine, mizoribine, mycophenolate mofetil, leflunomide, cyclophosphamide
• Depletion or inactivation of cell populations (down-regulation of the antigen on the cell surface); anti-CD3 antibody (OKT3), anti-CD52 (CAMPATH 1H)
• Depletion of activated T-cells (expressing IL-2 receptors): anti-CD25 antibodies, either humanized (daclizumab) or chimeric (basiliximab).

Drug side-effects are quite common. CsA and FK-506 share side-effects like nephrotoxicity, neurotoxicity and glucose intolerance. Both drugs have increased neurotoxicity when administered intravenously, and cyclosporine also can cause gum hypertrophy and increase of body and facial hair. Main side-effects of rapamycins are thrombocytopenia and hyperlipidemia. Main side-effects of mizoribine and mycophenolate are bone marrow depression and gastro-intestinal toxicity especially diarrhoea. Azathioprine shows bone marrow depression and liver toxicity. Side-effects of corticosteroids are Cushing's syndrome, growth stunting, bone necrosis, diabetes, and gastric ulcers.

Transplant patients normally receive combinations of drugs in order to exploit synergy, e.g., between rapamycins and calcineurin inhibitors. However, the active agents each have side-effects, either related or unrelated to their immunosuppressive properties, which can be additive in combination. Also, there can be pharmacokinetic interaction with other drugs either at the absorbtion metabolism or at the excretion level, thereby significantly affecting blood levels and drug exposure.

Polyclonal anti-lymphocyte reagents have beem on the market since the mid-1960s (ATG, ALG) and they kill or inhibit lymphocytes. The antibodies bind to many different sites on the cell surface. Upon administration there may be a first dose cytokine-release syndrome varying from mild headache and feeling unwell, to severe collapse of the circulation. This can be prevented in most cases by a bolus steroid dose given 30–60 min before administration of the globulin. The anti-CD3 antibody was the first mouse monoclonal antibody approved for clinical use in the mid-1980s. A cytokine-release syndrome can also be observed for this antibody, which can be quite severe. Therefore anti-CD3 treatment should be done within a prophylactic steroid bolus. The

Table 1. Main immunosuppressants presently on the market or in advanced clinical development

Compound	Trade name	Mechanism of action
Xenobiotics		
Cyclosporine	Neoral	calcineurin inhibitor
FK506, tacrolimus	Prograf	calcineurin inhibitor
Rapamycin, sirolimus	Rapamune	inhibitor of growth factor-driven cell proliferation
RAD, everolimus	Certican	inhibitor of growth factor-driven cell proliferation
Cyclophosphamide		inhibitor of cell proliferation
Methotrexate		inhibitor of cell proliferation: anti-inflammatory
Azathioprine	Imuran	inhibitor of cell proliferation
Mizoribine	Bredinin	inhibitor of inosine monophosphate dehydrogenase
Mycophenolate mofetil	Cellcept	inhibitor of inosine monophosphate dehydrogenase
Leflunomide	Arava	inhibitor of dihydroorotate dehydrogenase
15-Deoxyspergualin	Spanidin	inhibitor of cell differentiation
Biologicals		
OKT3	Orthoclone-OKT3	T-cell depletion
CD25 antibody, basiliximab	Simulect	depletion of CD25-positive T-cells
CD25 antibody, daclizumab	Zenapax	depletion of CD25-positive T-cells
CD4 antibody		depletion of CD4-positive cells
CD52 antibody	Enlimomab	depletion of leukocytes
anti-TNFα antibody	Remicade	TNF blockade
CTLA4-Ig		inhibition of costimulation

Data modified from reference [10]

humanized or chimeric anti-CD25 antibodies have been on the market since the late 1990s for use in induction immunosuppression. They are without side-effects, notably, no cytokine-release syndrome.

The anti-CD52 antibody (CAMPATH 1H) has been introduced in the clinic as treatment for leukemia/lymphoma [11]. It is also used as treatment for autoimmune diseases. It is not yet registered as an immunosuppressant in transplantation. The CD52 antigen is a peptide linked to a membrane glyco-protein present on all lymphocytes, monocytes and macrophages. CAMPATH 1H causes marked depletion of lymphocytes: the depletion of CD4$^+$ cells may persist for years. Following the protocol presented below it has potential application to achieve "almost tolerance".

The future: tolerance

From the patient's point of view the objective of transplantation is for an organ graft which functions for many years and restores health without the burden of drug side-effects. In the attempt to achieve this objective, the clinician should aim at the best matched donor, minimal ischaemia, skilful surgery and immuno-suppression designed to avoid all known side-effects of these agents, preferably used in such a way that a tolerant state of graft acceptance develops which elim-inates the need for continuous life-long maintenance immunosuppression. Some patients with liver grafts have achieved this goal. The world's longest survivor after liver grafting, now 25 years post-transplantation, has taken no immunosuppression for the past 15 years [12]. Several patients with accepted bone marrow grafts who developed renal failure have had kidney grafts from the bone marrow donor without the need for further immunosuppression.

Probably there are several potential routes to "operational tolerance". It has to be emphasized that there is currently no *in vitro* test to determine whether or not a patient could stop immunosuppression, and enter or maintain a toler-ant state. This might be ultimately required to avoid the worry that specific graft rejection in patients off immunosuppression and with stable graft func-tion could occur, for instance precipitated by an intercurrent immunological stimulus like a viral infection (flu) or an allergic reaction.

One approach aimed at achieving operational tolerance with a relatively short follow-up in recipients with cadaveric renal allografts has been called "almost" or the Latin *prope* tolerance [13]. On return from surgery, the patients are given an intravenous dose of 20 mg anti-CD52 antibody CAMPATH 1H and the next day a second and final dose; subsequently no immunosuppression is given for 48 h, and thereafter the patients are maintained on monotherapy with half-dose CsA to produce blood trough levels around 100 ng/ml. The lymphocyte counts fall close to zero for 1 month and then recover slowly. Infection prophylaxis is the same as for patients receiving standard immuno-suppression. Of 31 consecutive cases treated this way no renal allografts have been lost to rejection. One patient with severe heart failure died of this condi-tion with a functioning allograft at 11 months; the remaining 30 patients are alive with functioning grafts. There have been five cases of acute rejection, all of which responded to steroid bolus therapy. Infections have been comparable to those expected on standard therapy and there have been no malignancies. Serum creatinine levels have remained stable with no evidence of chronic rejection so far. The results are encouraging, especially for the patients off steroids and receiving non-toxic doses of cyclosporine. The protocol was derived by extrapolation from animal experiments and clinical data on the use of CAMPATH 1H in patients with auto-immune diseases. Although many vari-ations of this protocol could be devised using the same or alternative agents, a clinical randomised trial is currently underway using the above protocol com-pared with standard immunosuppression. *Prope* tolerance could be a step on the road to true "operational tolerance".

References

1 Billingham B, Medawar (1956) Antigenic stimulus in transplantation immunity. *Proc Trans R Soc* 2nd Bulletin 239: 375
2 Schwartz R, Damashek W (1959) Drug induced immunologic tolerance. *Nature* 183: 1682
3 Calne RY (1960) The rejection of renal homografts: Inhibition in dogs by 6-mercaptopurine. *Lancet* 1: 417–418
4 Calne RY (1961) Inhibition of the rejection of renal homographs in dogs by purine analogues. *Transplant Bull* 28: 445–461
5 Murray JE, Merrill JP, Harrison JH et al (1963) Prolonged survival of human kidney homografts by immunosuppressive drug therapy. *N Engl J Med* 268; 1315
6 Waksman BH, Arbouys S, Arnason BG (1961) The use of specific "lymphocytye antisera" to inhibit hypersensitive reactions of the delayed type. *J Exp Med* 114: 997
7 Woodruff MFA, Anderson NF (1963) Effect of lymphocyte depletion by thoracic duct fistula and administration of anti-lymphocytic scrum on the survival of skin homografts in rats. *Nature* 200: 702
8 Calne RY, Rolles K, White DJG, Thiru S, Evans DB, McMaster P, Dunn DC, Craddock GN, Henderson RG, Aziz S et al (1979) Cyclosporin A initially as the only immunosuppressant in 34 recipients of cadaveric organs: 32 kidneys, 2 pancreases, and 2 livers. *Lancet* 2: 1033–1036
9 Winter G, Milstein C (1991) Man-made antibodies. *Nature* 349: 293–299
10 Schuurman H-J, Zenke G, Schreier MH (1999) Immunosuppressives: transplant rejection inhibitors and cytotoxic drugs. *In*: FP Nijkamp, MJ Parnham (eds): *Principles of Immunopharmacology*. Birkhäuser Verlag, Basel, Chapter C8: 337–360
11 Hale G, Dyer MJ, Clark MR, Phillips JM, Marcus R, Riechmann L, Winter G, Waldmann H (1988) Remission induction in non-Hodgkin lymphoma with reshaped human monoclonal antibody CAMPATH-1H. *Lancet* 2: 1394–1399
12 Starzl TE, Demetris AJ, Trucco M (1996) Cell migration, chimerism, and graft acceptance, with particular reference to the liver. *In*: RW Busuttil, GB Klintmalm (eds): *Transplantation of the liver*. WB Saunders, London, 274–287
13 Calne R, Friend P, Moffatt S, Bradley A, Hale G, Firth J, Bradley J, Smith K, Waldmann H (1998) Prope tolerance, perioperative Campath 1H, and low-dose cyclosporin monotherapy in renal allograft recipients. *Lancet* 351: 1701–1702

Immunosuppressive drugs

Modern Immunosuppressives
ed. by H.-J Schuurman, G. Feutren and J.-F. Bach
© 2001 Birkhäuser Verlag/Switzerland

Cyclosporine: role of pharmacokinetics

Gary A. Levy[1], Gerard F. Murphy[2] and Paul A. Keown[3]

[1] Multi Organ Transplant Program, Toronto General Hospital, University Health Network, 621 University Avenue, NU-10-116, Toronto, ON, Canada M5G 2C4
[2] Novartis Pharmaceuticals Canada, 385 Boul. Bouchard, Dorval, PQ H9S 119, Canada
[3] Vancouver General Hospital, 855 West 12th Ave., Vancouver, BC V5Z 1M9, Canada

Introduction

The introduction of the immunosuppressive agent cyclosporine (CsA) in the early 1980s was a major advance both in our understanding of the pathogenesis and treatment of allograft rejection [1, 2]. The use of CsA resulted not only in a marked reduction in the incidence of acute cellular rejection, increased patient and graft survival in renal transplant recipients, who previously had been treated with azathioprine and prednisone, but also allowed for the establishment of successful liver, heart, pancreas, lung and small bowel transplant programs.

Incomplete, unpredictable and inconsistent absorption from the previous galenic formulation of CsA, Sandimmune, limited the clinical use of this agent in transplantation [3]). The pharmacokinetic problems were reflected in our inability to define optimal doses to maximize the efficacy and minimize toxicity, especially nephrotoxicity (low therapeutic index). It has been suggested that low intra- and inter-patient variability and a high bioavailability is essential for therapeutic monitoring to be of use [4, 5]. Bioavailability is defined as the rate and extent to which the active drug ingredient or therapeutic moiety is absorbed from a drug product and becomes available at the site of drug action. With Sandimmune, bioavailability is erratic and ranges from 3% to 50%; furthermore, it is profoundly influenced by bile flow, food, gastrointestinal motility, use of concomitant drugs and changes in these factors over time post-transplant [6–8]. This variability has been shown to be an important risk factor for the development of acute and chronic rejection and nephrotoxicity [9–11]. The presence of cytochrome P (CYP) 450 3A4 isoenzymes in the gastrointestinal tract has been shown to be a major reason for the poor and variable bioavailability of Sandimmune. Factors influencing CYP450 will have an effect on metabolic clearance of the drug. Enzyme inducers (phenobarb, steroids, rifampicin) and inhibitors (ketoconazole, erythromycin) will affect bioavailability. Tissue activity of the CYP450 3A4 enzyme changes over time post-transplant and may play a role in determining CsA levels in organs at steady-state.

The initial use of Sandimmune was not associated with therapeutic drug monitoring (TDM) strategies. However, problems with nephrotoxicity were soon recognized and the concept of individualizing the dose based on a target trough level ($C_{min}0$) was established. It was assumed that monitoring of $C_{min}0$ would be the most reproducible value reflecting drug exposure, and least likely to be affected by drug absorption and distribution phases [12, 13]. Unfortunately, this assumption has proven to be inaccurate. The impact of diurnal variation leading to delayed absorption in the overnight dosing interval resulted in variation in $C_{min}0$ within the same patient and at the same dose [3, 14].

Another issue which has confounded the data is the lack of a practical, uniform measure of CsA parent compound in blood samples. Initial assays of serum samples utilized polyclonal antibodies which recognized both the parent molecule and its metabolites [15]. Metabolic profiles following administration of CsA may differ in different organ groups and may vary over time post-transplantation reflecting changes in hepatic function and biliary excretion of metabolites. The introduction of assays in whole blood utilizing monoclonal antibodies with greater specificity for parent compound has largely, but not entirely solved this problem [16]. The gold standard (high pressure liquid chromatography, HPLC) is impractical in the clinical setting. Presently, the multiplicity of assays with varying crossreactivity with metabolites has impeded standardization of target levels.

To address some of these deficiencies, a new microemulsion formulation of Cyclosporine, Neoral, has been developed [17]. This formulation incorporates Cyclosporine in a microsuspension preconcentrate with a surfactant, lipophilic and hydrophilic solvents and a hydrophilic cosolvent forming a self-stabilizing microemulsion in aqueous media. Using this preparation, Cyclosporine is rapidly and more completely absorbed from Neoral by the gastrointestinal tract so that blood concentrations reach a higher peak concentration (C_{max}) within a shorter time to reach maximum concentration (T_{max}) than with Sandimmune [18]. Importantly, dispersion of the microemulsion formulation within the intestinal tract does not rely in emulsification with bile salts. Cyclosporine is therefore absorbed from the small intestine more uniformly from Neoral than from Sandimmune, providing a closer correlation between dose and exposure assesed as area under the time-concentration curve (AUC) and trough blood levels of CsA ($C_{min}0$), and less inter- and intra-patient variation [19, 20]. Furthermore, Koravik et al. [21] have shown that Neoral provides superior within-day consistency of CsA pharmacokinetics compared to Sandimmune. At steady-state in stable renal transplant recipients, there is a more stable concentration time profile over the two dosing intervals which may explain the superior relationship of $C_{min}0$ and AUC, for Neoral [21]. However, the correlation between $C_{min}0$ and AUC although markedly better for Neoral than Sandimmune, is still insufficient to reflect AUC by itself [22].

The molecular basis of immunosuppressive effects of CsA has now been identified [23–25]. Once CsA enters the cell, it binds to a ubiquitous intracellular protein, cyclophilin. This binary complex is the active drug which engages calcineurin [26], a widely distributed calcium-activated serine phosphatase, and inhibits its activity. Inhibition of calcineurin activity prevents the activation of transcription factors such as nuclear factor for activated T-cells (NFAT) which are essential for the induction of interleukin 2 and probably other T-cell responses to antigen. Calcineurin activity is the rate-limiting step for the activation of primary human T-lymphocytes. Cyclosporine produces incomplete calcineurin inhibition in lymphocytes of CsA-treated patients [27]. In *de novo* renal transplants, peak CsA levels of early post-dose produce 70–90% calcineurin inhibition. Calcineurin inhibition closely correlated with the rise and fall of CsA levels with no lag time. Repeated measurements in *de novo* renal transplant patients showed similar inhibition to the first dose of Cyclosporine with no adaptation over time. It has been speculated that calcineurin inhibition might be greater in some tissues due to drug accumulation which may have implications for organ toxicity (Phil Halloran, personal communication). From *in vivo* studies in liver patients, it has been shown that blood CsA levels do not reflect tissue levels [28]. Thus, local levels may influence the biological response in different organs at the same ambient blood levels.

Additional studies in renal transplant patients receiving CsA for 1 month, have shown a relationship between renal function over the dosing interval and the rise and fall of CsA levels. The nadir of glomerular filtration rate occurred 2–4 h after maximal CsA levels (4–6 h post-dose) and returned to baseline by the end of the 12-h dosing interval. Similar results occurred with renal plasma flow, hypoperfusion occurred 2–4 h after peak blood concentrations were reached, and returned to within the normal range in the subsequent 6 h which may reflect the falling CsA levels with corresponding restoration of calcineurin activity. It has been postulated that excessive renal synthesis of endothelin was the cause of renal hypoperfusion [29].

The introduction of Neoral as a superior formulation of CsA has led to an evaluation of the traditional approach to therapeutic drug monitoring of cyclosporine based on trough levels ($C_{min}0$) [30]. The improved and more consistent AUCs seen in patients taking Neoral as compared with Sandimmune have been demonstrated in several studies in *de novo* renal [31–36], liver [37–41], lung [42], and cardiac transplant recipients [43]. Furthermore, several open-labeled studies have also documented a significant reduction in the incidence of acute cellular rejection in Neoral-treated *versus* Sandimmune-treated *de novo* renal and liver transplant recipients, which strongly supports the important influence of consistent and enhanced bioavailability of CsA on clinical outcomes in transplant recipients [44].

The influence of CsA pharmacokinetics on clinical outcomes using Neoral has reawakened interest in the utility of monitoring blood concentrations of cyclosporine. Furthermore, it has stimulated exploration of other therapeutic monitoring strategies with a focus on sparse-sampling-derived AUCs and single point sampling taken in the early post-dose period using methods to provide better efficacy and reduced toxicity profiles. The focus of this chapter will be to describe the emerging evidence that a relationship exists between pharmacokinetics and clinical outcomes.

Therapeutic drug monitoring strategies

For drugs with a low therapeutic index (narrow window between efficacy and toxicity) which are used in critically ill patients, whose status is changing over time, it has been suggested that TDM is essential [45]. To this end, applied pharmacokinetics, that is, a strategy by which dosing regimens for patients are guided by repeated measurements of plasma/whole blood drugs concentrations, must be adopted. Thus, if the drug concentration is not within the "target concentration range", the dose is adjusted accordingly. Drug concentrations above the target range are defined as toxic and below the range as subtherapeutic. The use of pharmacokinetics has been established for a number of drugs and conditions and this topic has been extensively reviewed by Spector et al. [45].

Assumptions are implicit in the use of target concentration strategies. The first is that the target concentration strategy used to adjust drug doses decreases variability in blood drug concentration. A second assumption is that there is a clear relationship between blood drug concentration and the drug's pharmacologic effects. The first assumption includes drug dissolution, absorption, distribution and excretion, which all contribute to variability in the relationship between drug dose and blood concentration. The second includes all factors that contribute to variability in the relationship between plasma drug concentration and pharmacologic effect. It has been recognized that large interindividual variations exist in the relationship between the dose of the drug and drug concentration. The magnitude of these inter individual variations can be as high as forty-fold in some instances. As a consequence of this, the same dose of the drug given to different patients can produce high levels in some, the desired level in others and subtherapeutic (low) levels in many individuals. A number of studies have shown that repeated pharmacokinetic studies can reduce inter- and intra-patient variability in blood drug concentrations, thus allowing the investigator to select appropriate doses of drug for a particular patient. Furthermore, even if the appropriate drug level is reached, the pharmacologic effect within the patient may vary over time due to changes in age, diet, alterations in plasma binding protein levels and activity, the presence of metabolites and the use of other drugs which can affect the metabolism, binding and elimination of the drug.

It has been suggested that certain criteria must be fulfilled for the effective use of pharmacokinetics (Tab. 1). Comparisons of Sandimmune and Neoral suggests that pharmacokinetics can be more effectively utilized with Neoral due to its more consistent absorption profile although pharmacokinetic data, especially in the early post-transplantation period are lacking to derive definitive conclusions about the use of TDM and Cyclosporine A. In the use of other

Table 1. Criteria for use of target concentration strategies

Criteria	Sandimmune	Neoral
Appropriate assay	HPLC	HPLC
Significant interindividual and intraindividual variability in drug absorption elimination and distribution	++++	+
Adequate pharmacokinetic data available	+	+++
Pharmacologic effect is proportional to blood drug concentration	not known	not known
A narrow range between efficacy and toxicity	+	+
Constant pharmacologic effect over time	not known	not known
Studies done to define therapeutic and toxic drug ranges	no	no

From [45]
HPLC - high pressure liquid chromatography
+   - positive
+++   - very positive
++++ - markedly positive

drugs, however, simple routine measurements of a single parameter have rarely been successfully utilized to monitor critical drugs such as Cyclosporine A.

Importance of pharmacokinetics to clinical outcomes

Use of $C_{min}0$ (trough concentration)

Initial TDM of CsA utilized samples drawn at trough, namely, the time immediately before the next dose is administered ($C_{min}0$) [3]. This was chosen as it was thought to be the most reproducible value, least likely to be affected by drug absorption and distribution. On examination of $C_{min}0$ records from patients experiencing toxic complications of CsA therapy, a serum trough level of 250 ng/ml was established as the upper limit of the putative therapeutic window. The lower limit of the therapeutic window was assumed to correspond to the dose of CsA necessary to cause a 50% inhibition of an *in vitro* mixed lymphocyte reaction and was found to be 100 ng/ml [12]. A correlation was found between the incidence of acute cellular rejection episodes and the number of days required to achieve the target level (100 ng/ml). Patients who achieved the target range early had a markedly reduced incidence and severity of rejection

[12]. Thus, based on clinical experience, the apparent therapeutic window for trough serum CsA levels (assessed by radioimmunoassy) in the immediate post-transplantation period was 100–250 ng/ml. However, when re-analyzed by HPLC, the level in whole blood was found to be 100–150 ng/ml. However, this target did not take into consideration variable CsA pharmacodynamics and the presence of drugs which might affect metabolism of CsA or directly cause nephrotoxicity.

Using, these "guidelines" transplant centers successfully instituted CsA regimes with acceptable rejection rates and toxicity profiles. While Neoral has improved bioavailability and pharmacokinetic parameters, studies undertaken in renal, heart, liver and lung patients using $C_{min}0$ strategies have not uniformly shown that improved pharmacokinetics translate to improved clinical outcome, namely a reduction in the incidence of acute cellular rejection. In multicentered trials in lung, heart, heart-lung, kidney and liver patients, the institution of Neoral in *de novo* transplant recipients was associated with high C_{max}, earlier T_{max}, and higher AUC in comparison to patients receiving Sandimmune. Furthermore, in all studies there was markedly less inter- and intra-patient variability and a closer correlation between $C_{min}0$ and AUC. In studies involving liver transplant recipients, dependence on bile was markedly less in patients who received Neoral, and target trough levels could be achieved without the need for intravenous CsA [44]. A number of controlled open and blinded studies, primarily in renal and liver patients, have now been undertaken to test the hypothesis that the improved pharmacokinetic profiles associated with Neoral would result in a reduction in the incidence of acute cellular rejection [31–41]. In some of these studies, Neoral clearly was superior to Sandimmune with increased drug exposure, less intra- and inter-patient variability in pharmacokinetic profiles, and a highly statistical reduction in the incidence of rejection without incremental toxicity [31, 32, 40, 41]. In a multinational renal study, the number of patients experiencing acute rejection was significantly reduced for the Neoral group (44.2% *versus* 60.5%; $p = 0.04$), and significantly fewer patients experienced multiple episodes of rejection (12.8% *versus* 22.2%; $p = 0.028$) [31]. However, these results were not universal, and in many cases increased or equivalent rejection rates were observed in patients who received Neoral and Sandimmune (Tab. 2). On further analysis, simultaneous administration of intravenous CsA with Neoral negated the benefit and these patients had significantly more rejection episodes than patients not receiving intravenous CsA [32]. These data suggest that important pharmacokinetic parameters including ability to achieve high C_{max} may be important in freedom from rejection [30]. It is also clear from these studies that although the relationship between $C_{min}0$ and AUC is markedly improved with Neoral ($r^2 = 0.80$), it is still not sufficient to allow its use to predict total exposure (AUC) [30]. Furthermore, data is emerging to suggest that absorption of Neoral in the early postoperative period is still unpredictable using trough level strategies.

Thus, from these studies it has been suggested that the $C_{min}0$ value as a monitoring tool for CsA therapy may not be sufficient to maximize immune

Table 2. Incidence of rejection in patients receiving Neoral/Sandimmune

Organ	Reference	Study design	Incidence of rejection (%)		
			Neoral	Sandimmune	P
Renal	Barone [33]	db/mc	37	30	n.s.
	Frei [36]	db/mc	44	51	n.s.
	Keown [31]	db/mc	44	61	<0.05
	Korn [35]	nb/mc	36	56	n.s.
	Lodge [32]	nb/mc	32	46	<0.05
	Niese [34]	db/mc	42	65	n.s.
Liver	Donovan [37]	db/mc	63	59	n.s.
	Gradziadei [38]	b/sc	53	56	n.s.
	Grant [39]	nb/mc	54	33	n.s.
	Otto [40]	db/mc	48	53	<0.05
	Pinson [41]	nb/mc	56	87	<0.05

db - double-blind
nb - non-blinded
mc - multi-centered
sc - single-centered
n.s.- not significant
numbers in brackets [] refer to reference citation

suppression while at the same time minimize toxicity. It has been suggested that alternative TDM methods may be required to determine more sensitive and more predictive pharmacokinetic markers for optimal management of CsA therapy.

Use of alternative strategies

Total exposure (area under the curve, AUC)

It has been suggested that full AUC monitoring is the most sensitive and precise indicator of drug exposure [46]. With CsA, this was first demonstrated by Lindholm and Kahan to assess the importance of cyclosporine pharmacokinetics on renal graft outcome and acute rejection episodes [47]. A number of pivotal studies were performed with Sandimmune utilizing pre- and post-transplant whole-blood cyclosporine pharmacokinetic profiles from patients undergoing renal transplantation, which demonstrated that large inter- and intraindividual variability in the CsA pharmacokinetic parameters bioavailability and clearance rate correlated with poor patient and graft outcome [48].

Several important relationships were suggested between CsA pharmacokinetic parameters and outcome and incidence of acute cellular rejection after kidney transplantation. Post transplant bioavailability (AUC) values less than 25% of the cohort and clearance values greater than 1500 ml/min were especially associated with high rates of rejection and poor graft survival. Patients with average concentration of CsA greater than 550 ng/ml during their first oral study in the early post transplantation period had low incidences of acute rejection.

Additional studies were performed at the University of Texas involving 204 adult renal transplant patients. Based upon pharmacokinetic profiles that were obtained over a 5-year period in patients receiving Sandimmune, it was found that intra-patient variability of greater than 20% over time was a significant risk factor for the development of chronic rejection. These studies demonstrated that many patients who had a high CsA pharmacokinetic variability early in the postoperative period continued to exhibit this variability even 8 years post transplantation. Furthermore, using mathematical modeling, this group and others were able to define variability thresholds for development and freedom of chronic rejection. In those patients with low variability 10-year graft survival and patient survival exceeded 90%, whereas when the variability was high graft survival and patient survival was only 57%. Studies recently undertaken in patients who received Neoral have now shown lower intra-patient variability of AUC than in those patients who received Sandimmune, thus suggesting that monitoring of AUC will be more effective and may be achievable by sparse sampling algorithms [49, 50]. These studies collectively suggested than $C_{min}0$ is not sensitive enough to predict for freedom from rejection and that multiple time point measurements may be required for optimal management of CsA therapy using Neoral.

Sparse sampling algorithms: AUC

The use of sparse sampling models for estimation of CsA AUC values was instituted by a number of investigators [51, 52]. In an analysis of full AUC profiles from renal transplant patients, it was shown that three sampling points taken at 3, 8 and 10 h post-CsA dose could estimate the full AUC with 99% accuracy. When the algorithm was adapted to cardiac transplant recipients the relationship held. On further analysis of stable renal transplant recipients, samples taken at 1.5 and 5 h predicted AUC with a 95% accuracy (Tab. 3). If sampling times were limited to 4 h or less after drug administration, the best combination, 1 and 4 h post-dose, had an error prediction of 24%. If three sampling time points were chosen, the best combination, 0, 1 and 3 h post-dose, had a 23% prediction error. Further analysis of sparse sampling strategies by Johnston et al. [50–52] showed that the same concepts could be utilized for all organ systems, adult and pediatric.

A recent study in *de novo* renal transplant recipients compared the accuracy and utility of a sparse sample algorithm (2 and 6 h post-dose) to predict full AUC, and found this to be better in stable patients ($r^2 = 0.97$) than in *de novo* patients ($r^2 = 0.92$). It was suggested that the poorer correlation in the early post-transplantation period was due to delayed gastric emptying and distur-

Table 3. Relationship between sparse sampling algorithms and AUC (0–12 h) using Neoral

Predictor	r^2
C0 + C1 + C2 + C3 + C4	.971
C0 + C1 + C2 + C3	.969
C0 + C1 + C2 + C4	.971
C0 + C1 + C3 + C4	.966
C0 + C2 + C3 + C4	.922
C0 + C1 + C2	.967
C0 + C1 + C3	.964
C0 + C2 + C3	.912
C0 + C1 + C4	.957
C0 + C2 + C4	.901
C0 + C1	.856
C0 + C2	.900
C0 + C3	.842
C0	.723
C1	.592
C2	.755
C3	.777
C4	.844

Studies undertaken in 55 stable renal transplant patients on two separate occasions [49].

bances in gastrointestinal motility. Thus in the early post-transplantation peri-od the T_{max} would be more prolonged, gradually decreasing by 2 weeks post-transplantation. Based upon these results, it was suggested that full AUC mon-itoring might be necessary in the first few weeks post-transplantation with institution of sparse sample strategies for long-term monitoring of CsA [50].

In a study recently conducted at Dalhousie University, Halifax, Canada, a strong association between freedom from rejection and AUC levels using sparse sample algorithms in adult *de novo* renal transplant recipients was demonstrated [53]. Immune suppression consisted of Neoral and prednisone and AUC was calculated based on samples collected at 0,1,2,3 and 4 h post dose. In this study, $C_{min}0$ (trough) correlated poorly with both AUC_{0-12} and AUC_{0-4} and freedom from rejection, whereas in patients who achieved AUC measured for the first 4 h of the dosing interval (AUC_{0-4}) of 4500–5500 µg·h/l acute cellular rejection was markedly attenuated without a significant increase in toxicity.

A study was recently conducted in Canada to examine the role of AUC monitoring in stable renal transplant recipients. One thousand and ninety seven (1097) stable renal transplant recipients on Sandimmune in 14 Canadian cen-ters were randomized to treatment with Neoral or Sandimmune. In those patients who were converted to Neoral, the absorption of CsA was more rapid and complete during the first 4 h of the dosing interval, resulting in almost

40% greater exposure. There was a close correlation between AUC_{0-4} and AUC over the entire 12-h dosage interval for both formulations of CsA, making AUC_{0-4} a good predictor of total CsA exposure. Patients previously on Sandimmune with low absorption who were randomized to receive Neoral showed a marked increase in drug exposure by 3 and 6 months post-transplantation, whereas there was no change in those who continued to receive Sandimmune. It was concluded that a limited sampling strategy utilizing samples at the pre-dose and post-dose trough levels provided an excellent correlation with AUC, particularly for those patients who were receiving Neoral ($r^2 = 0.94$ Neoral *versus* $r^2 = 0.89$ Sandimmune).

Concentration 2 h after drug intake (C2)

Prospective studies, primarily in liver transplant recipients, have demonstrated that absorption of Neoral is relatively independent of bile flow and food intake and provides increased Cyclosporine bioavailability (AUC) with a higher C_{max} and no increase in toxicity [54, 55]. Recent open-label studies using Neoral in liver transplant recipients have suggested that the improved pharmacokinetics of Neoral may allow for improved clinical outcomes including a reduction in the incidence of acute cellular rejection [44]. To examine this, a prospective randomized double-blind multicenter trial was undertaken in Canada to compare two treatment groups for incidence of acute cellular rejection, correlation between CsA pharmacokinetics and clinical events and requirement for intravenous CsA to achieve target levels [56].

Rejection rates in the Neoral-treated patients who achieved C_{max} values greater than 800 ng/ml or AUC_{0-6} greater than 3300 µg·h/l were 28.6% and 33.3% respectively (Fig. 1). A similar relationship was seen in patients who received Sandimmune, however, as compared with Neoral fewer patients receiving Sandimmune achieved high C_{max} or AUC values. In patients who received Neoral, C2 proved to be an excellent surrogate marker of AUC_{0-6} and C_{max} ($r^2 = 0.93$), whereas the relationship of C2 to AUC in the Sandimmune group was not as good ($r^2 = 0.73$). No relationship between C0 (trough level) and freedom from rejection was observed in either group, even when C0 approached or exceeded 450 ng/ml. The relationship of C2 with C_{max} was less strong early in the postoperative period (<5 days), but was excellent thereafter.

The data sets were divided into four equal quartiles of $C_{min}0$ ranges (<250 ng/ml; 250–300; 300–400 and greater than 400 ng/ml). In none of the quartiles was there a trend towards freedom from acute rejection and increase in $C_{min}0$ values (Tab. 4). Conversely, when C_{max} quartiles were examined for incidence of rejection, there was significant reduction in the incidence of rejection in patients who achieved higher C_{max}. The relationship was similar for patients who received either Sandimmune or Neoral, but only reached statistical significance in the Neoral group (70% of the highest quartile were on

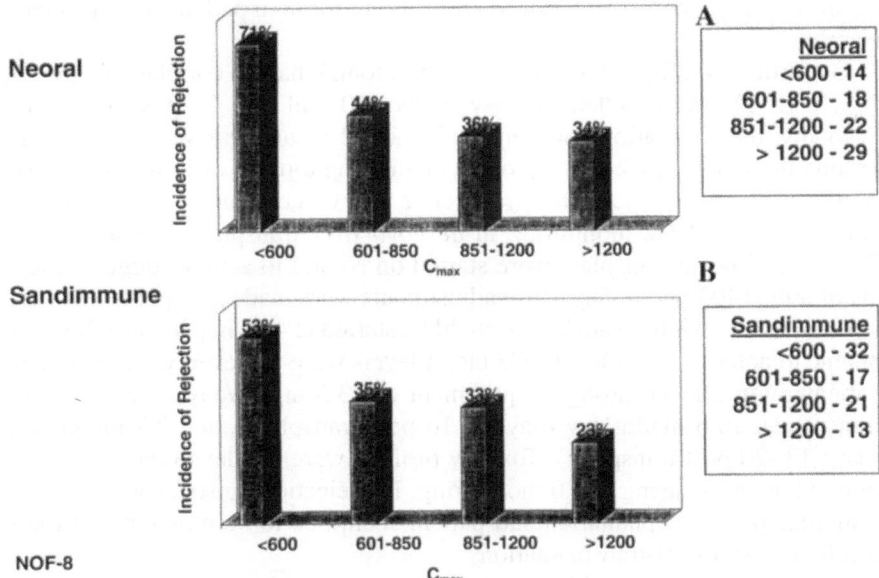

Figure 1. Relationship of rejection between C2 and C_{max}. Liver patients were treated with (A) Neoral or (B) Sandimmune. Retrospectively patients were divided into four equal C_{max} quartiles and incidence of rejection analyzed (Study NOF-8).

Table 4. Relationship of pharmacokinetic parameters and graft rejection

Parameter	Week	Quartile	Neoral			Sandimmune		
			n/N	%	P	n/N	%	P
C_{max}	2	1	10/14	71.4		15/29	51.7	
		2	8/19	42.1	0.019	8/23	34.8	0.087
		3	8/23	34.8		7/19	36.8	
		4	9/29	31.0		3.13	23.1	
AUC	2	1	9/13	69.2		17/30	56.7	
		2	8/18	44.4	0.026	6/24	25.0	0.060
		3	9/25	36.0		7/17	41.2	
		4	9/29	31.0		3/13	23.1	
C0	2	1	11/21	52.4		9/22	40.9	
		2	8/20	40.4	0.417	7/22	31.8	0.894
		3	7/23	30.4		9/19	47.4	
		4	9/21	42.9		8/21	38.1	

The quartiles were developed by dividing patients into four groups based on CsA levels.
Data from Study NOF-8 [56].

Neoral). This reflects the enhanced absorption profile in patients who received Neoral.

On further examination of the data, it was found that the correlation between C_{max} and C2 was excellent on day 3, day 10 and day 21 post transplant. Secondly, the correlation between AUC and C2 values was very strong, suggesting the utility of C2 as a surrogate monitoring tool for cyclosporine TDM.

Recently, a small open-label prospective trial was conducted to examine the clinical utility of C2 monitoring in *de novo* liver transplant recipients [57]. Patients following transplant were started on Neoral to achieve target C2 levels of 800–1400 ng/ml. Oral dose adjustments were made if target levels were not achieved and intravenous CsA could be started at 48 h in patients who were unable to achieve target levels. C2 target levels were achieved with 48 h in all patients with a mean dosage requirement of 13.5 mg/kg/day (days 1–5 post transplant), 10.6 mg/kg/day (days 6–10 post transplant), and 8.7 mg/kg/day (days 13–20 post transplant). Toxicity profiles were similar to those reported in previous trials using $C_{min}0$ monitoring. No rejection episodes were seen at 6 months post-transplantation and patients continue to be monitored at these levels at 1-year post-transplantation.

These studies thus provided an important pharmacokinetic correlation of C2 and AUC with acute rejection incidence in liver transplant recipients. Not only was the sampling point C2 an accurate predictor of the full AUC for the Neoral-treated patients, but there was also a correlation between C2 concentrations and incidence of acute rejection in both treatment arms. The data clearly emphasize the greater utility of C2 over $C_{min}0$ in *de novo* liver transplant recipients on Neoral dosing. However, these results further suggest that for the full beneficial effects, monitoring of AUC in the early post-transplantation period may be necessary with later monitoring of C2 at a time when the patients' pharmacokinetic profiles have stabilized.

Use of Neoral in pediatric patients

There are few reports of the use of Neoral in pediatric transplant patients. However, two recent reports have demonstrated similar improvement in absorption and pharmacokinetics in pediatric liver patients who were malabsorbing CsA or who had severe cholestasis [58, 59]. No additional adverse effects were seen despite an increase in C_{max} and AUC similar to what has been reported in adults. More recently, it has been demonstrated in a direct comparison between Neoral and Sandimmune that pediatric patients who received Neoral had a marked reduction in the incidence of acute cellular rejection and time to first rejection episodes [60].

Conclusions and discussion

Although CsA trough level monitoring ($C_{min}0$) has developed over the past 20 years as the standard of practice for patient management, a more accurate measure of a pharmacokinetic parameter which predicts clinical outcome is necessary (Fig. 2) [30, 61]. Previous reports have suggested that the AUC is the most sensitive predictor of outcomes such as freedom from acute rejection and graft survival at 1 year post-transplantation in adult renal and liver transplant recipients [3, 13, 46]. Furthermore, intrapatient variability in AUC has been shown to be a major risk factor in the development of chronic rejection in renal transplant recipients. With Sandimmune, the relationship between $C_{min}0$ (trough) and AUC was not sufficient to allow the use of this single time point to predict total exposure (AUC) of CsA. Even though the relationship between $C_{min}0$ and AUC with Neoral is better, studies have shown that the correlation is still not sufficient to allow the use of $C_{min}0$ as a marker for AUC [49, 52, 56].

Investigators have suggested that full AUC monitoring may be necessary in the early postoperative period although this may prove impractical. Full AUC monitoring requires several blood samples to be taken over the 12–24 h dosing interval. AUC measurements may be manipulated to derive the average blood concentration for the dosing interval as the quotient of the AUC and the dose interval [3, 9, 30].

The sparse sample algorithm is a novel way of predicting AUC without the need for extensive blood monitoring [49–51]. It has been shown that by using two or three points a full AUC may be deduced. This approach may be more practical and a sufficiently accurate estimation of AUC with Neoral in all transplant groups. Initial data in renal, and liver patients have supported such a contention.

Investigations into the use of alternative single time points that are measures of AUC has suggested that either C2 or C6 alone or together might be sufficient, although clearly pharmacokinetic data is not available in all organ systems and in the early post-transplantation period, when variability is greatest, to firmly draw this conclusion [30]. In a study in stable renal transplant patients, two-point sampling (C0 and C2) had a high correlation with AUC_{0-12} using Neoral [30, 56]. Poor absorbers on Sandimmune experienced marked improvement in CsA absorption when converted to Neoral [62]. Furthermore, patient pharmacokinetic variability declined with Neoral usage. In *de novo* renal transplant patients, early in the post-transplant period, C_{max} was delayed and a few patients exhibited secondary peaks. In contrast to stable patients, two-point algorithms had a poorer correlation with AUC, however, three-point measurements C0, C2 and C3 were excellent predictors of AUC_{0-12} ($r^2 > 0.90$). These anomalies resolved over the first 2 weeks post-transplant [49].

Studies using other drugs have shown that the rate of bioavailability is as important as bioavailability (AUC) in determining effectiveness (minimal inhibitory concentration) [45]. Thus, although two drugs may have an identi-

Evolution of therapeutic drug monitoring for cyclosporine A

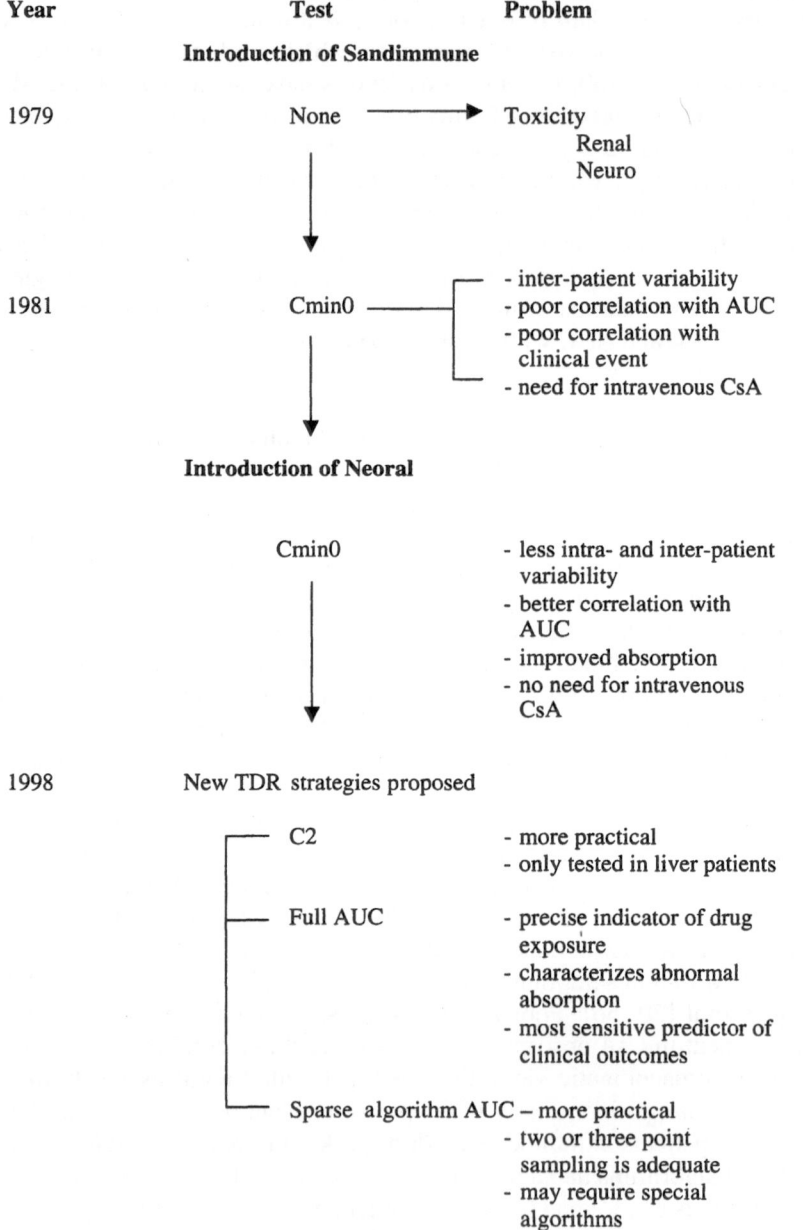

Figure 2. Evolution of therapeutic drug monitoring for cyclosporine A

cal AUC, this does not necessarily mean that they result in comparable blood level curves, as the rate determines the time (T_{max}) and height of the peak (C_{max}) which are important determinants of drug effectiveness. C_{max} may correlate with pharmacodynamic measurements and in particular inhibition of calcineurin activity which has been shown to be an important determinant of freedom from rejection.

In liver transplant patients, studies have suggested that C2, as a surrogate marker for C_{max} and/or AUC, might predict freedom from rejection [30, 56]. However, early post-transplantation, it has become apparent that in some patients C2 may not be predictive of either C_{max} or AUC and thus for the individual patient this single time measurement may not prove satisfactory.

Another important consideration in any drug monitoring strategy is the choice of the measuring assay and source of the samples to be assayed. Today, there are a number of assays using monoclonal specific antibodies to measure CsA (Tab. 5). When compared with HPLC, it is apparent that measurements from many of these assays do not give an accurate measure of parent drug. This is especially true early in the postoperative period following liver transplantation, but large variations can also be seen in heart, lung and renal patients. Furthermore, the variation not only is seen at $C_{min}0$, but also at C2 and other time points after dosing. Studies have suggested that whole blood measurements of CsA may over- or under-estimate the amount of parent CsA in the target tissue. These studies demonstrated that freedom from rejection and toxicity correlated better with tissue levels of CsA than whole blood levels [29, 63, 64]. Thus, if we are going to adopt a strategy to measure CsA which will provide a better clinical correlate, it is essential that transplant centers adopt a similar measurement approach and that this measurement tool reflect appropriate tissue target levels.

For over two decades now, we have empirically used $C_{min}0$ to monitor CsA levels in an attempt to maximize efficacy and minimize toxicity. It is clear from pharmacokinetic studies that use of this monitoring strategy is not sufficient as a tool for either of these clinical outcomes. The variability in absorption and early metabolism of Sandimmune impeded work to develop alternative TDM strategies.

In conclusion, the introduction of Neoral with a more consistent pharmacokinetic profile has re-awakened interest in establishing effective TDM strategies to maximize the clinical use of this agent. Studies are now ongoing to

Table 5. Comparison of assays for cyclosporine relative to HPLC

HPLC	1.00
EMIT	1.15
TDX (FPIA)	1.4
INKSTAR (RIA)	1.3–1.4

Values are at C_{min} only

evaluate the role of full AUC monitoring and sparse sampling strategies to find more effective ways of monitoring CsA based immunosuppression. This will be especially important as new immunosuppressive agents and combination strategies are being considered.

References

1　Kahan B (1989) Cyclosporine. *N Engl J Med* 321: 1725–1738
2　Borel JF, Bauman G, Chapman I, Donatach P, Fahr A, Mueller EA, Vigouret JM (1996) *In vivo* pharmacological effects of ciclosporin and some analogues. *Adv Pharm* 35: 115–246
3　Kahan BD (1985) Individualization of cyclosporine therapy using pharmacokinetic and pharmacodynamic parameters. *Transplantation* 40: 457–469
4　Grevel J (1986) Absorption of Cyclosporine A after oral dosing. *Transplant Proc* 18: 9–15
5　Ohlman S, Lindholm A, Hagglund H, Sawe J, Kahan BD (1993) On the intraindividual variabililty and chronobiology of cyclosporine pharmacokinetics in renal transplantation. *Eur J Clin Pharmacol* 44: 265–269
6　Lemaire M, Fahr A, Maurer G (1990) Pharmacokinetics of cyclospor*In*: Inter-and intra-individual variations and metabolic pathways. *Transplant Proc* 22: 1110–1112
7　Mehta MU, Venkataramanan R, Burchardt GJ, Starzl TE (1988) Effect of bile on cyclosporin absorption in liver transplant patients. *Brit J Clin Pharmacol* 25: 579–581
8　Naoumov NV, Tredger JM, Steward CM (1989) Cyclosporin A pharmacokinetics in liver transplant recipients in relation to biliary T-tube clamping and liver dysfunction. *Gut* 30: 391–396
9　Lindholm A, Kahan BD (1993) Influence of cyclosporine pharmacokinetics, trough concentrations and AUC monitoring on outcome after kidney transplantation. *Clin Pharmacol Ther* 54: 205–218
10　Best NG, Trull AK, Tan KKC, Hue KL, Spiegelhalter DJ, Gore SM, Wallwork J (1992) Blood cyclosporin concentrations and the short term risk of lung rejection following heart-lung transplantation. *Brit J Clin Pharmacol* 34: 315–320
11　Kovarik JM, Mueller EA, Richard F, Niese D, Halloran PF, Jeffery J, Paul LC, Keown PA (1996) Evidence for earlier stabilization of cyclosporine pharmacokinetics in *de novo* renal transplant patients receiving a microemulsion formulation. *Transplantation* 62: 759–763
12　Kahan BD, Wideman C, Ried M, Gibbons S, Jarowenko M, Flechner S, Van Buren CT (1984) The value of serial serum trough cyclosporine levels in human renal transplantation. *Transplant Proc* 16: 1195–1199
13　Kahan BD, Van Buren CT, Lin SN, Ono Y, Agostino G, LeGrue SJ, Boileau M, Payne WD, Kerman RH (1982) Immunopharmacologic monitoring of cyclosporin A-treated recipients of cadaveric kidney allografts. *Transplantation* 34: 36–45
14　Cunningham C, Gavin MP, Whiting PH, Burke MD, Macintyre F, Thomson AW, Simpson JG (1984) Serum cyclosporin levels, hepatic drug metabolism and renal tubulotoxicity. *Biochem Pharmacol* 33: 2857–2861
15　Donatsch P, Abisch E, Hornberger M, Traber R, Trapp M, Voges R (1981) A radioimmunoassay to measure cyclosporin A in plasma and serum samples. *J Immunoassay* 2: 19–32
16　Niederberger W, Schaub P, Beveridge T (1980) High-performance liquid chromatographic determination of cyclosporin A in human plasma and urine. *J Chromatogr* 182: 454–458
17　Vonderscher J, Meinzer A (1994) Rationale for the development of Sandimmun Neoral. *Transplant Proc* 26: 2925–2927
18　Coukell AJ, Plosker GL (1998) Cyclosporin Microemulsion (Neoral): A pharmacoeconomic review of its use compared with standard cyclosporin in renal and hepatic transplantation. *Pharmacoeconomics* 14: 691–708
19　Kovarik JM, Mueller EA, Van Bree JB, Arns W, Renner E, Kutz K (1994) Within-day consistency in cyclosporine pharmacokinetics from a microemulsion formulation in renal transplant patients. *Ther Drug Monit* 16: 232–237
20　Mueller EA, Kovarik JM, Van Bree JB, Lison AE, Kutz K (1994) Pharmacokinetics and tolerability of a microemulsion formulation of cyclosporine in renal allograft recipients – a concentration-controlled comparison with the commercial formulation. *Transplantation* 57: 1178–1182

21 Kovarik JM, Mueller EA, Van Bree JB, Fluckiger SS, Lange H, Schmidt B, Boesken WH, Lison AE, Kutz K (1994) Cyclosporine pharmacokinetics and variability from a microemulsion formulation – A multicenter investigation in kidney transplant patients. *Transplantation* 58: 658–663
22 Levy GA (1999) Relationship of pharmacokinetics to clinical outcomes. *Transplant Proc* 31: 1654–1658
23 Halloran P (1998) Calcineurin inhibition – relationship to cyclosporin blood concentration. *Focus Med* 13: 15–18
24 Batiuk TD, Kung L, Halloran PF (1997) Evidence that calcineurin is rate-limiting for primary human lymphocyte activation. *J Clin Invest* 100: 1894–1901
25 Batiuk TD, Pazderka F, Halloran PF (1995) Calcineurin activity is only partially inhibited in leukocytes of cyclosporine-treated patients. *Transplantation* 59: 1400–1404
26 Batiuk TD, Urmson J, Vincent D, Yatscoff RW, Halloran PF (1996) Quantitating immunosuppression. *Transplantation* 61: 1618–1624
27 Batiuk TD, Pazderka F, Enns J, De Castro L, Halloran PF (1996) Cyclosporine inhibition of leukocyte calcineurin is much less in whole blood than in culture medium. *Transplantation* 61: 158–161
28 Sandborn WJ, Lawson GM, Krom RA, Wiesner RH (1992) Hepatic allograft cyclosporine concentration is independent of the route of cyclosporine administration and correlates with the occurrence of early cellular rejection. *Hepatology* 15: 1086–1091
29 Perico N, Ruggenenti P, Gaspari F, Mosconi L, Benigni A, Amuchastegui CS, Gasparini F, Remuzzi G (1992) Daily renal hypoperfusion induced by cyclosporine in patients with renal transplantation. *Transplantation* 54: 56–60
30 Keown P, Kahan BD, Johnston A, Levy G, Dunn SP, Cittero F, Grino JM, Hoyer PF, Wolf P, Halloran PF (1998) Optimization of cyclosporine therapy with new therapeutic drug monitoring strategies: Report from the international Neoral TDM advisory consensus meeting (Vancouver, November 1997). *Transplant Proc* 30: 1645–1649
31 Keown P, Niese D (1998) Cyclosporine microemulsion increases drug exposure and reduces acute rejection without incremental toxicity in de novo renal transplantation. *Kidney Int* 54: 938–944
32 Lodge JPA, Pollard SG (1997) Neoral vs. Sandimmune: interim results of a randomized trial of efficacy and safety in preventing acute rejection in new renal transplant recipients. *Transplant Proc* 29: 272–273
33 Barone G, Bunke CM, Choc Jr, MG, Hricik DE, Jin JH, Klein JB, Marsh CL, Min DI, Pescovitz MD, Pollak R et al (1996) Safety and tolerability of Neoral vs Sandimmune: 1-year data in primary renal allograft recipients. *Transplant Proc* 28: 2183–2186
34 Niese D (1995) A double-blind randomized study of Sandimmun Neoral *versus* Sandimmun in new renal transplant recipients: results after 12 months. *Transplant Proc* 27: 1849–1856
35 Korn A, Farber L, Maibucher A, Buchholz B, Offermann G (1997) Long-term experience with Sandimmun Neoral: results in de novo and stable renal transplant patients after 24-month treatment. *Transplant Proc* 29: 2945–2947
36 Frei U, Taesch S, Niese D (1994) Use of Sandimmun Neoral in renal transplant patients. International Sandimmun Neoral study group. *Transplant Proc* 26: 2928–2931
37 Donovan J (1998) OLN 354 Study Group. A randomized, double-blind study of Neoral vs. Sandimmune in primary liver transplant recipients with two year follow up. *Transplantation* 65: S14
38 Gradziadei IW, Wiesner RH, Marotta PJ, Porayko ML, Dahlke LJ, Wilson SM, Steers JL, Krom RA (1997) Neoral compared to Sandimmune is associated with a decrease in histologic severity of rejection in patients undergoing primary liver transplantation. *Transplantation* 64: 726–731
39 Grant D, Rochon J, Levy GA (1996) Comparison of the long-term tolerability, pharmacodynamics, and safety of Sandimmune and Neoral in liver transplant recipients. Ontario liver transplant study group. *Transplant Proc* 28: 2232–2233
40 Otto MG, Mayer AD, Clavien PA, Cavallari A, Gunawardena KA, Mueller EA (1999) Randomised trial of cyclosporin microemulsion (Neoral) *versus* conventional cyclosporine in liver transplantation. MILTON study. Multicentre international study in liver transplantation. *Transplantation* 66: 1632–1640
41 Pinson CW, Chapman WC, Wright JK, Hunter EB, Awad JA, Raiford RS, Payne JL, Geevarghese S, Blair TK, Van Buren DH (1998) Experience with Neoral *versus* Sandimmune in primary liver transplant recipients. *Transplant Int* 11: S278-S283
42 Trull AK, Steel L, Sharples L, Stewart S, Parameshwar J, McNeil K, Wallwork J (1999) Randomised, trough blood cyclosporine concentration-controlled trial to compare the pharmacodynamics of Sandimmune and Neoral in de novo lung transplant recipients. *Ther Drug Monit* 21: 17–26

43 Best NG, Trull AK, Tan KKC, Hue KL, Spiegelhalter DJ, Gore SM, Wallwork J (1992) Blood cyclosporin concentrations and the short-term risk of lung rejection following heart-lung transplantation. *Brit J Clin Pharmacol* 34: 513–520

44 Levy GA, Rasmussen A, Mayer AD, Jamieson NV, Neuhaus P (1997) Neoral in *de novo* liver transplantation: adequate immunosuppression without intravenous cyclosporine. *Liver Transplant Surg* 3: 571–77

45 Spector R, Park GD, Johnson GF, Vessell ES (1988) Therapeutic drug monitoring. *Clin Pharmacol Ther* 43: 345–353

46 Kahan BD (1998) Pharmacokinetics of cyclosporin formulations and their relationship to clinical outcomes. *Focus Med* 13: 3–6

47 Lindholm A, Kahan BD (1993) Influence of cyclosporine pharmacokinetics, trough concentrations and AUC monitoring on outcome after kidney transplantation. *Clin Trials Ther* 54: 205–228

48 Kahan BD, Welsh M, Schoenberg L, Tutzky LP, Katz SM, Urbauer DL, Van Buren CT (1996) Variable oral absorption of cyclosporine. A biopharmaceutical risk factor for chronic renal allograft rejection. *Transplantation* 62: 599–606

49 Primmett DRN, Levin M, Kovarik JM, Mueller EA, Keown PA (1998) Cyclosporine monitoring in patients with renal transplants: Two- or three-point methods that estimate area under the curve are superior to trough levels in predicting drug exposure. *Ther Drug Monit* 20: 276–283

50 Johnston A (1998) Sparse-sampling- a practical method for measurement of AUCs. *Focus Med* 13: 7–10

51 Johnston A, Sketris I, Marsden JT, Galustian CG, Fashola T, Taube D, Pepper J, Holt DW (1990) A limited sampling strategy for the measurement of cyclosporine AUC. *Transplant Proc* 22: 1345–1346

52 Johnston A, Kovarik JM, Mueller EA, Holt DW (1996) Predicting patients' exposure to cyclosporin. *Transplant Int* 9 suppl 1: S305-S307

53 Mahalti K, Belitsky P, Sketris I, West K, Panek R (1999) Neoral monitoring by simplified sparse sampling area under the concentration-time curve: its relationship to acute rejection and cyclosporine nephrotoxicity early after kidney transplantation. *Transplantation* 68: 55–62

54 Freeman D, Grant D, Levy G, Rochon J, Wong PY, Altraif A, Asfar S (1995) Pharmacokinetics of a new oral formulation of cyclosporine in liver transplant recipients. *Ther Drug Monit* 17: 213–216

55 Levy G, Rochon J, Freeman D, Wong PY, Banks L, Roach C, Engel K, Grant D (1994) Cyclosporine neoral in liver transplant recipients. *Transplant Proc* 26: 2949–2952

56 Grant D, Kneteman N, Tchervenkov J, Roy A, Murphy G, Tan A, Hendricks L, Guilbault N, Levy G (1999) Peak cyclosporine levels (Cmax) correlate with freedom from liver graft rejection: results of a prospective, randomized comparison of Neoral and Sandimmune for liver transplantation (NOF-8). *Transplantation* 67: 1133–1137

57 Levy GA (1998) Two-hour cyclosporin concentration (C2) as a monitoring tool for Neoral. *Focus Med* 13: 19–22

58 Superina RA, Strong DK, Acal LA, DeLuca E (1994) Relative bioavailability of Sandimmune and Sandimmune Neoral in pediatric liver transplant recipients. *Transplant Proc* 26: 2979–2980

59 Alvarez F, Atkison P, Grant D, Jones A, Kim P, Kneteman N, Laurin L, Martin S, Paradis K, Shapiro J et al (1998) NOF-11: a one-year randomized double-blind comparison of Neoral *versus* Sandimmune in pediatric liver transplantation. *Transplant Proc* 30: 1961

60 Alvarez F, Atkison PR, Grant DR, Guilbault N, Jones AB, Kim PS, Kneteman NM, Laurin L, Martin SR, Murphy GF et al (2000) NOF-11: a one-year pediatric randomized double-blind comparison of neoral *versus* sandimmune in orthotopic liver transplantation. *Transplantation* 69: 10–16

61 Halloran P (1998) Introduction and goals. *Focus Med* 13: 1–2

62 Keown P, Landsberg D, Halloran P, Shoker A, Rush D, Jeffery J, Russell D, Stiller C, Muirhead N, Cole E et al (1996) A randomized, prospective multicenter pharmacoepidemiologic study of cyclosporine microemulsion in stable renal graft recipients. *Transplantation* 62: 1744–1752

63 Stepkowski SM, Goto S, Ito T, Reynolds K, Didlake R, Kim EK, Kahan BD (1989) Prolongation of heterotopic heart allograft survival by local delivery of continuous low-dose cyclosporine therapy. *Transplantation* 47: 17–23

64 Belitsky P, Ghose T, Givner M, Rowden G, Pope B (1986) Tissue distribution of cyclosporine A in the mouse: a clue to toxicity? *Clin Nephrol* 25: S27-S29

Modern Immunosuppressives
ed. by H.-J Schuurman, G. Feutren and J.-F. Bach
© 2001 Birkhäuser Verlag/Switzerland

Tacrolimus

Suphamai Bunnapradist[1] and Gabriel Danovitch[2]

[1] Kidney Transplant Program, Cedars-Sinai Medical Center, 8635 W. 3rd Street, Suite 590 W, Los Angeles, CA 90048, USA
[2] Renal Transplantation Unit, Department of Nephrology, UCLA Medical Centre, 10833 Le Conte Avenue, Los Angeles, CA 90024, USA

Introduction

Tacrolimus (FK-506) is a macrocyclic lactone antibiotic that was discovered in soil samples in 1984 by Kino et al. [1]. It is derived from *Streptomyces tsukubaensis*. It was first used clinically in recipients of liver transplant who were suffering ongoing rejection despite cyclosporin (CsA)-based immunosuppression [2]. Numerous studies now confirm beneficial immunosuppressive effects of tacrolimus as a *de novo* agent for acute rejection prophylaxis and rescue therapy in a variety of solid organ transplants [3–7]. It is also effective in prevention and treatment of graft *versus* host disease in bone marrow transplant recipients [8] and in a variety of autoimmune diseases such as atopic dermatitis [9]. Tacrolimus was approved by the Food and Drug Administration for the prevention of acute rejection in liver transplantation in 1994, and for kidney transplantation in 1997.

Mechanism of immunosuppressive action [10]

To better understand the mechanisms of immunosuppression, it is prudent to review the normal, unimpaired response of the immune system to foreign antigens. T-cell activation is an orderly series of events which begins when T-cell antigen receptor binds to a suitable peptide plus a major histocompatibility complex antigen (so-called signal 1). Proteins on antigen-presenting cells are needed to provide costimulation (so-called signal 2). The stimulation activates protein tyrosine kinases, which in turn initiate three key signaling pathways from the T-cell antigen receptor to the cytosolic cytoplasm. One of these is the calcium-calcineurin pathway. The rise in intracellular calcium following stimulation provides calcium to bind to subunit B of calcineurin and calmodulin, which binds to calcineurin subunit A. These changes induce a conformation change as calcineurin is activated. The calcineurin phosphatase activity is necessary for dephosphorylation (and subsequent activation) of the cytoplasmic form of the nuclear factor of activated T-cells (so-called NFAT). Calcineurin inhibitors prevent nuclear translocation of this factor and subsequent production of interleukin-2 (IL-2) resulting in immunosuppressive properties. After binding *via* the pipecolic portion of the molecule to their respective intercellular cytoplasmic immunophilin proteins (FK-binding protein, FKBP), particularly FKBP12, and cyclophilin, tacrolimus and CsA inhibit the generation of T-cell regulatory proteins critical for upregulation of DNA transcription of mRNAs for IL-2 and other proinflammatory cytokines including IL-3, IL-4, interferon-γ, tumor necrosis factor, granulocyte-macrophage colony-stimulating factor, as well as proto-oncogenes such as *ras, myc* and *rel.* Tacrolimus (but not CsA) seems to enhance antigen-induced apoptosis in murine thymocytes and peripheral T-cells. The data on transforming growth factor-β is controversial, but this factor is upregulated in the model of chronic tacrolimus nephrotoxicity [11, 12].

Pharmacokinetic properties [13]

Tacrolimus displays wide inter- as well as intra-individual pharmacokinetic variability in both kidney and liver transplant patients. The adverse effects of tacrolimus correlate better with trough concentration than with dose. The oral bioavailability ranges from 4 to 93% (mean about 25%) and the half-life from 5.5 to 16.6 h (mean 8.7 h). At 1 to 4 h after an oral dose of 0.15 mg/kg, the peak plasma concentration is 0.4 to 3.7 ng/ml. Both the rate and the extent of absorption are reduced with food intake. Since neither cholestasis nor impaired biliary function influence the absorption of orally administered tacrolimus, intravenous administration of tacrolimus is not necessary during the early postoperative period after liver transplantation, despite T-tube biliary diversion.

Tacrolimus is extensively distributed throughout the body, with a high affinity to formed blood elements; the whole blood concentrations are 11–114 (mean 15) times higher than the plasma concentration. Tacrolimus is primarily metabolized by the liver and to a lesser extent by the gut, by cytochrome P450 (CYP450) 3A4 isoenzymes to at least 15 metabolites which each has variable immunosuppressive activity. Marked hepatic dysfunction reduces the clearance, but not the absorption of tacrolimus: therefore, dosage reduction is necessary in severe liver disease. Tacrolimus is metabolized largely by hydrosylation and demethylation and the main excretory pathway is *via* the bile. Less than 1% of parent compound is renally excreted: dose adjustment is not necessary in the clinical settings of either renal dysfunction or dialysis treatment. Tacrolimus crosses the placenta and can be detected in breast milk. Furthermore, tacrolimus shows pharmacokinetic interactions with other CYP 3A4 substrates that increase the concentration of each drug. Tacrolimus is highly protein-bound, but in contrast to CsA it is not significantly associated with the lipoprotein portion.

In theory, the combination of tacrolimus and rapamycin is contraindicated given the potential antagonistic property due to competitive inhibition of the FKBP receptors but a clinical study showed the beneficially effects of the combination regimen [14]. The combination of CsA and tacrolimus is clearly contraindicated not only due to the severe pharmacokinetic interaction, but also to the immunosuppressive antagonism between these two agents [15]. This combination potentiates the toxic side-effects of the individual drugs particularly the nephrotoxicity, a potentiation that explains the observations of "conversion nephrotoxicity" upon switching from a CsA- to a tacrolimus-based regimen. It is recommended that a 12- to 20-h period elapses after CsA is discontinued before starting tacrolimus.

Dosage forms, dosing and therapeutic drug monitoring [13]

Tacrolimus is currently available for both intravenous (5 mg/ml in a 1 ml vial) and oral (0.5, 1 mg and 5 mg capsules) administration. For continuous intravenous infusion, initial tacrolimus doses are 0.01–0.1 mg/kg/d; when taken orally a total of 0.1–0.3 mg/kg/day is administered in divided doses every 12 h. The oral route is preferred due to high incidence of nephrotoxicity when the intravenous route is used. It is rarely necessary to employ the intravenous route in clinical solid organ transplantation.

To achieve blood concentrations similar to those of adults, children have a higher dose requirement (0.03–0.1 mg/kg/d for the intravenous or 0.15–0.3 mg/kg/d for the oral route) due to their propensity for a higher rate of CYP 3A4 metabolism. Pediatric patients may benefit from an overlap of intravenous and oral drug administration to avoid suboptimal trough concentrations during the early post-transplantation period. African-American patients may require higher doses of tacrolimus than either Caucasian or Asian patients to achieve the target drug level [16].

Only liquid chromatography/tandem mass spectrometry methods can precisely quantify tacrolimus parent compound in whole bloood [17]. However, in response to the technical difficulty performing these assays, two commercial kits have been developed to monitor tacrolimus concentrations. Both kits use the same monoclonal antibody, a reagent that detects not only parent compound but also an array of metabolites. The IMx tacrolimus assay (Abbott Laboratories, North Chicago, IL) is a microparticle enzyme immunoassay, and the Pro-Trac test (INCSTAR, Minneapolis, MN) is an enzyme-linked immunosorbent assay [18]. The advantages of the microparticle enzyme immunoassay over the enzyme-linked immunosorbent assay include simpler sample preparation, fully- rather than semi-automated analysis, and a faster procedure time of 30 min compared to 3 to 4 h. However, because the microparticle enzyme immunoassay has a major limitation of low sensitivity (5–10 ng/ml), the more sensitive enzyme-linked immunosorbent assay (0.2 ng/ml) is preferable for monitoring the patients receiving low doses of tacrolimus.

The optimal therapeutic ranges for tacrolimus drug concentrations during the induction, acute rejection prophylaxis, and maintenance phases of immunosuppression are unknown. The US multicenter study [3] of the correlation between tacrolimus concentrations and episodes of toxicity and rejection among 120 kidney transplant patients reported that optimal efficacy occurred with tacrolimus trough concentrations of 5–15 ng/ml. Trough concentrations below 5 ng/ml were associated with a 30% incidence of acute rejection episodes, and those above 15 ng/ml were associated with a 45% incidence of adverse events and a 3% incidence of rejection episodes.

Toxic side-effects

The most common adverse events associated with tacrolimus therapy are neurotoxic effects. Tremor is the most common neurologic adverse effect and usually improves upon dose reduction. Headache, seizures, coma, reversible cortical blindness and posterior leukoencephalopathy are occasionally reported. Gastrointestinal side-effects such as nausea and diarrhoea are also common. Renal dysfunction and new-onset diabetes mellitus represent more serious and more frequently encountered toxicities. In the early clinical trial, the incidence of post-transplant diabetes mellitus (PTDM) was significantly higher for the tacrolimus cohort group than for the CsA-treated group (19% *versus* 4% respectively, $p < 0.001$). The incidence of PTDM was three times higher among African-american patients than among Caucasian patients. Unfortunately, the majority (80%) of African-american patients continuously required insulin treatment beyond 2 years post-transplantation, possibly related to the higher tacrolimus doses in African-americans to achieve target whole blood drug concentrations [16]. Risk factors for PTDM include older age, African-American race, obesity and family history of diabetes. African-American patients did not experience an increased incidence of other tacrolimus-related adverse effects. Subsequent large trials indicate that the incidences of new-onset diabetes are lower and comparable to those seen in CsA-treated patients, when early and aggressive tacrolimus dose-reduction is performed. The incidence may be higher in liver transplantation and is surprisingly lower in simultaneous pancreas-kidney patients who receive tacrolimus rescue therapy.

Hypertension, a common side-effect of CsA therapy, appears to be less frequent with tacrolimus but this effect attenuates after 3 years. The acute allograft nephropathy seen with tacrolimus, and CsA are usually reversed within 12–24 h after the dose is withheld or reduced although it may take longer for tacrolimus toxicity to resolve. Nephrotoxity is usually manifested as a symptomatic rise in serum creatinine and serves as the diagnosis of exclusion. Isometric vacuolization in the renal tubule is compatible with calcineurin inhibitor toxicity, but is not diagnostic. One study suggests that an increase in CsA dose results in reduction of serum creatinine and resolution of histopathology in case of concomitant borderline rejection and isometric vacuolization [19]. Tacrolimus and CsA appear to produce similar degrees of clinical and histopathological evidences of nephrotoxicity upon long-term administration, namely, arteriolar hyalinosis and striped interstitial fibrosis. Hyperkalemia, hypomagnesemia and hyperuricemia are also common and may necessitate treatment. Tacrolimus has a less lipemic effect than CsA. Results from the US South-Eastern Organ Procurement Group suggested that tacrolimus conversion in renal transplant patients is usually safe and effective [20]. Both CsA and tacrolimus can cause thrombotic microangiopathy, which is a rare, but an important cause of renal allograft loss [21].

Tacrolimus, like some macrolides, is reported to cause QT prolongation and cardiac arrhythmia especially after intravenous administration [22]. Tacrolimus is not associated with hypertrichosis or gingival hyperplasia, which are not-uncommon cosmetic side-effects of CsA therapy; however, tacrolimus can produce alopecia especially with high serum trough levels [23]. These common cosmetic side-effects can lead to non-compliance, especially in teenage patients. Data from liver transplantation demonstrated that pregnancy is usually safe especially after 2 years of stable graft function [24].

Review of clinical trials of tacrolimus in solid organ transplantation

Primary de novo therapy

Liver transplantation

The US and European open-label multicenter trials [25–27] found similar 1-year recipient and hepatic allograft survival rates among groups of patients treated with either tacrolimus or the original oil-based Sandimmune formulation of CsA as the primary immunosuppressant. In a 5-year follow-up report, Wiesner [25] described similar recipient and graft survival rates for tacrolimus-based treatment (79% and 71.8%, respectively) and for CsA-based treatment (73.1% and 66.4%, respectively). However, the tacrolimus cohort showed a lower rate of acute rejection episodes than the Sandimmune group (68% versus 76%, respectively, $p < 0.001$) as well as a lower rate of steroid-resistant rejection episodes (19% versus 36%, respectively, $p < 0.001$). Patients in both treatment groups showed a low incidence of late steroid-resistant acute rejection episodes, or death or rejection-related graft loss [28]. Data on recurrent disease as causes of allograft dysfunction are inconclusive. However, improved patient survival was observed in hepatitis C patients who received tacrolimus (79% versus 60% in the CsA group, respectively).

Kidney transplantation

The US [3] and European [28] open-label multicenter randomized parallel-group studies showed similar 1-year recipient and graft survival rates for the tacrolimus- and CsA-treated groups. Both studies used steroids and azathioprine as part of the immunosuppressive regimen, while the US study also included antibody induction. In both the US and European study the acute allograft rejection episodes were lower for tacrolimus (30.7% and 25.9%, respec-

tively) than for CsA (46.4% and 45.7%, respectively: both $p < 0.001$).
Corticosteroid-resistant rejection occurred in 11.3% of tacrolimus-treated
patients and 21.6% of CsA-treated recipients ($p = 0.001$). However, the rates
of occurrence of chronic allograft rejection reactions did not differ significantly between tacrolimus-treated and CsA-treated patients (5.2% and 9.3%,
respectively). At 3 years post-transplantation, UNOS data did not show a significant advantage of tacrolimus in terms of long-term graft survival [29]. In a
European study on high-risk patients defined as showing a high panel-reactive
antibody and/or previous transplant function less than a year, tacrolimus
showed a lower incidence of biopsy-proven acute rejection (31.8%) and higher graft survival (86%) compared to CsA (54.2 and 72%, respectively) at 1
year post-transplantation. A single-center prospective randomized study comparing tacrolimus and Neoral (a microemulsion formulation of cyclosporine)
as primary immunosuppression in cadaveric renal transplantation suggests that
tacrolimus appeared to be effective with a similar side-effect profile as Neoral
after a 3-month follow-up. Long-term data are not available [30]. The addition
of azathioprine to a regimen comprising tacrolimus and steroids did not seem
to improve graft survival or reduce acute rejection episodes [31]. A single-center prospective randomized trial of 208 patients receiving either tacrolimus
with prednisone or tacrolimus with prednisone and mycophenolate showed a
lower incidence of rejection at 1 year in the triple-therapy group (27% *versus*
44% in the double-therapy group, $p = 0.014$): there was no statistically significant difference in graft survival. The incidence of cytomegalovirus infection
was higher in the triple therapy group (16.7 *versus* 8.5% in the double-therapy group) but this was not statistically significant [32].

Pancreas transplantation
Despite aggressive immunosuppressive regimens, acute rejection remains the
major cause of morbidity and graft failure in pancreas transplant recipients at
1 and 5 years post-transplantation. The incidences of graft loss due to rejection
at 1 and 5 years post-transplantation are 6% and 13%, respectively, for simultaneous pancreas-kidney transplants, 32% and 68% for pancreas transplants
alone, and 29% and 79% for pancreas after kidney transplantation [33].
Shaffer et al. [34] observed a beneficial effect of tacrolimus in two simultaneous pancreas-kidney transplant recipients suffering from refractory rejection
without impairing long-term pancreas graft function. Hariharan et al. [35] presented a long-term follow-up of a cohort of 12 patients who underwent conversion from CsA to tacrolimus due to CsA-induced vasculopathy with persistent rejection in the kidney biopsy of four of these patients despite treatment
at therapeutic CsA levels. Renal graft function stabilized without changes in
blood glucose concentration, hemoglobin A1c and C-peptide levels. The findings also showed a non-significant tendency toward a lower rate of recurrent
acute rejection episodes.
    Gruessner et al. [33] reported the 6-month data from a multicenter, open-
label study of 154 pancreas allograft recipients, which either received tacro-

limus *de novo* ($n = 82$) or were converted from CsA to tacrolimus for anti-rejection or rescue therapy ($n = 61$) or for other reasons ($n = 11$). The median tacrolimus starting dose was 4 mg/d orally to achieve a median blood trough concentration of 12 ng/ml. Among patients treated *de novo* 66% were simultaneous pancreas-kidney graft recipients who, as a group, displayed a patient survival rate of 90% and a pancreas graft survival rate of 87% at 6 months post-transplantation. For comparison, an arbitrary *post hoc* "matched-pair" analysis showed a 70% graft survival rate among an historical cohort of CsA-treated recipients ($p = 0.04$). The *de novo* tacrolimus group showed a 35% rate of reversible rejection episodes within the first 6 months. The most commonly reported adverse events were neurotoxicity (16%), nephrotoxicity (13%), and/or gastrointestinal toxicity (9%); new-onset insulin-dependent diabetes mellitus was not observed. Among the group of patients treated for rejection, 72% had undergone simultaneous pancreas-kidney transplantation. At 6 months post-transplantation, this subgroup showed patient and graft survival rates of 91% and 90%, respectively, with a 44% rate of recurrent acute rejection episodes within 6 months despite conversion. Compared to *de novo* patients, those converted to tacrolimus for rescue purposes had a higher incidence of adverse reactions, namely neurotoxicity (23%), nephrotoxicity (25%), and gastrointestinal toxicity (21%). New-onset insulin-dependent diabetes was noted in one patient, which interestingly displayed good exocrine function; however, two patients had to be reconverted to CsA due to persistent hyperglycemia.

The first long-term safety and efficacy study of tacrolimus in pancreas transplant patients came from the University of Pittsburgh group. Sixty patients, including simultaneous pancreas-kidney transplant recipients ($n = 55$), recipients of pancreas transplant alone ($n = 4$), and recipients of a pancreas after kidney transplantation ($n = 1$), underwent induction therapy consisting of tacrolimus and steroids without antibody induction therapy. The majority of the patients also received azathioprine. Graft survival at 6 months and 1, 2 and 3 years post-transplantation was 88%, 82%, 80% and 80%, respectively, for pancreas grafts and 98%, 96%, 93% and 91%, respectively, for kidney transplants. Complete tapering of steroids was possible in 31 (65%) of the 48 patients with a functioning pancreas.

Heart transplantation
In a US multi-center trail 88 primary heart transplant were randomized to tacrolimus or CsA in addition to azathioprine and corticosteroids. At 6 months post-transplantation, the survival rate was 93% in the tacrolimus group compared to 91% in the CsA group. Hypertension was less in tacrolimus-treated patients (52% *versus* 79% in the CsA group) and mean cholesterol levels were lower in the patients receiving tacrolimus (181 *versus* 233 mg/dl in the CsA group). The histologic grading as determined by endomyocardial biopsy did not differ between the groups.

The European Multicenter Tacrolimus Heart Pilot Study group found no significant difference between the tacrolimus- and CsA-treatment groups in either the incidence of acute rejection episodes or the graft/patient survival rates at 1 year post-transplantation. The rate of freedom from acute rejection episodes was 26.3% in the tacrolimus-treated group and 18.5% in the CsA-treated group (not statistically significant), and graft survival rates were 79.6% and 92.9%, respectively ($p = 0.0125$). Although fewer patients in the tacrolimus group required antihypertensive therapy compared to the CsA group (59.5% and 87.5%, respectively, not statistically significant), the overall rates of adverse effects, including infections, impaired renal function (31.5% and 21.4%, respectively), and/or glucose intolerance (7.0% and 4.3%, respectively) did not differ significantly between the groups. Although cardiac biopsy specimens from tacrolimus-treated patients showed a greater percentage of inflamed fragments and a higher rejection grade than those from CsA-treated patients within the first 30 days post-transplantation, specimens collected during the late post-transplantation period (275 to 548 days) showed the reverse. However, cardiac allograft biopsy histopathology in the later phase did not differ between patients treated with tacrolimus and those treated with CsA-based therapy and antibody induction [43].

Lung transplantation

Keenan et al. [36] reported a prospective randomized trial of tacrolimus *versus* CsA in 133 adults receiving single- or double-lung transplants who also received steroids and azathioprine. Tacrolimus treatment resulted in a modest but not significant reduction in the incidence of acute rejection episodes per 100 patient-days when compared to an historical cohort treated with CsA (0.85 and 1.09, respectively, $p = 0.07$). The authors observed that obliterative bronchiolitis, a major cause of long-term morbidity and mortality after lung transplantation, was detected in significantly fewer patients in the tacrolimus group than in the historical CsA group at 1 year follow-up (22% *versus* 38%, $p = 0.025$). However, the 1- and 2-year graft survival rates were similar in the two treatment groups.

Graft-versus-host disease (GVHD)

A few multicenter randomised studies compared tacrolimus with or without methotrexate to CsA-methotrexate in the prevention of GVHD in related-donor and unrelated-donor bone marrow transplants. The usual starting dose of tacrolimus is 0.03 to 0.05 mg/kg/d given continuously. One study [8] showed a significantly lower incidence of grade II-IV acute GVHD in patients who received tacrolimus. There was no relationship between the whole blood level of tacrolimus and the rate of acute GVHD, although nephrotoxicity increased significantly when whole blood levels exceeded 20 ng/ml. The incidences of nephrotoxicity ranged between 32% and 93% in related-donor transplants, and between 63% and 88% in unrelated-donor transplants. Although CsA-methotrexate is more effective than CsA alone, tacrolimus in combination with low dose of methotrexate was also effective and did minimize mucosal toxicity.

Rescue therapy

Rescue therapy include conversion from CsA to tacrolimus in the treatment of rejection or because of side-effects.

Liver transplantation

Conversion from CsA to tacrolimus as rescue therapy in hepatic allograft recipients who experienced steroid-resistant rejection or early chronic rejection processes was reported to confer both histological and biochemical improvements in allograft function [4, 37]. For example, an anecdotal report in 64 patients which were presumably diagnosed with acute rejection at the time of study entry, described "normalization" of mean serum levels of total bilirubin and transaminases within 6 months after conversion. In contrast, patients diagnosed with chronic rejection at study entry ($n = 113$) showed "normalization" of bilirubin, but had persistently elevated serum transaminase levels at 6 months after conversion. Following conversion to tacrolimus therapy, 47% of patients showed a deterioration in the pathologic findings [37]. This may be explained by the inhibitory effect of tacrolimus on synthesis of transforming growth factor-β.

Renal transplantation

Rescue therapy for refractory acute kidney transplant rejection has been examined in two non-randomized US trials which showed similar results [5, 38]. Patient survival was 94 and 93%, respectively, and graft survival rate was 74% and 75%, respectively. Prior to conversion from CsA to tacrolimus the majority of patients had been unresponsive to corticosteroids with or without administration of antilymphocyte antibody agents. Tacrolimus therapy was initated at a median of 4.3 months post-transplantation. Two factors appeared to influence the success of tacrolimus rescue therapy: the preconversion serum creatinine level as an index of kidney damage, and the time post-transplantation. Not surprisingly, successful conversion was more common in patients that had low serum creatinine values at the time of tacrolimus conversion, as well as in patients converted before 6 months post-transplantation (75% *versus* 50%, $p = 0.006$). Jordan et al. [38] claimed that 13 of 28 patients (46%) that were on dialysis at the time of conversion had functioning grafts at a mean follow-up of 37 months. This was achieved without a significantly higher incidence of infection of malignancy. Tacrolimus has never been shown to stabilize or reverse chronic rejection. Other uses of rescue therapy include conversion due to side-effects such as thrombotic microangiopathy with or without plasmapheresis [21].

Heart transplantation

Tacrolimus rescue therapy has been reported in 16 heart and 15 lung transplant recipients [7] that were converted due to CsA intolerance, the occurrence of acute rejection episodes, or the presence of histopathologic changes suggestive of humoral rejection. Among the heart transplant recipients, all patients and grafts were surviving at the time of the report (mean 183 ± 65 days). Only 20% of heart transplant recipients were free from rejection episodes after conversion to tacrolimus. Among the lung transplant recipients, the patient and graft survival rates at a mean survival time of 169 ± 86 days were 67% and 60%, respectively. Following conversion, 80% of the lung transplant patients did not experience rejection episodes.

Tacrolimus *versus* cyclosporine: which agent to use? [39]

The evaluation of tacrolimus and CsA in most studies reported to date is not necessarily comparable to current immunosuppressive regimens. Most trials compared tacrolimus to the original oil-based CsA formulation (Sandimmune) rather than the recently introduced microemulsion formulation (Neoral). The introduction of the microemulsion formulation addressed major limitations of the oil-based CsA preparation, namely the highly variable, partial, and bile-dependent gastrointestinal absorption. The replacement of Sandimmune by Neoral has significantly reduced the incidence of acute rejection episodes in some liver and kidney transplant recipients, but the results are not universal [30, 40]. This aside, the reduced incidence could mitigate at least some of the apparent differences between CsA- and tacrolimus-based regimens. The impact of this new preparation on the incidence of chronic rejection or nephrotoxicity is not yet well studied. The addition of mycophenolate, rapamycin and IL-2 receptor antagonists to calcineurin inhibitor regimens is expected to decrease this gap further.

The selection of Neoral or tacrolimus as the baseline calcineurin-inhibitor in primary rejection prevention is generally based on physician's preferences, baseline metabolic profiles such as hyperlipidemia, patient intolerance to the side-effect profile of either one of the agents (such as the neurotoxicity of tacrolimus or the cosmetic effects of CsA), and/or ill-defined pharmacodynamic resistance to the agent used *de novo*. Tacrolimus is shown to be more effective than CsA in high immunologic risk groups such as in patients considered for retransplantation or patients with high pre-transplant panel-reactive antibodies [41]. For rescue therapy, tacrolimus presents a viable alternative in addition to mycophenolate or antibody treatment, or after failed antibody treatment.

References

1 Kino T, Hatanaka H, Hashimoto M, Nishiyama M, Goto T, Okuhara M, Kohsaka M, Aoki H, Imanaka H (1987) FK-506, a novel immunosuppressant isolated from a *Streptomyces*. I. Fermentation, isolation, and physico-chemical and biological characteristics. *J Antibiot* 40: 1249–1255

2 Starzl TE, Todo S, Fung J, Demetris AJ, Venkataramman R, Jain A (1989) FK-506 for liver, kidney, and pancreas transplantation. *Lancet* 2: 1000–1004

3 Pirsch JD, Miller J, Deierhoi MH, Vincenti F, Filo RS (1997) A comparison of tacrolimus (FK506) and cyclosporine for immunosuppression after cadaveric renal transplantation. FK506 Kidney Transplant Study Group [see comments]. *Transplantation* 63: 977–983

4 Sher LS, Cosenza CA, Michel J, Makowka L, Miller CM, Schwartz ME, Busuttil R, McDiarmid S, Burdick JF, Klein AS et al (1997) Efficacy of tacrolimus as rescue therapy for chronic rejection in orthotopic liver transplantation: a report of the U.S. Multicenter Liver Study Group. *Transplantation* 64: 258–263

5 Woodle ES, Thistlethwaite JR, Gordon JH, Laskow D, Deierhoi MH, Burdick J, Pirsch JD, Sollinger H, Vincenti F, Burrows L (1996) A multicenter trial of FK506 (tacrolimus) therapy in refractory acute renal allograft rejection. A report of the Tacrolimus Kidney Transplantation Rescue Study Group. *Transplantation* 62: 594–599

6 Woodle ES, Thistlethwaite JR, Gordon JH (1996) Tacrolimus therapy for refractory acute renal allograft rejection: a prospective multicenter trial. Tacrolimus Kidney Transplantation Rescue Study Group. *Transplant Proc* 28: 3163–3164

7 Mentzer RM Jr, Jahania MS, Lasley RD (1998) Tacrolimus as a rescue immunosuppressant after heart and lung transplantation. The U.S. Multicenter FK506 Study Group. *Transplantation* 65: 109–113

8 Ratanatharathorn V, Nash RA, Przepiorka D, Devine SM, Klein JL, Weisdorf D, Fay JW, Nademanee A, Antin JH, Christiansen NP et al (1998) Phase III study comparing methotrexate and tacrolimus (prograf, FK506) with methotrexate and cyclosporine for graft-*versus*-host disease prophylaxis after HLA-identical sibling bone marrow transplantation. *Blood* 92: 2303–2314

9 Bieber T (1998) Topical tacrolimus (FK506): a new milestone in the management of atopic dermatitis [editorial comment]. *J Allergy Clin Immunol* 102: 555–557

10 Thomson AW, Bonham CA, Zeevi A (1995) Mode of action of tacrolimus (FK506): molecular and cellular mechanisms. *Ther Drug Monit* 17: 584–591

11 Shihab FS, Bennett WM, Tanner AM, Andoh TF (1997) Mechanism of fibrosis in experimental tacrolimus nephrotoxicity. *Transplantation* 64: 1829–1837

12 Zhang JG, Walmsley MW, Moy JV, Cunningham AC, Talbot D, Dark JH, Kirby JA (1998) Differential effects of cyclosporin A and tacrolimus on the production of TGF-beta: implications for the development of obliterative bronchiolitis after lung transplantation. *Transplant Int* 11 Suppl 1: S325-S327

13 Venkataramanan R, Swaminathan A, Prasad T, Jain A, Zuckerman S, Warty V, McMichael J, Lever J, Burckart G, Starzl T (1995) Clinical pharmacokinetics of tacrolimus. *Clin Pharmacokinet* 29: 404–430

14 Vu MD, Qi S, Xu D, Wu J, Fitzsimmons WE, Sehgal SN, Dumont L, Busque S, Daloze P, Chen H (1997) Tacrolimus (FK506) and sirolimus (rapamycin) in combination are not antagonistic but produce extended graft survival in cardiac transplantation in the rat. *Transplantation* 64: 1853–1856

15 Vathsala A, Goto S, Yoshimura N, Stepkowski S, Chou TC, Kahan BD (1991) The immunosuppressive antagonism of low doses of FK506 and cyclosporine. *Transplantation* 52: 121–128

16 Neylan JF (1998) Racial differences in renal transplantation after immunosuppression with tacrolimus *versus* cyclosporine. FK506 Kidney Transplant Study Group. *Transplantation* 64: 515–523

17 Taylor PJ, Jones A, Balderson GA, Lynch SV, Norris RL, Pond SM (1996) Sensitive, specific quantitative analysis of tacrolimus (FK506) in blood by liquid chromatography-electrospray tandem mass spectrometry. *Clin Chem* 42: 279–285

18 Brunet M, Pou L, Torra M, Lopez R, Rodamilans M, Corbella J (1996) Comparative analysis of tacrolimus (FK506) in whole blood liver transplant recipients by PRO-TRAC enzyme-linked immunosorbent assay and microparticle enzyme immunoassay IMX methods. *Ther Drug Monit* 18: 706–709

19 Randhawa PS, Saad RS, Jordan M, Scantlebury V, Vivas C, Shapiro R (1999) Clinical significance of renal biopsies showing concurrent acute rejection and tacrolimus-associated tubular vacuolization. *Transplantation* 67: 85–89

20 McCune TR, Thacker LRII, Peters TG, Mulloy L, Rohr MS, Adams PA, Yium J, Light JA, Pruett T, Gaber AO et al (1998) Effects of tacrolimus on hyperlipidemia after successful renal transplantation: a Southeastern Organ Procurement Foundation multicenter clinical study.

Transplantation 65: 87–92

21 Grupp C, Schmidt F, Braun F, Lorf T, Ringe B, Muller GA (1998) Haemolytic uraemic syndrome (HUS) during treatment with cyclosporin A after renal transplantation – is tacrolimus the answer? [editorial] *Nephrol Dialysis Transplant* 13: 1629–1631

22 Hodak SP, Moubarak JB, Rodriguez I, Gelfand MC, Alijani MR, Tracy CM (1998) QT prolongation and near fatal cardiac arrythmia after intravenous tacrolimus administration: a case report. *Transplantation* 66: 535–537

23 Shapiro R, Jordan ML, Scantlebury VP, Vivas C, McCauley J, Johnston J, Fung JJ, Starzl TE (1998) Alopecia as a consequence of tacrolimus therapy. *Transplantation* 65: 1284

24 Rayes N, Neuhaus R, David M, Steinmuller T, Bechstein WO, Neuhaus P (1998) Pregnancies following liver transplantation – how safe are they? A report of 19 cases under cyclosporine A and tacrolimus. *Clin Transplant* 12: 396–400

25 Wiesner RH (1998) A long-term comparison of tacrolimus (FK506) *versus* cyclosporine in liver transplantation: a report of the United States FK506 Study Group. *Transplantation* 66: 493–499

26 Pichlmayr R, Winkler M, Neuhaus P, McMaster P, Calne R, Otto G, Williams R, Groth CG, Bismuth H (1997) Three-year follow-up of the European Multicenter Tacrolimus (FK506) Liver Study. *Transplant Proc* 29: 2499–2502

27 McDiarmid SV, Busuttil RW, Ascher NL, Burdick J, D'Alessandro AM, Esquivel C, Kalayoglu M, Klein AS, Marsh JW, Miller CM et al (1995) FK506 (tacrolimus) compared with cyclosporine for primary immunosuppression after pediatric liver transplantation. Results from the U.S. Multicenter Trial. *Transplantation* 59: 530–536

28 Mayer AD, Dmitrewski J, Squifflet JP, Besse T, Grabensee B, Klein B, Eigler FW, Heemann U, Pichlmayr R, Behrend M et al (1997) Multicenter randomized trial comparing tacrolimus (FK506) and cyclosporine in the prevention of renal allograft rejection: a report of the European Tacrolimus Multicenter Renal Study Group. *Transplantation* 64: 436–443

29 Katznelson S, Cecka JM (1996) Immunosuppressive regimens and their effects on renal allograft outcome. *Clin Transplant* 61: 361–371

30 Morris-Stiff G, Ostrowski K, Balaji V, Moore R, Darby C, Lord R, Jurewicz WA (1998) Prospective randomised study comparing tacrolimus (Prograf) and cyclosporin (Neoral) as primary immunosuppression in cadaveric renal transplants at a single institution: interim report of the first 80 cases. *Transplant Int* 11 Suppl 1: S334–S336

31 Shapiro R, Jordan ML, Scantlebury VP, Vivas C, Fung JJ, McCauley J, Randhawa P, Demetris AJ, Irish W, Jain A et al (1995) A prospective, randomized trial of FK506/prednisone vs FK 506/azathioprine/prednisone in renal transplant patients. *Transplant Proc* 27: 814–817

32 Shapiro R, Jordan ML, Scantlebury VP, Vivas C, Gritsch HA, Casavilla FA, McCauley J, Johnston JR, Randhawa P, Irish W et al (1998) A prospective, randomized trial to compare tacrolimus and prednisone with and without mycophenolate mofetil in patients undergoing renal transplantation: first report. *J Urol* 160: 1982–1986

33 Gruessner RW, Burke GW, Stratta R, Sollinger H, Benedetti E, Marsh C, Stock P, Boudreaux JP, Martin M, Drangstveit MB et al (1996) A multicenter analysis of the first experience with FK506 for induction and rescue therapy after pancreas transplantation. *Transplantation* 61: 261–273

34 Sutherland DE, Gruessner A (1995) Pancreas transplantation in the United States as reported to the United Network for Organ Sharing (UNOS) and analyzed by the International Pancreas Transplant Registry. *Clin Transplant* 59: 49–67

35 Hariharan S, Munda R, Cavallo T, Demmy AM, Schroeder TJ, Alexander JW, First MR (1996) Rescue therapy with tacrolimus after combined kidney/pancreas and isolated pancreas transplantation in patients with severe cyclosporine nephrotoxicity. *Transplantation* 61: 1161–1165

36 Keenan RJ, Konishi H, Kawai A, Paradis IL, Nunley DR, Iacono AT, Hardesty RL, Weyant RJ, Griffith BP (1995) Clinical trial of tacrolimus *versus* cyclosporine in lung transplantation. *Ann Thorac Surg* 60: 580–585

37 Sher LS, Cosenza CA, Petrovic LM, Rojter S, Hoffman A, Lopez RR, Meehan M, Pan SH, Vierling J, Makowka L (1996) Tacrolimus (FK506) for rescue of chronic rejection following orthotopic liver transplantation. *Transplant Proc* 28: 1011–1013

38 Jordan ML, Naraghi RN, Shapiro R, Smith D, Vivas CA, Scantlebury VP, Gritsch HA, McCauley J, Randhawa P, Demetris AJ et al (1997) Five-year experience with tacrolimus rescue for renal allograft rejection. *Transplant Proc* 29: 306

39 Danovitch GM (1997) Cyclosporin or tacrolimus: which agent to choose? *Nephrol Dialysis Transplant* 12: 1566–1568

40 Otto MG, Mayer AD, Clavien PA, Cavallari A, Gunawardena KA, Mueller EA (1998) Randomized trial of cyclosporine microemulsion (neoral) *versus* conventional cyclosporine in liver transplantation: MILTON study. Multicentre International Study in Liver Transplantation of Neoral. *Transplantation* 66: 1632–1640

41 Hauser IA, Neumayer HN (1998) Tacrolimus and cyclosporine efficacy in high-risk kidney transplantation. European Multicentre Tacrolimus (FK506) Renal Study Group. *Transplant Int* 11 Suppl 1: S73-S77

Modern Immunosuppressives
ed. by H.-J Schuurman, G. Feutren and J.-F. Bach
© 2001 Birkhäuser Verlag/Switzerland

The potential role of immunosuppressive macrocyclic lactones

Johnny C. Hong and Barry D. Kahan

Division of Organ Transplantation, Department of Surgery, The University of Texas Medical School at Houston, 6431 Fannin Street, Suite 6.240, Houston, TX 77030, USA

Macrocyclic lactones: a group of unique antibiotics

Macrocyclic lactones are lipophilic molecules bearing a large 12-, 14-, or 16-membered lactone ring substituted with hydroxyl, methyl, and ethyl groups, as well as carbonyl functions with one, two, or three carbohydrate fragments. The first compound of this class, pikromycin, was isolated by Brockman et al. in 1950 [1]. The past three decades have witnessed the development and extensive use of a group of medium-to-narrow-spectrum antibiotic macrocyclic lactones: erythromycin, oleandomycin, leucomycin (kitasamycin), josamycin (leucomycin A$_3$), acetylspiramycin, and midemycin.

Although as a class these agents are considered to be well tolerated in man [2], their side-effect profile includes most commonly gastrointestinal intolerance, as well as hepatotoxicity, ototoxicity, and dermatologic effects. Less commonly reported reactions include pancreatitis, cardiovascular toxicity, hemolytic anemia, and psychotic reactions. Of great interest are the apparently idiosyncratic, adverse cardiac toxicities. Intravenous administration of either tacrolimus [3, 4] or erythromycin, particularly in women [5–7], has been associated with the electrocardiographic sign of lengthening of the rate-correlated QT interval. This alteration may lead to torsades de pointes ventricular arrhythmia, in similar fashion as potassium channel blockers such as quinidine and amiodarone. Furthermore, co-administration of astemizole, cisapride, pimozide or terfenadine may increase the proclivity of macrocyclic lactones to produce cardiac side-effects.

Macrocyclic lactones display three pharmacokinetic limitations. First, low and variable bioavailability may result from several factors: namely, the sensitivity of these drugs to gastric acid, incomplete absorption from the intestine, and first-pass hepatic metabolism. Second, these drugs show variable binding to plasma proteins, ranging between 10 and 93% at therapeutic concentrations. Third, macrocyclic lactones display widespread drug-drug interactions with co-administered pharmaceuticals. These interactions frequently affect serum concentrations, the nature of the effect being dependent upon the action of the macrolide upon cytochrome P (CYP) 450 3A isozymes. Drugs such as rifamycin that act only as inducers of P450 3A isozymes but do not form inhibitory complexes with them, frequently cause rapid oxidization and elimination of macrocyclic lactones. In contrast, troleandomycin and erythromycin derivatives act initially as inducers, and later as inhibitors of CYP450 3A due to complex formation. Following induction of CYP450 3A, the macrocyclic lactone metabolite nitrosoalkane binds to P450 iron (II), forming an inactive iron-metabolite complex, which is stable despite the presence of degrading enzymes. Persistence of the complex leads to accumulation of inactive CYP450. Thus macrocyclic lactones can cause abnormally high plasma levels and prolonged half-lives of drugs that are also metabolized by the CYP 450 3A isozyme system.

This chapter describes two natural microbial products, tacrolimus (FK506, Prograf TRL) and sirolimus (rapamycin, RAPA; Wyeth-Ayerst, Princeton, NJ), which were isolated from the soil actinomycetes *Streptomyces tsukubaensis* and *Streptomyces hygroscopicus*, respectively (Fig. 1a and 1b). Both agents are poorly absorbed from the gastrointestinal tract and widely distributed throughout the body upon binding to cytoplasmic FK-binding proteins (FKBP, molecular weight 10–11 kDa), a family of cis-trans prolyl peptidyl isomerases. Although TRL and RAPA display immunosuppressive efficacy in clinical transplantation, they also show appreciable toxicities. Already, a TRL analog, indolyl-ascomycin (ASC), has been synthesized in an attempt to improve the therapeutic efficacy of TRL. Indolyl-ASC has a lower affinity for cytosolic FKBPs, and thereby seems to act selectively in cells with high concentrations of FKBP12 such as lymphocytes, when compared to cells with a lower ratio of FKBP12-to-calcineurin content (e.g., brain cells) [8]. Studies in animal models seem to support this hypothesis: ASC retains immunosuppressive potency with apparently reduced nephrotoxicity, neurotoxicity, and/or gastrointestinal system dysfunction [9]. However, these findings have not yet been applied to human transplantation in clinical trials.

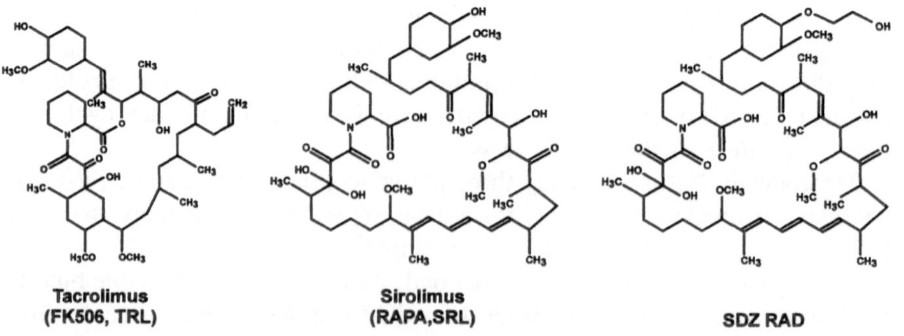

Tacrolimus (FK506, TRL)   **Sirolimus (RAPA,SRL)**   **SDZ RAD**

Figure 1. Structures of the immunosuppressive macrolides tacrolimus, rapamycin and RAD.

Tacrolimus

Introduction

Discovered in 1984 by Goto et al. [10], the macrocyclic lactone antibiotic tacrolimus (TRL, Prograf; Fujisawa U.S.A., Inc, Deerfield, IL) is derived from *Streptomyces tsukubaensis. In vitro*, TRL displays 50–100-fold greater immunosuppressive potency than cyclosporine (CsA). Although the original report on TRL therapy described the "salvage" of liver allografts in patients suffering ongoing rejection despite CsA-based immunosuppression [11], numerous studies now suggest beneficial immunosuppressive effects of TRL as a *de novo* agent for acute rejection prophylaxis in a variety of solid organ transplants. TRL was approved by the Food and Drug Administration for use in liver transplantation in 1994, and for kidney transplantation in 1997.

Mechanism of immunosuppressive action

On the one hand, TRL and RAPA are structurally related macrocyclic lactones (Fig. 1) that mediate distinct immunosuppressive effects on T-cell activation. On the other hand, although chemically distinct from the cyclic endecapeptide CsA, TRL exhibits a common mechanism of action with CsA to interrupt the antigen-driven signal transduction pathway (Fig. 2). After binding *via* the pipecolic portion of the molecule to their respective intercellular cytoplasmic immunophilin proteins – FKBP (particularly FKBP12) and cyclophilin – , TRL and CsA inhibit the generation of T-cell regulatory proteins critical for upregulation of DNA transcription of mRNAs for interleukin-2 (IL-2) and other pro-inflammatory cytokines, including IL-3, IL-4, interferon-γ, tumor

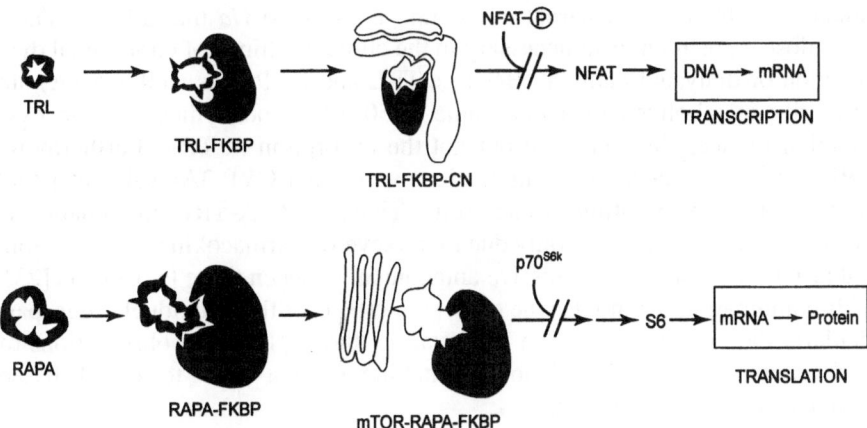

Figure 2. Comparison of the mechanisms of action of TRL *versus* RAPA.

necrosis factor-α, granulocyte-macrophage colony-stimulating factor, as well as proto-oncogenes such as *ras, myc and rel* [12, 13]. The calcineurin phosphatase activity is necessary for dephosphorylation (and subsequent activation) of the cytoplasmic form of nuclear factor of activated T-cells. In contrast, both TRL and CsA seem to enhance the expression of transforming growth factor-β (TGF-β). This cytokine not only has immunosuppressive effects, possibly at least in part mediated by cell cycle arrest in the G phase *via* p21, but also seems to predispose to the progression of renal allograft fibrosis [14]. Although TRL (but not CsA) seems to enhance antigen-induced apoptosis in murine thymocytes and peripheral T-cells [15], it is not clear whether its greater potency is due to this or to another unique immunosuppressive effect.

Pharmacokinetic properties

TRL displays wide inter- as well as intra-individual pharmacokinetic variations in both kidney and liver transplant patients [16, 17]. The adverse effects of TRL correlate better with trough concentration than with dose [18]. The oral bioavailability ranges from 4 to 93% (mean about 25%) [19], and the half-life from 5.5 to 16.6 h (mean 8.7 h). At 1 to 4 h after an oral dose of 0.15 mg/kg, the peak plasma concentration is between 0.4 and 3.7 ng/mL. Both the rate and the extent of absorption are reduced with food intake. Since neither cholestasis nor impaired biliary function influence the absorption of orally administered TRL, intravenous administration of TRL is unnecessary during the early post-operative period after liver transplantation, despite T-tube biliary diversion [20].

Tacrolimus is extensively distributed throughout the body, with a high affinity to formed blood elements. Whole blood concentrations are 11–114 times higher than the content in the plasma fraction [21, 22]. Since the main excretory pathway for TRL metabolites is biliary and the majority of drug is cell-bound, less than 1% of parent compound is excreted *via* the kidneys. Thus, drug-dose adjustment is unnecessary in the clinical settings of either renal dysfunction or dialysis treatment. Because TRL and RAPA (as well as CsA) are primarily metabolized by cytochrome P450 3A4 isoenzymes, hepatic dysfunction reduces the clearance but not the absorption of TRL. Furthermore, TRL shows pharmacokinetic interactions with other CYP 3A4 substrates that increase the concentration of each drug. Thus, the CsA-TRL combination is clearly contraindicated, not only due to the severe pharmacokinetic interaction, but also to the immunosuppressive antagonism between these two agents [23]. This combination potentiates the toxic side-effects of the individual drugs, particularly the nephrotoxicity – a potentiation that explains the observations of "conversion nephrotoxicity" upon switching from a CsA- to a TRL-based immunosuppression regimen.

Dosage forms, dosing, and therapeutic drug monitoring

TRL is currently available for both intravenous (5 mg/mL in a 1 mL vial) and oral (1 mg and 5 mg capsules) administration. For continuous intravenous infusion, initial TRL doses are 0.01–0.1 mg/kg/day; when taken orally, a total of 0.1–0.3 mg/kg/day is administered in divided doses every 12 h.

To achieve blood concentrations similar to those of adults, children have a higher dose requirement (0.03–0.1 mg/kg/day intravenous or 0.15–0.3 mg/kg/day orally) due to their propensity for greater rates of CYP450 3A4 metabolism. Pediatric patients may benefit from an overlap of intravenous and oral drug administration to avoid suboptimal trough concentrations during the critical first 2 weeks post-transplantation. In addition, just as with CsA therapy, African-American patients may require higher doses of TRL than either Caucasian or Asian recipients.

Only liquid chromatography/tandem mass spectrometry methods can precisely quantify TRL parent compound in whole blood [24]. However, in response to the awkwardness of these methods, two commercial kits have been developed to monitor TRL concentrations. Both kits use the same monoclonal antibody, a reagent that detects not only parent compound, but also an array of metabolites. The IMx tacrolimus assay (Abbott Laboratories, North Chicago, IL) is a microparticle enzyme immunoassay, and the Pro-Trac test (DiaSorin, Stillwater, MN) is an enzyme-linked immunosorbent assay. The advantages of the microparticle enzyme immunoassay over the enzyme-linked immunosorbent assay include simpler sample preparation, fully (rather than semi-) automated analysis, and a faster procedure time of 30 min (compared to 3 to 4 h). However, because the microparticle enzyme immunoassay has a major limitation of low sensitivity (5–10 ng/mL), the more sensitive enzyme-linked immunosorbent assay (0.2 ng/mL) is preferable for monitoring patients receiving low doses of TRL [25].

Unfortunately, the optimal therapeutic ranges for TRL drug concentrations during the induction, acute rejection prophylaxis, and maintenance phases of immunosuppression are unknown. The US multicenter study [18] of the correlation between TRL concentrations and episodes of toxicity and rejection among 120 kidney transplant patients reported that optimal efficacy occurred with TRL trough concentrations of 5–15 ng/mL. Trough concentrations below 5 ng/mL were associated with a 30% incidence of acute rejection episodes, and those above 15 ng/mL with a 45% incidence of adverse events and a 3% incidence of rejection episodes.

Toxic side-effects

The most common adverse events associated with TRL therapy are neurotoxic: tremor, seizures, coma, and headache. Although a significant proportion of patients complain of nausea and diarrhea, renal dysfunction and new onset diabetes mellitus represent more serious and more frequently encountered toxicities. The incidence of post-transplant diabetes mellitus (PTDM) is significantly higher for the TRL-treated cohort groups than for the CsA-treated cohort groups (19% *versus* 4% respectively; $p < 0.001$) [26]. The incidence of PTDM was three times higher among African-American patients than among Caucasian patients [27]. Unfortunately, the majority (80%) of afflicted African-American patients continuously required insulin treatment beyond 2 years post-transplantation, possibly due to the need for higher TRL doses to achieve target whole-blood drug concentrations in this racial group [28, 29]. However, African-American patients did not experience an increased incidence of other TRL-related adverse effects. TRL and CsA appear to produce similar degrees of clinical and histopathological evidences of nephrotoxicity upon long-term administration, namely arteriolar hyalinosis and striped interstitial fibrosis [30, 31]. In contrast to the greater degree of neurotoxicity and incidence of PTDM associated with TRL therapy, hypertension, a common side-effect of CsA therapy, has been reported less frequently with TRL in some [32], but not other [26] studies. Similarly, lower cholesterol levels under TRL therapy when compared to CsA therapy have been reported inconsistently. TRL is not associated with hypertrichosis or gingival hyperplasia, not-uncommon cosmetic side-effects of CsA therapy; however, TRL can produce alopecia [33] (Tab. 1).

Table 1. Comparison of selected adverse events with tacrolimus and cyclosporine [26]

Adverse event	TRL ($n = 205$)	CsA ($n = 207$)	p value
Nephrotoxicity	45.5% (93)	41.5% (86)	NS
Neurotoxicity (tremor)	53.6% (111)	33.8% (70)	0.001
Hypertension	49.8% (102)	52.2% (108)	NS
Post-transplant diabetes mellitus	19.9% (30)	2.90% (6)	0.001
Hyperlipidemia	30.7% (63)	38.2% (79)	NS
Hypercholesterolemia	7.80% (16)	14.5% (30)	NS
Alopecia	10.7% (22)	0.97% (2)	0.001
Hirsutism	0.49% (1)	8.7% (18)	0.001
Gingivitis	1.46% (3)	8.7% (18)	0.001

NS, not statistically significant

Current applications of Tacrolimus in solid organ transplantation

Primary de novo therapy

Liver transplantation: The US and European open-label multicenter trials [34–38] observed similar 1-year recipient and hepatic allograft survival rates among groups of patients treated with either TRL or the original oil-based Sandimmune formulation of CsA as the primary immunosuppressive drug

Table 2. Randomized controlled clinical trials on efficacy of tacrolimus- (TRL-) versus cyclosporine- (CsA-) based immunosuppressive therapy in liver transplantation

Reference	No. of patients	Duration (years)	Survival rates (%)						Acute rejection episodes (%)		
			Patient			Graft					
			TRL	CsA	p	TRL	CsA	p	TRL	CsA	p
U.S. trials											
Multicenter [35]	529	1	88	88	NS[b]	82	79	NS	59	65	0.002
Fung [36]	154	4	84	84	NS	ND[c]	ND	ND	63.8	83	0.003
Wiesner Multicenter [34]	529	5	79	73.1	NS	71.8	66.4	NS	68	76	<0.001
European trials											
Kling [38]	121	1	90.2	96.7	NS	88.5	91.7	NS	34.4	33.3	NS
Multicenter [37]	545	1	82.9	77.5	NS	77.5	72.6	NS	40.5	49.8	0.04

[a] Acute rejection rates between 1 and 5 years followup.
[b] NS = not significant.
[c] ND = no data reported.

(Tab. 2). In a 5-year follow-up report, Wiesner [34] described similar recipient and graft survival rates for TRL- (79%, 71.8%) *versus* Sandimmune CsA-based (73.1%, 66.4%) therapies. Compared with the Sandimmune group, the TRL cohort showed a lower rate of acute rejection episodes (68% *versus* 76%, $p < 0.001$) as well as a lower rate of steroid-resistant rejection episodes (19% *versus* 36%, $p < 0.001$) during the first year after transplant. Thereafter patients in both treatment groups showed a low incidence of late, steroid-resistant acute rejection episodes, (4.9% *versus* 6.3%, not statistically significant), of death or of rejection-related graft losses [34].

Kidney transplantation: Using TRL rather than Sandimmune CsA in conjunction with azathioprine and steroids, the US and European open-label multicenter randomized parallel-group studies showed similar 1-year recipient and graft survival rates. The acute allograft rejection episodes [26, 39] were lower in both studies for TRL (30.7% or 25.9%) than for Sandimmune (46.4% or 45.7%; both $p < 0.001$; Tab. 3). Rejection episodes resistant to increased doses of steroids occurred in 11.3% of TRL and 21.6% of CsA recipients ($p = 0.001$). However, the rates of occurrence of chronic allograft rejection reactions did not differ significantly between TRL- and CsA-treated patients (5.2% *versus* 9.3%) [39].

Pancreas transplantation: Despite aggressive immunosuppressive regimens, acute rejection reactions remain the major cause of morbidity and graft failure among pancreas transplant recipients at 1 and 5 years post-transplantation. The incidences of graft loss due to rejection, respectively, are 6% and 13% for simultaneous pancreas-kidney transplants, 32% and 68% for pancreas transplants alone, and 29% and 79% for pancreas after kidney transplantation [40]. Shaffer et al. [41] observed a beneficial effect of TRL in two simultaneous pancreas-kidney recipients suffering from refractory rejection without impairing long-term pancreas graft function. Hariharan et al. [42, 43] presented a long-term follow-up of a cohort of 12 patients who underwent conversion from CsA to TRL due to CsA-induced vasculopathy upon renal biopsy; four of these patients also experienced persistent rejection despite treatment with therapeutic CsA levels. Renal graft function stabilized without changes in blood glucose concentration, hemoglobin A_{1c}, and C-peptide levels. The findings also showed a non-significant tendency toward a lower rate of recurrent acute rejection episodes. Teroaka et al. [44] claimed beneficial effects of TRL among patients with relapsing rejection episodes after combined pancreas-kidney transplants.

Gruessner et al. [45] reported the 6-month data from a multicenter open-label study of 154 pancreas allograft recipients treated with TRL *de novo* ($n = 82$), or converted from CsA to TRL for anti-rejection, rescue therapy ($n = 61$), or for other reasons ($n = 11$). The median TRL starting dose was 4 mg/day orally, seeking to achieve a blood trough concentration of 12 ng/mL. Among patients treated *de novo*, 66% were simultaneous pancreas-kidney

Table 3. Randomized controlled clinical trials on efficacy of tacrolimus- (TRL-) *versus* cyclosporine (CsA-) based immunosuppressive therapy in conjunction with aza-thioprine and prednisone in renal transplantation

Reference	No. of patients	Duration (years)	Survival rates (%)							Acute rejection episodes (%)		
			Patient			Graft					
			TRL	CsA	p	TRL	CsA	p	TRL	CsA	p
U.S. Multicenter	412	1	95.6	96.6	NS	91.2	87.9	NS	30.7	46.6	0.001
European Multicenter	448	1	93	96.5	NS	82.5	86.2	NS	25.9	45.7	0.001

NS, not significant

recipients who, as a group, displayed a patient survival rate of 90% and a pancreas graft survival rate of 87% at 6 months. For comparison, an arbitrary *post hoc* "matched-pair" analysis showed a 70% graft survival rate among an historical cohort of CsA recipients ($p = 0.04$). The *de novo* TRL group showed a 35% rate of reversible rejection episodes within the first 6 months post-transplantation. The most commonly reported adverse events were neurotoxicity (16%), nephrotoxicity (13%), and/or gastrointestinal toxicity (9%); new-onset insulin-dependent diabetes mellitus was not observed. Among the group of patients treated for rejection indications, 72% had undergone simultaneous pancreas-kidney transplantation. At 6 months, this subgroup showed patient and graft survival rates of 91% and 90%, respectively, with a 44% rate of recurrent acute rejection episodes within 6 months despite conversion. Compared to *de novo* patients, those converted to TRL for rescue purposes had a higher incidence of adverse reactions, namely, neurotoxicity (23%), nephrotoxicity (25%), and gastrointestinal toxicity (21%). New-onset insulin-dependent diabetes was noted in one recipient, who, interestingly, displayed good exocrine function; however, two patients were reconverted to CsA due to persistent hyperglycemia.

Heart transplantation: An initial pilot US trial revealed a higher incidence of patients treated *de novo* with TRL to be free from acute rejection episodes than a cohort treated with Sandimmune CsA (47% *versus* 22%, $p = 0.01$) [46]. However, the incidence of patients free from rejection episodes was similar for TRL treatment when compared to Sandimmune CsA plus antilymphocyte induction therapy (47% *versus* 53.1%). Patient survival rates did not differ between the three cohorts, and no patients required discontinuation of TRL due to side-effects.

In contrast, the European Multicenter Tacrolimus Heart Pilot Study group [47] found a similar incidence of acute rejection episodes and graft as well as patient survival rates at 1 year for TRL and CsA treatment groups. The rates of freedom from acute rejection episodes were 26.3% for TRL and 18.5% for CsA ($p = 0.444$), with graft survival rates of 79.6% and 92.9%, respectively ($p = 0.125$). Although fewer patients in the TRL compared with the CsA group required antihypertensive therapy (59.5% *versus* 87.5%, not statistically significant), the overall rates of adverse effects including infections, impaired renal function (31.5% *versus* 21.4%) and/or glucose intolerance (7.0% *versus* 4.3%) did not differ significantly. Although cardiac biopsy specimens of TRL-treated patients showed a greater percentage of inflamed fragments and a higher rejection grade than those of CsA-treated patients within the first 30 days post-transplant, specimens collected during the late transplant period (275 to 548 days) showed the reverse. However, the cardiac allograft biopsy histopathology in the later phase did not differ between patients treated with TRL and those with CsA-based therapy and antibody induction [48].

Lung transplantation: Keenan et al. [49] reported that TRL treatment seemed modestly but not significantly to reduce the incidence of acute rejection episodes per 100 patient-days compared with an historical cohort treated with Sandimmune CsA (0.85 *versus* 1.09, $p = 0.07$). The authors observed that obliterative bronchiolitis, a major cause of long-term morbidity and mortality after lung transplantation, was detected in significantly fewer patients in the TRL group compared to the historical Sandimmune CsA group (21.7% *versus* 38%, $p = 0.025$). However, the 1- and 2-year graft survival rates were similar in the two treatment groups.

Rescue therapy

Liver transplantation: Conversion from Sandimmune CsA to TRL as rescue therapy in hepatic allograft recipients who experienced steroid-resistant rejection or early chronic processes was reported to confer both histological and biochemical improvements in allograft function [50–52]. For example, an anecdotal report in 64 patients presumably diagnosed with acute rejection at the time of study entry described "normalization" of mean serum levels of total bilirubin and transaminases within 6 months after conversion. In contrast, patients diagnosed with chronic rejection at entry ($n = 113$) showed "normalization" of bilirubin, but persistently elevated serum transaminase levels at 6 months. Following conversion to TRL therapy, 47% of patients showed improvement in liver biopsy histology, while 17% showed deterioration in the pathologic findings [53].

Kidney transplantation: Rescue therapy for refractory kidney transplant rejection has been examined in two nonrandomized US trials. Patient and graft survival rates were 94% and 93%, and 74% and 75%, respectively [54, 55]. Prior to conversion from Sandimmune CsA to TRL, the majority of patients had been unresponsive to increased doses of steroids with or without administration of antilymphocyte antibody agents. TRL therapy was initiated at a median of 4.3 months post-transplantation. Two factors appeared to influence the success of TRL rescue therapy, namely the pre-conversion serum creatinine level as an index of kidney damage and the time post-transplantation. Not surprisingly, successful conversion was more common in patients that had low serum creatinine values at the time of TRL inception, as well as in patients converted before 6 months post-transplantation (75% *versus* 50%, $p = 0.006$). Jordan et al. [54] claimed that 13 of 28 (46%) patients that were on dialysis at the time of conversion had functioning grafts at a mean follow-up of 37 months.

Heart transplantation: TRL rescue therapy has been reported in 16 heart and 15 lung transplant recipients [56] that were converted due to CsA intolerance, to the occurrence of acute rejection episodes, or to the presence of histopathologic changes suggestive of humoral rejection. Among the heart transplant recipients, all patients and grafts were surviving at the time of the report (mean

183 ± 65 days). Only 20% of heart transplant recipients were free from rejection episodes post-TRL conversion. Among the lung transplant recipients, the patient and graft survival rates at a mean time of 169 ± 86 days were 67% and 60%, respectively. Following conversion, 80% of the lung transplant patients did not experience rejection episodes.

Tacrolimus or cyclosporine: which agent to use?

The comparisons of clinical outcomes under TRL- *versus* CsA- based immunosuppressive therapies in studies published to date are irrelevant to current practice. All these trials compared TRL to the original oil-based (Sandimmune) rather than the recent microemulsion formulation of CsA (Neoral; Novartis, Basel, Switzerland). The introduction of the microemulsion formulation addressed major limitations of the oil-based CsA preparations: namely, highly variable, partial, and bile-dependent gastrointestinal absorption. As would be anticipated, Neoral substitution for Sandimmune has significantly reduced the incidence of acute rejection episodes [57]. This reduced incidence undoubtedly mitigates at least some of the apparent differences between CsA- and TRL-based regimens. This concern is supported when one compares the rejection rate of 30.7% under TRL-steroid with the 24% rate among the patients treated with Neoral-azathioprine-Prednisone in the blinded multicenter USA Phase III clinical trial [58].

The selection of CsA or TRL as the baseline calcineurin-inhibitor is presently based on physician preference, patient intolerance to the side-effect profile of either agent (such as the neurotoxicity of TRL or the cosmetic effects of CsA), and/or ill-defined pharmacodynamic resistance to the agent used *de novo*.

Sirolimus

Cellular mechanism of immunosuppressive action

Sirolimus (rapamycin RAPA) is a macrocyclic lactone product of *Streptomyces hygroscopicus,* which was discovered in the soil of the Vai Atari region of Rapa Nui (Easter Island) [59–61]. RAPA has a unique mechanism of action, namely, to inhibit enzymes regulating progression through the G_1 phase of the cell cycle, thereby inhibiting cytokine-driven cell proliferation and maturation [62]. This potent, novel immunosuppressant has been shown in animal models not only to prolong allograft survival [63], but also to interact synergistically with CsA [64]. RAPA blocks Ca^{2+}-dependent and Ca^{2+}-independent events during the G_1 phase of the cell cycle, including transduction of the signals delivered by IL-2, IL-3, IL-5 and IL-6. To a lesser degree, RAPA blocks signals delivered by fibroblast growth factor, stem cell factor, platelet-derived growth factor, colony stimulating factor and insulin growth factor. When added *in vitro*, RAPA (1–300 nM) inhibits a variety of mitogen- and antigen-driven B- and T-lymphocyte proliferative responses, but does not block effector cytotoxic T-cell action.

RAPA blocks T-cell maturation and inhibits B-cell responses and immunoglobulin (Ig) production both *in vitro* and *in vivo*. At concentrations of 1 nM, RAPA inhibits the stimulation of DNA synthesis by B-cells; at concentrations of 10 nM, RAPA inhibits IgM, IgA, and IgG secretion by B-cells that have been stimulated with *Staphylococcus aureus* or soluble CD40 ligand. These effects on T- and B-cells occur at RAPA concentrations 10- to 100-fold lower than those required to inhibit the cytotoxic actions of natural killer, lymphokine-activated killer, and antibody-dependent cytotoxic cells.

The initial claim that RAPA inhibits cytokine-driven cell proliferation and maturation by reducing the cell surface expression of IL-2 or IL-4 receptors on mitogen-activated T-cells, has not been confirmed. Rather, RAPA interrupts post-receptor events by forming active complexes with FKBP. This complex probably inhibits several molecular effectors, the most prominent of which seems to be a phosphatidyl-inositol kinase denoted as mammalian target of rapamycin (mTOR) that enzymatically regulates the phosphorylation status of several sarcoma (src)-like, receptor-type, and cell-cycle-dependent kinases, as well as intracellular phosphatases. One important molecular target of this FKBP-12-RAPA-mTOR complex is $p70^{S6}$ kinase, which hyperphosphorylates the 40S ribosomal protein $p70^{S6}$ (but not the $p85^{S6k}$ variety). Inhibition of this hyperphosphorylation, an essential step in G_1 progression, occurs at the same concentrations as those required for RAPA to block cell proliferation [65, 66]. In addition, RAPA, perhaps *via* an effect on mTOR, increases the stability of $p27^{kip}$, thus inhibiting the action of downstream serine-threonine protein kinases ($p34^{cdc2}$) and preventing the generation of two factors that control the rate of T-cell progression into the S phase of the cell cycle, namely, the active $p34^{cdc2}$-cyclin D heterodimeric complex that forms the critical "maturational-promoting factor" and the cyclin-dependent kinase cdk2, the catalytic partner of cyclin E.

Mechanism of induction of long-term unresponsiveness in transplanted hosts

In addition to the apparent effects of RAPA treatment on T-cell maturation, a unique action on B-cells seems to mediate the long-term unresponsiveness produced in rodent models even after cessation of treatment. Unlike rats treated with CsA, which induces a state of anergy among cytotoxic T-lymphocytes (CTL), rats rendered tolerant by RAPA have CTL-precursor frequencies equal to those observed in virgin rats [67]. In addition, splenic and lymph node T-cells adoptively transfer unresponsiveness after CsA, but not after RAPA treatment. In contrast, the transfer of B-cells or serum IgG_{2c} fractions from RAPA-treated rats induces a state of donor-specific unresponsiveness that is mediated by non-complement-fixing antibodies that are alloantigen-, not anti-idiotype-, specific. Interestingly, the cells that infiltrate the heart allografts of unresponsive RAPA-treated recipients showed preferential expression of the T-helper 2 phenotype by increased levels of IL-4 and IL-10, rather than the T-helper 1 phenotype (IL-2), as documented by profiles of their mRNA transcripts.

Because RAPA was believed to act by inhibiting cytokine receptor signal transduction, and because little is known about cytokine regulation of Ig class switching in rats, we conducted further experiments in mice. RAPA treatment did not affect the action of IL-4 to promote the switch from the μ (IgM) to the γ_1 (IgG$_1$) heavy chain, but did inhibit the ability of interferon-γ to switch to γ_{2a} (IgG$_{2a}$) and γ_3 (IgG$_3$), and of TGF-β to switch to γ_{2b} (IgG$_{2b}$) and α (IgA). Alloantigen-specific IgM antibody production was halved, and γ_{2a}, γ_{2b}, and γ_3 production was almost completely abrogated. In contrast, the levels of non-complement-binding γ_1 isotype antibodies increased, peaking between days 56 and 100. The graft sites contained increased levels of γ_1, but not μ, γ_{2a}, γ_{2b}, or γ_3 mRNA transcripts, as well as amplified levels of IL-4, and diminished levels of IL-2, mRNA transcripts. The allo-unresponsiveness was transferred to irradiated (200 rad) secondary recipients by serum and B-cells, but not by T-cells. Thus, RAPA in mice directly, or *via* promotion of IL-4 synthesis, diverts Ig-isotype switching toward the appearance of donor-specific blocking γ_1 antibodies.

Pharmacokinetic properties of RAPA

RAPA has an oral bioavailability of about 15% and an average terminal half-life between 57 and 62 h. After a single oral dose of $1-34$ mg/m^2, the whole blood concentration peaked between $0.8-3$ h and, in about 70% of the patients, peak concentrations occurred within 1 h. There was a good correlation ($r = 0.94$) between the trough and the area-under-the-concentration-time-curve (AUC) concentrations, suggesting that the trough level is a good indicator of total drug exposure [68, 69].

RAPA is extensively distributed in tissues, with a volume of distribution of $5.6-16.7$ L/kg in stable renal transplant recipients [70]. RAPA whole blood concentration is far higher than plasma concentrations, because 94.5% is bound to red blood cells, 1% to lymphocytes and granulocytes, and only 3.1% to plasma.

RAPA is metabolized by CYP450 3A isoenzymes. The large inter-subject variability in the clearance of orally administered RAPA may owe to the impact of both CYP3A4 and the multidrug action efflux pump P-glycoprotein, which are located in small intestinal enterocytes [71]. Not only is there an 11-fold inter-individual variation in the intestinal content of CYP3A4 proteins, but also both CYP3A4 and P-glycoprotein activity are affected by co-administered drugs [72, 73].

Although the wide inter-subject variation displayed by RAPA is shared by CsA and TRL, RAPA shows a more extensive partitioning in tissue and red blood cells resulting in a greater delay to steady-state concentrations and a relatively long terminal half-life that permits once-daily dosing [69].

Dosage forms and regimens

The primary clinical trials of RAPA utilized an oil-based liquid formulation that requires refrigeration for stabilization of the drug suspension: however, a solid RAPA tablet was recently introduced [74]. A pharmacokinetic comparison of the liquid and the pill formulation was performed in 12 renal transplant recipients who had been receiving liquid for more than 1 year. Concurrent 12-hour pharmacokinetic profiles of RAPA and CsA were conducted on the last dose of liquid and again at 2, 4, and 8 weeks post-conversion to the solid formulation. The only significant difference was a higher maximum concentration (C_{max}) after administration of the liquid compared with the solid formulation. There were no significant differences for the pharmacokinetic parameters of AUC_{0-12}, dose-corrected RAPA C_0, time to maximum RAPA concentration (t_{max}), relative oral bioavailability of liquid *versus* solid, or CsA AUC_{0-12}.

Several approaches may be employed to select RAPA dosing regimens. First, physician intuition may be guided by the assumption that drug doses sufficient to produce toxicity must indicate an adequate level of immunosuppression. However, this assumption is not entirely valid in the case of CsA therapy. Despite the occurrence of acute rejection episodes suggesting inadequate immunosuppression, CsA may produce renal injury particularly among allografts predisposed by virtue of elderly donor age, prolonged cold ischemia time, and/or operative misadventure. In the case of RAPA, we do not yet know whether the development of myelosuppressive or hyperlipidemic effects correlates with the drug's therapeutic effect. Furthermore, the toxic effects of RAPA may outlast its immunosuppressive effects, thus rendering patients susceptible to the emergence of breakthrough allograft rejection. In addition, the relationship between RAPA dosage and drug-induced toxicity has not been documented, with the exception of findings of a correlation between hypercholesterolemia and dose [75].

Trough concentration monitoring offers another option for choosing RAPA doses. In contrast to CsA, wherein trough blood concentration (C_0) measurements are not representative of overall drug exposure [76], trough RAPA concentrations correlate strongly with AUC measurements ($r^2 = 0.946$) [68]. However, trough level measurements by high-performance liquid chromatography with ultraviolet detection are expensive and are presently cumbersome, taking 22 min to perform, obstacles that may be addressed by an automated assay presently under development (IMx, Abbott Diagnostics, North Chicago, IL). Using the high-performance liquid chromatography method in Phase I/II trials, we observed that acute rejection prophylaxis was virtually guaranteed when the RAPA C_0 concentrations were maintained between 10 and 15 ng/mL and CsA exposure is set at average concentrations (the quotient of the AUC and the dosing interval) between 350–450 ng/mL, namely 40% lower than those used in CsA-steroid regimens [77]. The protocol of RAPA C_0 monitoring has been associated with only modest drug toxicity.

Serial measurements of drug exposure by pharmacokinetic profiles may also be useful in monitoring immunosuppressive therapy, based upon the evidence that intra-individual variation in CsA exposure is associated with an increased risk of chronic rejection. Although RAPA trough concentrations show a good overall correlation with AUC, this monitoring strategy may not be reliable for all patients. Full pharmacokinetic profiles are particularly useful during the initial 2 weeks of dosing, particularly in cases where patients are being treated with concomitant medications that affect CYP450 3A4 activity. Subsequently, an abbreviated sampling strategy [78] – aliquots of whole blood drawn at 0, 2, and 6 h – seems to reliably estimate the full AUC exposure (±15% prediction error). Preliminary evidence suggests that there is approximately a 25–30% degree of intra-individual variation in RAPA AUC over a 2-year period; however, the data base is not yet sufficiently robust to determine whether a higher degree of intra-individual variability of RAPA exposure predisposes toward the development of chronic rejection.

Pharmacodynamic monitoring may be performed using an efficacy parameter endpoint (e.g., acute rejection episodes), a toxicity parameter, or a surrogate laboratory measure of immunosuppressive activity (mTOR activity). During the early post-transplant phase myelosuppression may provide a convenient index of RAPA toxicity, since it occurs during the first month (as opposed to hyperlipidemia at 2 months), and since CsA as well as dietary indiscretions can produce hyperlipidemia. However, RAPA-induced myelosuppression occurs in only a minority of patients and may be obfuscated by concomitant treatment with the nucleoside inhibitors azathioprine or mycophenolate mofetil (MMF). A more robust assay would directly reflect the inhibitory effect of RAPA on its mTOR enzyme target or on the generation of a relevant intermediate product p70[S6] kinase, whose activity is necessary for microsomal protein synthesis to drive cell cycle progression through the G_1 phase. While these enzyme tests might be too complex for routine clinical use, they could provide at least an experimental index to link drug concentrations with immunosuppressive effects, and thereby yield reliable algorithms for RAPA dosing.

Despite the promising results from initial clinical trials, exact recommendations for either initial or maintenance dosing regimens, for therapeutic drug monitoring protocols, and for patient management are as yet unclear. To date, most clinical trials have sought to minimize RAPA toxicities by combining modest doses of the drug with CsA, thereby exploiting the synergistic interactions of the two agents. While Phase III trials have recently confirmed that 2.0 or 5.0 mg RAPA doses provide excellent prophylaxis of acute rejection episodes, some patients required dose reductions in response to toxic adverse events (see below). Contrariwise, there may be a need to increase the long-term RAPA dose to exploit its potential for chronic rejection [79]. Thus it is likely that at least in the near future, optimal results with this agent will depend upon the acumen of transplantation physicians to individualize the RAPA regimen.

Toxic side-effects

Phase II studies revealed that addition of RAPA to a CsA-based regimen only modestly increased the overall incidence of bacterial, viral, or fungal infections among recipients of living- [80] or cadaveric- [81] donor kidneys. Within a multi-center Phase IIB trial of RAPA addition to a CsA-Prednisone regimen, one center that did not administer prophylactic agents against *Pneumocystis carinii* reported six cases of the disease; therefore prophylactic treatment is now mandated for all patients. Although RAPA may increase the incidence of herpes simplex infections, the drug does not affect the occurrence or the severity of cytomegalovirus disease, despite the lack of routine prophylaxis for either infection in Phase II or III trials. Moreover, only three cases of post-transplant lymphoproliferative disease have occurred among the 300 patients treated with RAPA at our institution for periods of up to 5 years. All three cases occurred within 90 days and were associated with excessive immuno-suppression: namely, one second transplant recipient treated with high concentrations of RAPA and CsA, one elderly man with administration of OKT3 to provide a CsA holiday for renal allograft recovery, and one woman with renal allograft rejection refractory to murine OKT3, equine ATGAM, and rabbit thymoglobulin.

Cytopenias
As initially observed in the Phase I study [75], RAPA appears to interfere with the production of myeloid and erythroid elements particularly platelets. The changes usually occur during the first month, are modest in degree and resolve spontaneously. When dose reduction is required, there is usually a reversal of the toxic effect beginning on day 5, and requiring up to 14 days for full recovery.

In the Phase III trials, pre-transplant peripheral white blood cell counts below 3500/mm^3 or platelet counts below 100,000/mm^3 represented absolute contra-indications to entry. When these cell counts occurred post-transplantation, they signaled the need for more intense laboratory monitoring (Tab. 4). In cases of either extreme low counts or the need to continue RAPA therapy in the face of cytopenia(s), we have administered non-immunostimulatory cytokines – granulocyte colony stimulating factor, erythropoietin, or IL-11 – to counter drug-induced toxicity on granulocytes, erythrocytes, or platelets, respectively (Tab. 4). This strategy is based on our hypothesis that the

Table 4. Clinical management of the adverse effects of rapamycin therapy

Effect	Threshold for action	Countermeasure therapy
Thrombocytopenia	<100 000/mm^3	Dose reduction
	<50 000	Drug suspension
	<25 000	Neumega (50 µg/kg/d)
Absolute granulocytopenia	<2000/mm^3	Dose reduction
	<1500	Drug suspension
	<750	Neupogen 5 µg/kg/d (s.c. or i.v.)
Anemia	Hematocrit <32%	Epogen (6000 U, 3 times/week)
	Hematocrit <25%	Epogen (10 000 U, 3 times/week)
Hypertriglyceridemia	>300 ng/dl	Gemfibrozil 600 mg QD.
	>500 ng/dl	Gemfibrozil 600 mg bid; fish oil 2 tabs tid.
	>1000 ng/dl	Drug dose reduction
	>1500 ng/dl	Drug suspension
Hypercholesterolemia	With hypertriglyceridemia:	Pravastatin: dose proportionate to increase
	Without hypertriglyceridemia	Atorvastatin: dose proportionate to increase

myelodepression is due to RAPA inhibition of signal transduction *via* hematologic growth factor receptors that share the gp130 β chain with the lymphokine receptors that are the pharmacologic target of drug action. Although direct evidence is not available to clarify the issue, it appears that the presence of either concomitant cytomegalovirus infection or immunosuppressants that cause myelosuppression may exacerbate this toxicity of RAPA.

Hyperlipidemia
The most alarming side-effect of RAPA appears to be its tendency to increase serum lipids, an effect that may exacerbate CsA-induced hypercholesterolemia, as well as steroid-induced hypertriglyceridemia. Although the causes of the drug-induced hyperlipidemia are as yet unclear, it appears that RAPA interferes with lipid clearance from the blood possibly by inhibiting apolipoprotein action of lipolysis of low-density lipoproteins, and/or by disrupting signal transduction by insulin or insulin-like growth factors, thereby retarding the uptake of fatty acids. The toxic effect occurs in about 40 percent of renal transplant recipients generally during the second month post-transplantation. While diet instruction frequently ameliorates the condition, patients with triglyceride or cholesterol values about 300 mg% should receive countermeasure therapy (Tab. 4).

Patients with elevated serum cholesterol but not triglyceride levels are managed with administration of atorvastatin, which also has a mild effect to decrease serum triglycerides. When the triglycerides are also elevated, pravastatin is recommended since it has the least interaction with the CYP450 3A4 system and since it produces only modest rhabdomyolysis. Generally only modest 5–10 mg doses of pravastatin control the hypercholesterolemia. The hypertriglyceridemia is more difficult to manage due to the only modest activity of the fibrate and fish oil combination. It is rare for the serum triglyceride value to exceed 1000 mg%, the generally recognized threshold for the occurrence of pancreatitis, a complication that has not occurred in increased incidence among patients treated with RAPA. Although hypercholesterolemia has been implicated as a cause for cardiovascular complications – now the leading cause of mortality for patients under dual- and triple-drug regimens – and possibly for an increased incidence of chronic rejection [82, 83], the significance of RAPA-induced hypertriglyceridemia for further augmenting the incidence or severity of these complications is unclear.

Miscellaneous toxicities
RAPA displays little tendency to produce hepatotoxicity; only modest increases in serum glutamic-oxalic acid transaminase have been observed in randomized trials. There are anecdotal observations of delayed wound healing, of tendinitis, and of arthropathy, particularly in the heel. The incidence and significance of all of these side-effects are expected to be clarified upon analysis of the Phase III data comparing the clinical courses of patients in RAPA *versus* azathioprine (United States Trial) and RAPA *versus* placebo (Global Trial) trials.

Clinical results with RAPA therapy

Acute rejection prophylaxis
Phase I and II studies: Our Phase I study of 40 stable renal transplant recipients documented that CsA and RAPA have few overlapping toxicities. No nephrotoxic, hypertensive, or pharmacokinetic interactions between RAPA and CsA occurred during a 2-week treatment course [75]. Based on the Phase I results, we conducted an open-label single-center dose-escalation Phase I/II trial that examined the safety and efficacy of the *de novo* addition of RAPA to full therapeutic doses of CsA [80]. The first cohort of 20 patients was divided into groups of four patients and treated with ascending doses of RAPA (0.5, 1.0, 2.0, 3.0, and 5.0 mg/m^2/day) in combination with Prednisone according to our usual tapering schedule. Since only one patient experienced an acute rejection episode (an African-American recipient of a spousal transplant in the 0.5 mg/m^2/d dose group), and since we were concerned about the metabolic effects of long-term steroid treatment, we began to withdraw steroids (at a minimum of 5 months post-transplantation) from the immunosuppressive regimen of this cohort. There were no rebound acute rejection episodes. To test the possibility of early withdrawal of patients from Prednisone at either 1 week or 1 month post-transplantation, we treated two

additional cohorts of 10 patients each with 7 mg/m^2/day RAPA in addition to CsA and abbreviated courses of Prednisone. Only one rejection episode occurred in each cohort. Thus, among the 40 patients in this trial, there were three rejection episodes (two of which occurred among patients off steroids), yielding an overall 7.5% incidence of acute rejection episodes, a result that was significantly better than the 32% acute rejection rate in an historical CsA-Prednisone cohort [80]. Laboratory tests revealed that RAPA therapy increased the serum triglyceride and to a lesser extent cholesterol values, reduced the platelet and white blood cell counts, and produced a slower recovery of the hemoglobin content upon reversal of chronic renal failure. A greater incidence of adverse events in this trial appeared to be associated with RAPA trough concentrations >15 ng/mL. Overall the severity of the adverse events induced by RAPA seemed mild compared to the potency of the immunosuppressive effects.

A multi-center Phase II trial showed that addition of RAPA allowed doses of CsA in the Sandimmune formulation to be significantly reduced among non-African-American patients; despite the reduced CsA exposure, there was only a 12% incidence of acute rejection episodes [81]. Based on these findings, we have conducted a single-center *de novo* trial using markedly reduced doses of CsA to achieve target average blood concentrations of 250 ng/mL, rather than the usual CsA target of 550 ng/mL [77], with excellent prophylaxis of acute rejection episodes among cadaveric kidney recipients of all races (unpublished data).

Another Phase II multi-center trial compared immunosuppressive regimens including RAPA-azathioprine-Prednisone (41 patients) with that including CsA-azathioprine-Prednisone (42 patients). The incidences of acute rejection episodes diagnosed clinically or upon biopsy within 3 months of treatment, were 49% *versus* 43%, respectively [84]. Three graft losses occurred in the CsA group (one rejection and two thrombosis), and one in the RAPA group (rejection plus sepsis). No deaths occurred in either group. The laboratory abnormalities observed more frequently in the RAPA group included reduced leukocyte and platelet counts, and increased triglyceride and cholesterol levels; however, renal function in the RAPA cohort was at least transiently better than that among the CsA patients. These results suggest that RAPA may be as effective as CsA to prevent acute rejection episodes in renal transplant patients receiving azathioprine and steroids.

Phase III pivotal trials: The multicenter randomized blinded double-dummy clinical trial in 719 American renal transplant recipients compared the efficacy and safety of 2 mg/day ($n = 284$) or 5 mg/day ($n = 274$) RAPA to that of azathioprine ($n = 161$) in combination with a protocol-stipulated regimen of CsA Neoral and Prednisone [58]. Both doses of RAPA resulted in a significant reduction in the overall rate of efficacy failure at 6 months compared to azathioprine, namely 17.3% ($p = 0.003$), 17.9% ($p = 0.009$), and 29.2%, respectively. Not only was there a reduced incidence, but also a milder severity of the acute rejection episodes, as estimated by the Banff grade and by the number of patients who required antibody therapy to treat rejection episodes. Graft losses within 6 months occurred in 0.7% ($p = 0.016$), 2.8% (not statistically significant) and 2.5% of patients, respectively. Patient survival was similar across all treatment groups. The incidence of clinically important infections and of overall adverse events were similar in all groups, although elevated cholesterol and triglyceride levels were more common with RAPA, and thrombocytopenia was reported more frequently with 5 mg/day RAPA than with 2 mg/day RAPA or azathioprine.

The global multi-center randomized blinded single-dummy clinical trial in 576 recipients worldwide compared 2 mg/day ($n = 227$) or 5 mg/day ($n = 219$) RAPA with a placebo ($n = 130$). All groups received a baseline immunosuppressive regimen of CsA Neoral and steroids [85]. There was a reduction in the incidence of biopsy-proven rejection among the respective groups, namely 19% ($p = 0.076$), 11% ($p = 0.001$) and 37%, respectively. During the initial 6 months there were no differences in patient (95–98%) or graft survival (88–93%) rates among the three treatment groups. The overall severity of acute rejection was significantly lower among patients receiving 5 but not 2 mg/day RAPA when compared to placebo. Furthermore, the need for antibody therapy to treat steroid-resistant episodes of acute rejection was significantly reduced in the 2 mg/day RAPA group (2.2%) when compared to placebo (7.7%, $p = 0.025$). These two pivotal studies demonstrate that RAPA enhances the prophylactic effect of a CsA-Prednisone regimen in primary renal allograft recipients.

Refractory renal allograft rejection
Renal allograft rejection refractory to treatment with antilymphocyte antibodies almost inevitably progresses to transplant loss [86]. In a preliminary study of 13 adult patients, we defined refractory allograft rejection as the persistence of vascular rejection (Banff Grade IIB or III) on renal biopsy despite administration of both increased steroid doses, and at least one 14-day course of OKT3 and, in addition, a second 7-day course of OKT3 ($n = 13$), or a 14-day course of ATGAM ($n = 8$) and/or treatment with mycophenolate mofetil ($n = 5$). RAPA was initiated at 7 mg/m^2 for 5 days and continued thereafter at 5 mg/m^2. CsA doses were not changed; steroids were tapered or withdrawn as tolerated [87]. The actuarial 2-year patient survival was 85%; one patient succumbed to pre-existent congestive cardiomyopathy and one patient to sudden death of unknown cause, but with a functioning graft (creatinine 1.5 mg/dL). In addition, two other grafts were lost; one due to persistent rejection and one abandoned due to overwhelming, presumably infectious diarrhea. Prior to inception of RAPA therapy, the serum creatinine value at the end of the previous therapy and at the time of the confirmatory biopsy was 195% greater than the baseline value just prior to the acute episode. Among the nine patients with functioning grafts (70%) whose overall mean serum creatinine value after inception of RAPA was 2.15 mg/dL (range 1.4–4.0), five were also weaned from

steroids. There was no correlation between the response to RAPA and the baseline serum creatinine value or the previous anti-rejection regimen. These preliminary findings suggest that RAPA may represent a therapeutic alternative to reverse refractory allograft rejection episodes.

Steroid withdrawal

A recent study sought to assess the risks of withdrawal of steroids within 1 year from a *de novo* RAPA/CsA maintenance regimen. The data set included 75 patients, namely 40 recipients of HLA mismatched living donors (Phase IIA) and 35 recipients of cadaver (Phase IIB) donor renal transplants. The minimum follow-up periods were 18 and 12 months, respectively. The protocols stipulated steroid withdrawal within or at 1 month except when the patient had experienced an acute rejection episode or a medical contra-indication to continued participation, such as impaired renal function.

Among the 40 recipients in the Phase IIA Trial, eight patients were ineligible for steroid withdrawal [80]. Among the 32 recipients eligible for entry into the protocol, 25 were successfully withdrawn from steroids (78%), with two episodes of acute rejection occurring thereafter (8%). After a 6-month period of RAPA/CsA/Prednisone therapy, both patients who had experienced acute rejection episodes were successfully withdrawn the second time, such that all 25 patients were off steroids at 12 months and 24 were off steroids at 18 months minimum follow-up. One patient returned to steroid treatment due to a flare-up of her pre-existent lupus erythematosus. At 1 year, the patients who had been withdrawn from steroids showed significant reductions in white blood cell count, as well as serum cholesterol and triglyceride values (Tab. 5).

Among the 35 cadaver recipients, 27 were withdrawn (77%) [88]. There were four episodes of acute rejection after steroid withdrawal (15%), and four patients required re-initiation of steroid treatment due to medical reasons. Therefore, 19 patients (54%) were rejection- and steroid-free. The serum levels of triglycerides and cholesterol among recipients of cadaveric transplants

Table 5. One-year mean laboratory values of patients treated with regimens containing *versus* free of steroids

Donor	Treatment	n	Serum creatinine	Triglycerides	Cholesterol	White blood cell
Living	CsA-Pred	65	2.2	268	253	10.7
	RAPA-CsA	25	1.7	251[a]	244[b]	5.2[c]
	RAPA-CsA-Pred	7	2.3	365	278	5.8[c]
Cadaver	RAPA-CsA	19	1.7	361	260	5.8[c]
	RAPA-CsA-Pred	13	2.2	437	280	7.9

[a] $p = 0.02$
[b] $p = 0.05$
[c] $p < 0.001$

who had been withdrawn from steroids were not reduced, although the white blood cell counts were lower than those of RAPA/CsA/Prednisone-treated patients. Thus, steroid withdrawal from a RAPA/CsA regimen was possible in about 77% of transplant recipients; the success rates at 12 months were 78% in living- *versus* 70% in cadaveric-donor recipients.

Potential for prevention and/or treatment of chronic rejection
Chronic rejection has become the major limitation to long-term renal allograft success. Four observations suggest that RAPA may be useful for the prevention of chronic rejection [79]. First, RAPA inhibits growth factor-driven proliferation of endothelial and smooth muscle cells *in vitro*. Second, RAPA exerts a beneficial effect on vascular injury responses *in vivo*. Third, RAPA mitigates chronic rejection in rat models. Fourth, when used in combination with CsA in humans, RAPA reduces the incidence of acute rejection episodes, which are widely believed to forecast an increased risk of chronic rejection [89, 90]. Furthermore, RAPA administered at doses of 2–10 mg/day permits CsA dose-minimization during the early post-operative period, possibly mitigating CsA-induced renal dysfunction that possibly exacerbates other processes leading to chronic graft failure.

Clinical data in six different models suggest that RAPA blocks the action of cytokines critical to producing the immuno-obliterative vascular and bronchial lesions that serve as histopathologic hallmarks of chronic rejection. In one study, RAPA (but not TRL) prevented non-stimulated vascular smooth muscle cells from progressing from G_0 to G_1 [91], apparently due to inhibited retinoblastoma protein hyperphosphorylation associated with a decrease in $p33^{cdk2}$ activity. In another study, RAPA prevented established cultures of either bovine or human endothelial cells from displaying proliferation responses to cytokines ($IC_{50} = 8 \times 10^{-10}$ M), while TRL had no effect [92]. A third study revealed that the addition of RAPA to rat aortic smooth-muscle cell cultures undergoing stimulation induced by platelet-derived growth factor-BB ($IC_{50} = 5 \times 10^{-9}$ M), with or without insulin growth factor-I, blocked generation of the mRNA cap-binding protein, eukaryotic initiation factor eIF $4E_x$ [93]. This inhibitory effect was far greater than that obtained with TRL, mycophenolate mofetil, or leflunomide [94]. Fourth, RAPA blocked exogenous stimulation of cardiac fibroblasts by platelet-derived growth factor-AA [95]. Fifth, bronchial smooth muscle cells were not stimulated by platelet-derived growth factor in the presence of RAPA [96]. A sixth study showed that RAPA prevented insulin or insulin growth factor-I from triggering rat smooth muscle cell proliferation by inhibiting both leucine uptake and $p70^{S6k}$ activity [97].

Two studies suggest that RAPA dampens vascular injury responses *in vivo*. RAPA treatment reduced the degree of intimal thickening caused by balloon catheter arterial injury [98] to a greater extent than did mycophenolate mofetil; neither CsA nor TRL had any inhibitory effect. Modest (3 mg/kg, three times weekly) doses of RAPA reduced adventitial inflammatory infiltration, whereas CsA had this effect only at toxic (25 mg/kg, three times weekly) doses [99]. Thus, RAPA may blunt the restenosis response following angioplasty, as well as the arterial or venous proliferative responses at the sites of anastomoses between synthetic materials and native vessels.

RAPA also mitigates chronic rejection reactions in rat [100, 101], pig [100], and mouse [102] models. Schmid et al. [103] identified the degree of donor-recipient histo-incompatibility and the RAPA dose over the range of 0.5–2.0 mg/kg/day as determinants of the benefit of the drug on the development of transplant vasculopathy. While the lowest RAPA dose that was used in this study (0.5 mg/kg/day) was found to be effective, reducing the incidence of vasculopathy from $62 \pm 13\%$ to $25 \pm 15\%$ ($p < 0.005$), this daily dose would translate to approximately 35 mg/day in man, a dose that is considerably higher than the largest amount used chronically in renal transplant trials (5–10 mg/day) [80]. Thus, high doses of RAPA may be required to exploit its potency in chronic rejection settings, a suggestion that is supported by our initial analysis of the correlation between C_0 values and allograft attrition in long-term RAPA-treated recipients.

SDZ RAD

Our recent Phase I, randomized, blinded, placebo-controlled study assessed the safety profile and pharmacokinetics of a 4-week course of once-daily sequentially ascending doses (0.75, 2.5, or 7.5 mg/d) of RAD capsules in renal transplant recipients on a stable regimen of CsA Neoral and Prednisone [104]. RAD displayed a similar spectrum of side-effects as that observed with RAPA, namely an increased incidence of infections associated with the augmented immunosuppression and a dose-related occurrence of thrombocytopenia, hypercholesterolemia, and hypertriglyceridemia, particularly at the 7.5 mg dose. The pharmacokinetic parameters of RAD showed dose-proportionality with a good correlation between C_0 and AUC concentrations, but a moderate degree of drug accumulation (2.5-fold) at the 0.75 mg dose. The drug was absorbed rapidly, reaching a C_{max} within 2 h. It displayed a 16- to 19-h half-life, which is significantly shorter than that of RAPA and necessitates twice daily dosing. RAD concentrations reached a steady-state by 4 days. Preliminary kinetic-dynamic correlations indicate correlations between thrombocytopenia (but not hyperlipidemia) and AUC, C_{max}, and weight-adjusted dose. At the end of a 4-week course of simultaneous dosing, there was no evidence of a pharmacokinetic interaction between CsA and RAD. Controlled, multi-center trials are underway to assess the impact on clinical outcomes of the shorter half-life of RAD compared to RAPA in order to gauge whether RAD confers benefits related to its hydrophilicity: namely, less time to attain steady-state or, conversely, to dissipate its effects upon drug cessation relative to its RAPA parent compound.

Macrocyclic lactone agents in the matrix of new immunosuppressives

Interactions between RAPA and TRL or MMF

Upon introduction into clinical practice, RAPA is likely to be widely applied in drug combinations. Because of the potency of its interaction with CsA, one might suggest that combinations of another calcineurin inhibitor TRL with RAPA might also be synergistic. This combination was not extensively investigated during drug development, because *in vitro* assays suggested that the drugs antagonize each other's effects when either one is used in molecular excess [105]. However, *in vivo* studies claim that combinations of TRL and RAPA display more than additive interactions to prolong the survival of rat or mouse heart tissue allografts [106, 107]. Unfortunately these studies neither utilized rigorous methods to assess the drug interaction, nor included simultaneous drug concentrations to assess the contribution of pharmacokinetic interactions to the apparent prolongation of graft survival.

Clearly, a final assessment must await clinical trials comparing a TRL-RAPA with a Neoral-RAPA combination. Although these trials might be performed in concentration-controlled fashion, it is unfortunately difficult to imagine them being performed in blinded fashion. However, before embarking on such a trial, it should be noted that there may be a danger to conduct clinical trials based upon results of experimental animal studies conducted in less than a rigorous fashion. This danger is illustrated by the discrepancy between recent claims of synergy between MMF and RAPA based upon rat allograft survival [108] and the failure to observe a beneficial effect of a RAPA-MMF-Prednisone combination over a RAPA-azathioprine-Prednisone combination in a recent European multi-center randomized trial.

Interactions with anti-IL-2 receptor monoclonal antibodies

We have proposed a new immunosuppressive strategy, the cytokine paradigm (Fig. 3) [109]. In addition to CsA and RAPA, the paradigm includes the administration of either chimeric or humanized anti-IL-2 receptor monoclonal antibodies. Basiliximab (Simulect®, Novartis), a chimeric antibody, and daclizumab, a humanized reagent, bind to the α chain of the IL-2 receptor. These antibodies do not elicit the cytokine-release syndrome, and only rarely evoke the production of neutralizing antibodies. Administered in combination with CsA and steroid therapy, they reduced the severity of acute rejection episodes by about 30%, and produced minimal side-effects. Induction immunosuppression with anti-IL-2 receptor antibody and RAPA has been used in six patients to permit extended periods of freedom from the administration of CsA, which was subsequently introduced at low 50–100 mg twice daily doses upon resolution of the impaired function [110]. This beneficial effect should be further explored with longer courses of treatment with anti-IL-2 receptor antibody or

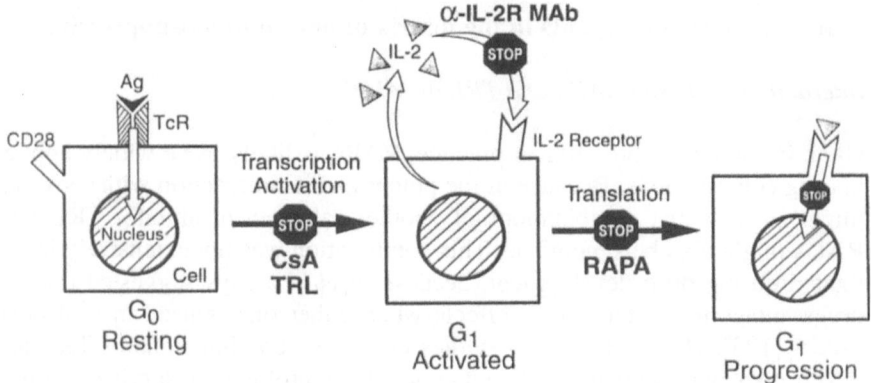

Figure 3. The cytokine paradigm: complementary sites of action of immunosuppressive drugs during lymphocyte activation. CsA and tacrolimus inhibit transcription of T-cell growth-promoting genes (e.g., IL-2). Anti-IL-2 monoclonal antibodies block binding of IL-2 to its receptor. RAPA blocks growth-factor-initiated signal transduction.

the use of selective receptor antagonists possibly designed akin to the IL-1 receptor antagonists presently in clinical use for treatment of rheumatoid conditions.

Interactions with experimental immunosuppressive drugs

Having discovered the synergistic interaction between RAPA and CsA, it is logical to search for a third agent that may enhance the synergistic interaction. Among the array of available agents, preclinical data suggest that the most likely candidates are FTY720, AG490, and c-raf antisense deoxynucleotides. FTY720 is a synthetic derivative of a sphingosine-like compound produced by the ascomycete *Isaria sinclairi*. The drug appears to selectively enhance the homing of lymphocytes to lymph nodes, thereby diverting them away from the graft. FTY720 displays a 10- to 100-fold-greater *in vivo* immunosuppressive potency than CsA. The molecular target of the drug's action is unknown. It may inhibit sphingolipid pathways leading to upregulated expression and/or cytoskeletal interactions of integrin cell surface markers; it may disrupt early events of lymphocyte signal transduction; and/or it may interact with intracellular intermediates leading to differentiation or apoptosis [111].

Because c-raf is a critical intermediate in both T-cell receptor and cytokine signal-transduction pathways, one might postulate that its blockade would inhibit organ allograft rejection. A recently designed antisense deoxynucleotide that specifically blocks protein translation by c-raf mRNA has been shown to prolong rat heart allograft survival and interact in supra-additive fashion with RAPA (unpublished data).

AG490 is a selective inhibitor of JAK3 kinase activity, which is linked to cytokine-driven signal transduction *via* the γ-chain of the IL-2 receptor. AG490 has been shown to prolong rat heart allograft survival. The drug may offer unique advances in immunosuppression since the γ-chain is selectively distributed on the family of IL-2, but not of non-lymphoid cytokine receptors. Ongoing studies seek to discern the relative advantages of these experimental agents in immunosuppressive combinations with RAPA and/or RAPA-CsA baseline treatments.

Concluding remarks

Macrocyclic lactones are becoming critical components of immunosuppressive drug regimens. While their common pipecolic acid structure permits binding to the immunophilin rotamase family of FKBPs, the ring structure determines their distinctive interactions with either the phosphatase calcineurin (TRL) or the kinase mTOR (RAPA or RAD). As a class, these drugs exhibit pharmacokinetic limitations including poor bioavailability, high inter-individual variability, and extensive drug-drug interactions. Furthermore, adverse drug reactions are frequent, and the individual therapeutic windows, narrow. Therefore, the most promising use of these agents in the coming millennium is likely to be as component(s) of multi-modality regimens that inhibit allo-activation at multiple steps in the development of cellular and humoral responses, as well as to block vasculopathic responses that contribute to chronic graft attrition.

The horizon of development of new immunosuppressive regimens depends upon the discovery of drugs with more selective mechanisms of action than the existent macrocyclic lactones. New calcineurin inhibitors should be developed to be selective for the molecular features of lymphoid *versus* renal isozymes, and signal transduction inhibitors, for the lymphoid-specific gamma as opposed to the shared β/gp130 chain activation pathways. Clinical therapy is likely to be revolutionized in the coming decade by these types of rational molecularly based drug-design strategies that understand and exploit the critical conformations within the macrocyclic lactones that were serendipitously discovered to have immunosuppressive properties.

References

1 Brockmann H, Henkel W (1950) Pikromycin, ein neues Antibiotikum aus Actinomycentin. *Naturwissenschaften* 37: 138
2 Eichenwald HF (1986) Adverse reactions to erythromycin. *Pediatr Infect Dis* 5: 147–150
3 Hodak SP, Moubarak JB, Rodriguez I, Gelfand MC, Alijani MR, Tracy CM (1998) QT prolongation and near fatal cardiac arrhythmia after intravenous tacrolimus administration: a case report. *Transplantation* 66: 535–537
4 Johnson MC, So S, Marsh JW, Murphy AM (1992) QT prolongation and Torsades de Pointes after administration of FK506. *Transplantation* 53: 929–930
5 Drici MD, Knollmann BC, Wang WX, Woosley RL (1998) Cardiac actions of erythromycin: influence of female sex. *JAMA* 280: 1774–1776

6 Antzelevitch C, Sun ZQ, Zhang ZQ, Yan GX (1996) Cellular and ionic mechanisms underlying erythromycin-induced long QT intervals and torsade de pointes. *J Amer Coll Cardiol* 28: 1836–1848

7 Guelon D, Bedock B, Chartier C, Haberer JP (1986) QT prolongation and recurrent "torsades de pointes" during erythromycin lactobionate infusion. *Amer J Cardiol* 58: 666

8 Dumont FJ, Koprak S, Staruch MJ, Talento A, Koo G, DaSilva C, Sinclair PJ, Wong F, Woods J, Barker J et al (1998) A tacrolimus-related immunosuppressant with reduced toxicity. *Transplantation* 65: 18–26

9 Peterson LB, Cryan JG, Rosa R, Martin MM, Wilusz MB, Sinclair PJ, Wong F, Parsons JN, O'Keefe SJ, Parsons WH et al (1998) A tacrolimus-related immunosuppressant with biochemical properties distinct from those of tacrolimus. *Transplantation* 65: 10–18

10 Goto T, Kino T, Hatanaka H, Nishiyama M, Okuhara M, Kohsaka M, Aoki H, Imanaka H (1987) Discovery of FK506, a novel immunosupressant isolated from *Streptomyces tsukubaensis*. *Transplant Proc* 19 (5 Suppl 6): 4–8

11 Starzl TE, Todo S, Fung J, Demetris AJ, Venkataramman R, Jain A (1989) FK506 for liver, kidney, and pancreas transplantation. *Lancet* 2: 1000–1004

12 Johansson A, Moller E (1990) Evidence that the immunosuppressive effects of FK506 and cyclosporine are identical. *Transplantation* 50: 1001–1007

13 Henderson DJ, Naya I, Bundick RV, Smith GM, Schmidt JA (1991) Comparison of the effects of FK506, cyclosporine A, and rapamycin on IL-2 production. *Immunology* 73: 316–321

14 Hutchinson IV (1997) The mode of action of Prograf (tacrolimus) and its significance for long-term graft survival. *New Horizons in Kidney Transplantation* 1: 22

15 Migita K, Eguchi K, Kawabe T, Tsukada T, Mizokami A, Nagataki S (1995) FK506 augments activation-induced programmed cell death of T lymphocytes *in vivo*. *J Clin Invest* 96: 727–732

16 Venkataramanan R, Swaminathan A, Prasad T, Jain A, Zuckerman S, Warty V, McMichael J, Lever J, Burckart G, Starzl T (1995) Clinical pharmacokinetics of tacrolimus. *Clin Pharmacokinet* 29: 404–430

17 Ihara H, Shinkuma D, Ichikawa Y, Nojima M, Nagano S, Ikoma F (1995) Intra- and interindividual variation in the pharmacokinetics of tacrolimus (FK506) in kidney transplant recipients – importance of trough level as a practical indicator. *Int J Urol* 2: 151–155

18 Laskow DA, Vincenti F, Neylan JF, Mendez R, Matas AJ (1996) An open-label, concentration-ranging trial of FK506 in primary kidney transplantation. *Transplantation* 62: 900–905

19 Jain AB, Abu-Elmagd K, Abdallah H, Warty V, Fung J, Todo S, Starzl TE, Venkataramanan R (1993) Pharmacokinetics of FK506 in liver transplant recipients after continuous intravenous infusion. *J Clin Pharmacol* 33: 606–611

20 Jain AB, Venkataramanan R, Cadoff E, Fung JJ, Todo S, Krajack A, Starzl TE (1990) Effect of hepatic dysfunction and T-tube clamping on FK506 pharmacokinetics and trough concentrations. *Transplant Proc* 22: 57–59

21 Jusko WJ, Thomson AW, Fung J, McMaster P, Wong SH, Zylber-Katz E, Christians U, Winkler M, Fitzsimmons WE, Lieberman R et al (1995) Consensus document: therapeutic monitoring of tacrolimus (FK506). *Ther Drug Monit* 17: 606–614

22 Jusko WJ (1995) Analysis of tacrolimus (FK506) in relation to therapeutic drug monitoring. *Ther Drug Monit* 17: 596–601

23 Vathsala A, Goto S, Yoshimura N, Stepkowski S, Chou TC, Kahan BD (1991) The immunosuppressive antagonism of low doses of FK506 and cyclosporine. *Transplantation* 52: 121–128

24 Zhang Q, Simpson J, Aboleneen HI (1997) A specific method for the measurement of tacrolimus on human whole blood by liquid chromatography/tandem mass spectrometry. *Ther Drug Monit* 19: 470–476

25 Alak AM (1997) Measurement of tacrolimus (FK506) and its metabolites: a review of assay development and application in therapeutic drug monitoring and pharmacokinetic studies. *Ther Drug Monit* 19: 338–351

26 Pirsch JD, Miller J, Deierhoi MH, Vincenti F, Filo RS (1997) A comparison of tacrolimus and cyclosporine for immunosuppression after cadaveric renal transplantation. *Transplantation* 63: 977–983

27 Neylan JF (1998) Racial differences in renal transplantation after immunosuppression with tacrolimus *versus* cyclosporine. FK506 Kidney Transplant Study Group. *Transplantation* 65: 515–523

28 Heifets M, Cooney G, Shaw L (1996) Ethnic differences in tacrolimus pharmacokinetics in renal

transplant candidates. *Annual Meeting of the American Society of Transplant Physicians*
29 Andrews PA, Sen M, Chang RW (1996) Racial variation in dosage requirements of tacrolimus. *Lancet* 348: 1446
30 Katari SR, Magnone M, Shapiro R, Jordan M, Scantlebury V, Vivas C, Gritsch A, McCauley J, Starzl T, Demetris AJ et al (1997) Clinical features of acute reversible tacrolimus (FK506) nephrotoxicity in kidney transplant recipients. *Clin Transplant* 11: 237–242
31 Randhawa PS, Shapiro R, Jordan ML, Starzl TE, Demetris AJ (1993) The histopathological changes associated with allograft rejection and drug toxicity in renal transplant recipients maintained on FK506. *Amer J Surg Pathol* 17: 60–68
32 Radermacher J, Meiners M, Bramlage C, Kliem V, Behrend M, Schlitt HJ, Pichlmayr R, Koch KM, Brunkhorst R (1998) Pronounced renal vasoconstriction and systemic in renal transplant patients treated with cyclosporine A *versus* FK 506. *Transplant Int* 11: 3–10
33 Shapiro R, Jordan ML, Scantlebury VP, Vivas C, McCauley J, Johnston J, Fung JJ, Starzl TE (1998) Alopecia as a consequence of tacrolimus therapy. *Transplantation* 65: 1284
34 Wiesner RH (1998) A long term comparison of tacrolimus (FK506) *versus* cyclosporine in liver transplantation: a report of the United States FK506 study group. *Transplantation* 66: 493–499
35 Anonymous (1994) A comparison of tacrolimus (FK506) and cyclosporine for immunosuppression in liver transplantation. The U.S. Multicenter FK506 Liver Study Group. *N Engl J Med* 331: 1110–1115
36 Fung J, Eliaziw M, Todo S, Jain A, Demetris AJ, McMichael JP, Starzl TE, Meier P, Donner A (1996) The Pittsburgh randomized trial of tacrolimus compared to cyclosporine for hepatic transplantation. *J Amer Coll Surg* 183: 117–125
37 Williams R, Neuhaus P, Bismuth H, McMaster P, Pichlmayr R, Calne R, Otto G, Groth C (1996) Two-year data from the European multicentre tacrolimus (FK506) liver study. *Transplant Int* 9 Suppl 1: S144–S150
38 Jonas S, Kling N, Bechstein WO, Blumhardt G, Lohmann R, Lobeck H, Neuhaus P (1995) Rejection episodes after liver transplantation during primary immunosuppression with FK506 or a cyclosporine-based regimen: a controlled, prospective, randomized trial. *Clin Transplant* 9: 406–414
39 Mayer AD, Dmitrewski J, Squifflet JP, Besse T, Grabensee B, Klein B, Eigler FW, Heemann U, Pichlmayr R, Behrend M et al (1997) Multicenter randomized trial comparing tacrolimus and cyclosporine in the prevention of renal allograft rejection: a report of the European Tacrolimus Multicenter Renal Study Group. *Transplantation* 64: 436–443
40 Gruessner A, Sutherland DE (1994) Pancreas transplant results in the United Network for Organ Sharing (UNOS) United States of America (USA) Registry compared with non-USA data in the International Registry. *Clin Transplant* 47–68
41 Shaffer D, Simpson MA, Conway P, Madras PN, Monaco AP (1995) Normal pancreas allograft function simultaneous pancreas kidney transplantation after rescue therapy with tacrolimus (FK506). *Transplantation* 59: 1063–1066
42 Hariharan S, Peddi VR, Munda R, Demmy AM, Schroeder TJ, Alexander JW, First MR (1997) Long-term renal and pancreas function with tacrolimus rescue therapy following pancreas transplantation. *Transplant Proc* 29: 652–653
43 Hariharan S, Munda R, Demmy TJ, Shroeder TJ, Alexander JW, First MR (1995) Conversion from cyclosporine to tacrolimus after pancreas transplantation. *Transplant Proc* 27: 2981–2982
44 Teroaka S, Babazono T, Koike T, Abe M, Kimikawa M, Shinkai M, Haruguchi H, Hirotani S, Kitajima K, Akamatsu M et al (1995) Effect of rescue therapy using FK506 on relapsing rejection after combined pancreas and kidney transplantation. *Transplant Proc* 27: 1335–1339
45 Gruessner RW, Burke GW, Stratta R, Sollinger H, Benedetti E, Marsh C, Stock P, Boudreaux JP, Martin M, Drangstveit MB et al (1996) A multicenter analysis of the first experience with FK506 for induction and rescue therapy after pancreas transplantation. *Transplantation* 61: 261–273
46 Pham SM, Kormos RL, Hattler BG, Kawai A, Tsamandas AC, Demetris AJ, Murali S, Fricker FJ, Chang HC, Jain AB et al (1996) A prospective trial of tacrolimus (FK 506) in clinical heart transplantation: intermediate-term results. *J Thorac Cardiovasc Surg* 111: 764–772
47 Reichart B, Meiser B, Vigano M, Rinaldi M, Martinelli L, Yacoub M, Banner NR, Gandjbakhch I, Dorent R, Hetzer R et al (1998) European Multicenter Tacrolimus (FK506) heart pilot study: one-year results – European Tacrolimus Multicenter Heart Study Group. *J Heart Lung Transplant* 17: 775–781
48 Tsamandas AC, Pham SM, Seaberg EC, Pappo O, Kormos RL, Kawai A, Griffith BP, Zeevi A,

Duquesnoy R, Fung JJ et al (1997) Adult heart transplantation under tacrolimus (FK506) immunosuppression: histopathologic observations and comparison to a cyclosporine-based regimen with lympholytic (ATG) induction. *J Heart Lung Transplant* 16: 723–734

49 Keenan RJ, Konishi H, Kawai A, Paradis IL, Nunley DR, Iacono AT, Hardesty RL, Weyant RJ, Griffith BP (1995) Clinical trial of tacrolimus *versus* cyclosporine in lung transplantation. *Ann Thorac Surg* 60: 580–585

50 Klintmalm GB, Goldstein R, Gonwa T, Wiesner RH, Krom RA, Shaw BW Jr, Stratta R, Ascher NL, Roberts JW, Lake J et al (1993) Use of Prograf (FK506) as rescue therapy for refractory rejection after liver transplantation. *Transplant Proc* 25 (1 Pt 1): 679–688

51 Sher LS, Cosenza CA, Michel J, Makowka L, Miller CM, Schwartz ME, Busuttil R, McDiarmid S, Burdick JF, Klein AS et al (1997) Efficacy of tacrolimus as rescue therapy for chronic rejection in orthotopic liver transplantation: a report of the U.S. Multicenter Liver Study Group. *Transplantation* 64: 258–263

52 Jain A, Fung J, Todo S (1996) More than six years actual follow-up: conversion from cyclosporine to tacrolimus for chronic liver allograft rejection. *Hepatology* 24: 181

53 Fung J, Todo S, Tsakis A, Demetris A, Jain A, Abu-Elmaged K, Alessiani M, Starzl TE (1991) Conversion of liver allograft recipients from cyclosporine to FK506-based immunosuppression: benefits and pitfalls. *Transplant Proc* 23: 14–21

54 Jordan ML, Naraghi R, Shapiro R, Smith D, Vivas CA, Scantlebury VP, Gritsch HA, McCauley J, Randhawa P, Demetris AJ et al (1997) Tacrolimus rescue therapy for renal allograft rejection – five-year experience. *Transplantation* 63: 223–228

55 Woodle ES, Thistlethwaite JR, Gordon JH, Laskow D, Deierhoi MH, Burdick J, Pirsch JD, Sollinger H, Vincenti F, Burrows L (1996) A multicenter trial of FK506 (tacrolimus) therapy in refractory acute renal allograft rejection. A report of the Tacrolimus Kidney Transplantation Rescue Study Group. *Transplantation* 62: 594–599

56 Mentzer RM Jr, Jahania MS, Lasley RD (1998) Tacrolimus as a rescue immunosuppressant after heart and lung transplantation. The U.S. Multicenter FK506 Study Group. *Transplantation* 65: 109–113

57 Keown P, Niese D (1988) Cyclosporine microemulsion increases drug exposure and reduces acute rejection without incremental toxicity in *de novo* renal transplantation. International Sandimmun Neoral Study Group. *Kidney Int* 54: 938–944

58 Kahan BD (2000) Efficacy of sirolimus compared with azathioprine for reduction of acute renal allograft rejection: a randomised multicentre study. The Rapamune US Study Group. *Lancet* 356: 194–202

59 Vezina C, Kudelski A, Sehgal SN (1975) Rapamycin (AY-22,989), a new antifungal antibiotic. I. Taxonomy of the producing streptomycete and isolation of the active principle. *J Antibiot* 28: 721–726

60 Sehgal SN, Baker H, Vezina C (1975) Rapamycin (AY-22,989), a new antifungal antibiotic. II. Fermentation, isolation and characterization. *J Antibiot* 28: 727–732

61 Eng CP, Sehgal SN, Vezina C (1984) Activity of rapamycin (AY-22,989) against transplanted tumors. *J Antibiot* 37: 1231–1237

62 Kuo CJ, Chung J, Fiorentino DF, Flanagan WM, Blenis J, Crabtree GR (1992) Rapamycin selectively inhibits interleukin-2 activation of p70 S6 kinase. *Nature* 358: 70–73

63 Stepkowski SM, Chen H, Daloze P, Kahan BD (1991) Rapamycin, a potent immunosuppressive drug for vascularized heart, kidney, and small bowel transplantation in the rat. *Transplantation* 51: 22–26

64 Kahan BD, Gibbons S, Tejpal N, Stepkowski SM, Chou TC (1991) Synergistic interactions of cyclosporine and rapamycin to inhibit immune performances of normal human peripheral blood lymphocytes *in vitro*. *Transplantation* 51: 232–239

65 Brown EJ, Albers MW, Shin TB, Ichikawa K, Keith CT, Lane WS, Schreiber SL (1994) A mammalian protein targeted by G1-arresting rapamycin-receptor complex. *Nature* 369: 756–758

66 Brown EJ, Beal PA, Keith CT, Chen J, Shin TB, Schreiber SL (1995) Control of p70 s6 kinase by kinase activity of FRAP *in vivo*. *Nature* 377: 441–446

67 Ferraresso M, Tian L, Ghobrial R, Stepkowski SM, Kahan BD (1994) Rapamycin inhibits production of cytotoxic but not noncytotoxic antibodies and preferentially activates Th2 cells that mediate long-term survival of heart allografts in rats. *J Immunol* 153: 3307–3318

68 Napoli KL, Kahan BD (1996) Routine clinical monitoring of sirolimus (rapamycin) whole-blood concentrations by HPLC with ultraviolet detection. *Clin Chem* 42: 1943–1948

69 Zimmerman JJ, Kahan BD (1997) Pharmacokinetics of sirolimus in stable renal transplant patients after multiple oral dose administration. *J Clin Pharmacol* 37: 405–415

70 Yatscoff RW, Wang P, Chan K, Hicks D, Zimmerman J (1995) Rapamyc*In*: distribution, pharmacokinetics, and therapeutic range investigations. *Ther Drug Monit* 17: 666–671

71 Lown KS, Mayo RR, Leichtman AB, Hsiao HL, Turgeon DK, Schmiedlin-Ren P, Brown MB, Guo W, Rossi SJ, Benet LZ et al (1997) Role of intestinal P-glycoprotein (mdr1) in interpatient variation in the oral bioavailability of cyclosporine. *Clin Pharmacol Ther* 62: 248–260

72 Wacher VJ, Wu CY, Benet LZ (1995) Overlapping substrate specificities and tissue distribution of cytochrome P450 3A and P-glycoprote*In*: implications for drug delivery and activity in cancer chemotherapy. *Mol Carcinogen* 13: 129–134

73 Hebert MF, Roberts JP, Prueksaritanont Benet LZ (1992) Bioavailability of cyclosporine with concomittant rifampin administration is markedly less than predicted by hepatic enzyme induction. *Clin Pharmacol Ther* 54: 453–457

74 Kelly PA, Napoli KL, Dunne C, Kahan BD (1997) Conversion from liquid to solid sirolimus formulations in stable renal allograft transplant recipients. *XVI Meeting of the American Society of Transplant Physicians* Abstract A236

75 Murgia MG, Jordan S, Kahan BD (1996) The side-effect profile of sirolimus: A phase I study in quiescent cyclosporine-prednisone-treated renal transplant patients. *Kidney Int* 49: 209–216

76 Grevel J, Welsh MS, Kahan BD (1989) Cyclosporine monitoring in renal transplantation: area under the curve monitoring is superior to trough-level monitoring. *Ther Drug Monit* 11: 246–248

77 Kahan BD, Welsh M, Rutzky LP (1995) Challenges in cyclosporine therapy: the role of therapeutic drug monitoring by area under the curve monitoring. *Ther Drug Monit* 17: 621–624

78 Kaplan B, Meier-Kriesche H-U, Napoli K, Kahan BD (1997) A limited sampling strategy for estimating sirolimus area-under-the-concentration-curve. *Clin Chem* 43: 539–540

79 Kahan BD (1998) The role of rapamycin in chronic rejection prophylaxis: a theoretical consideration. *Graft* 1 (2 Suppl II): 93

80 Kahan BD, Podbielski J, Napoli KL, Katz SM, Meier-Kriesche H-U, Van Buren CT (1998) Immunosuppressive effects and safety of a sirolimus/cyclosporine combination regimen for renal transplantation. *Transplantation* 66: 1040–1046

81 Kahan BD, Julian BA, Pescovitz MD, Vanrenterghem Y, Neylan J (1999) Sirolimus reduces the incidence of acute rejection episodes despite lower cyclosporine doses in caucasian recipients of mismatched primary renal allografts: a phase II trial. Rapamune Study Group. *Transplantation* 68: 1526–1532

82 Dimeny E, Fellstrom B, Larsson E, Tufveson G, Lithell H (1993) Hyperlipoproteinemia in renal transplant recipients: is there a linkage with chronic vascular rejection? *Transplant Proc* 25: 2065–2066

83 Dimeny E, Tufveson G, Lithell H, Larsson E, Siegbahn A, Fellstrom B (1993) The influence of pretransplant lipoprotein abnormalities on the early results of renal transplantation. *Eur J Clin Invest* 23: 572–579

84 Groth CG, Backman L, Morales JM, Calne R, Kreis H, Lang P, Touraine JL, Claesson K, Campistol JM, Durand D et al (1999) Sirolimus (rapamycin)-based therapy in human renal transplantation: similar efficacy and different toxicity compared with cyclosporine. Sirolimus European Renal Transplant Study Group. *Transplantation* 67: 1036–1042

85 MacDonald AS for the RAPAMUNEGlobal Study Group (1998) A randomized, placebo-controlled trial of rapamune in primary renal allograft recipients. Abstracts of the *Transplantation Society XXVII World Congress* Abstract 426

86 Slaton JW, Kahan BD (1996) Case report – sirolimus rescue therapy for refractory renal allograft rejection. *Transplantation* 61: 977–979

87 Kahan BD, Podbielski J, Van Buren CT (1998) Rapamycin for refractory renal allograft rejection. *XVII Annual Meeting of the American Society of Transplant Physicians* Abstract 711

88 Pescovitz MD, Kahan BD, Julian B, Neylan J, Chan G (1997) Sirolimus (SRL) permits early steroid withdrawal from a triple therapy renal prophylaxis regimen. *XVI Annual Meeting of the American Society for Transplant Physicians* Abstract 708

89 Almond PS, Matas A, Gillingham K, Dunn DL Payne WD Gores P Gruessner R Najarian JS (1993) Risk factors for chronic rejection in renal allograft recipients. *Transplantation* 55: 752–756

90 Kahan BD, Welsh M, Schoenberg L, Rutzky LP, Katz SM, Urbauer DL, Van Buren CT (1996) Variable oral absorption of cyclosporine. A biopharmaceutical risk factor for chronic renal allograft rejection. *Transplantation* 62: 599–606

91 Marx SO, Jayaraman T, Go LO, Marks AR (1995) Rapamycin-FKBP inhibits cell cycle regulators of proliferation in vascular smooth muscle cells. *Circ Res* 76: 412–417
92 Akselband Y, Harding MW, Nelson PA (1991) Rapamycin inhibits spontaneous and fibroblast growth factor beta-stimulated proliferation of endothelial cells and fibroblasts. *Transplant Proc* 23: 2833–2836
93 Graves LM, Bornfeldt KE, Argast GM, Krebs EG, Kong X, Lin TA, Lawrence JC Jr, (1995) cAMP- and rapamycin-sensitive regulation of the association of eukaryotic initiation factor 4E and the translational regulator PHAS-I in aortic smooth muscle cells. *Proc Natl Acad Sci USA* 92: 7222–7226
94 Mohacsi PJ, Tuller D, Hullinger B, Wijngaard PL (1997) Different inhibitory effects of immunosuppressive drugs on human and rat aortic smooth muscle and endothelial cell proliferation stimulated by platelet-derived growth factor or endothelial cell growth factor. *J Heart Lung Transplant* 16: 484–492
95 Simm A, Nestler M, Hoppe V (1997) PDGF-AA, a potent mitogen for cardiac fibroblasts from adult rats. *J Mol Cell Cardiol* 29: 357–368
96 Scott PH, Belham CM, al-Hafidh J, Chilvers ER, Peacock AJ, Gould GW, Plevin R (1966) A regulatory role for cAMP in phosphatidylinositol 3-kinase/p70 ribosomal S6 kinase-mediated DNA synthesis in platelet-derived-growth-factor-stimulated bovine airway smooth-muscle cells. *Biochem J* 318: 965–971
97 Obata T, Kashiwagi A, Maegawa H, Nishio Y, Ugi S, Hidaka H, Kikkawa R (1996) Insulin signaling and its regulation of system A amino acid uptake in cultured rat vascular smooth muscle cells. *Circ Res* 79: 1167–1176
98 Gregory CR, Huang X, Pratt RE, Nishio Y, Ugi S, Hidaka H, Kikkawa R (1995) Treatment with rapamycin and mycophenolic acid reduces arterial intimal thickening produced by mechanical injury and allows endothelial cell replacement. *Transplantation* 59: 655–661
99 Geerling RA, de Bruin RWF, Scheringa M, Bonthuis F, Jeekel J, Ijzermans JN, Marquet RL (1994) Suppression of acute rejection prevents graft arteriosclerosis after allogenic aorta transplantation in the rat. *Transplantation* 58: 1258–1263
100 Calne RY, Collier DS, Lim S, Pollard SG, Samaan A, White DJ, Thiru S (1989) Rapamycin for immunosuppression in organ allografting. *Lancet* 2: 227
101 Meiser BM, Billingham ME, Morris RE (1991) Effects of cyclosporin, FK506, and rapamycin on graft-vessel disease. *Lancet* 338: 1297–1298
102 Morris RE, Huang X, Gregory CR, Billingham ME, Rowan R, Shorthouse R, Berry GJ (1995) Studies in experimental models of chronic rejection: use of rapamycin (sirolimus) and isoxazole derivatives (leflunomide and its analogue) for the suppression of graft vascular disease and obliterative bronchiolitis. *Transplant Proc* 27: 2068–2069
103 Schmid C, Heemann U, Tilney NL (1997) Factors contributing to the development of chronic rejection in heterotopic rat heart transplantation. *Transplantation* 64: 222–228
104 Kahan BD, Wong RL, Carter C, Katz SH, Von Fellenberg J, Van Buren CT, Appel-Dingemanse S (1999) A phase I study of a 4-week course of SDZ-RAD (RAD) quiescent cyclosporine-prednisone-treated renal transplant recipients. *Transplantation* 68: 1100–1106
105 Dumont FJ, Melino MR, Staruch MJ, Koprak SL, Fisher PA, Sigal NH (1990) The immunosuppressive macrolides FK506 and rapamycin act as reciprocal antagonist in murine T-cells. *J Immunol* 144: 1418–1424
106 Vu MD, Qi S, Xu D, Wu J, Fitzsimmons WE, Sehgal SN, Dumont L, Busque S, Daloze P, Chen H (1997) Tacrolimus (FK506) and sirolimus (rapamycin) in combination are not antagositic but produce extended graft survival in caridac transplantation in the rat. *Transplantation* 64: 1853–1856
107 Chen H, Qi S, Xu D, Fitzsimmons WE, Bekersky I, Sehgal SN, Daloze P (1998) Combined effect of rapamycin and FK506 in prolongation of small bowel graft survival in the mouse. *Transplant Proc* 30: 2579–2581
108 Vu MD, Qi S, Xu D, Wu J, Peng J, Daloze P, Sehgal S, Leduc B, Chen H (1998) Synergistic effects of mycophenolate mofetil and sirolimus in prevention of acute heart, pancreas, and kidney allograft rejection and in reversal of ongoing heart allograft rejection in the rat. *Transplantation* 66: 1575–1580
109 Hong JC, Kahan BD (1998) Two paradigms for new immunosuppressive strategies in organ transplantation. *Curr Opin Organ Transplant* 3: 175
110 Hong JC, Kahan BD (1999) Use of anti-CD25 monoclonal antibody in combination with

rapamycin to eliminate cyclosporine treatment during the induction phase of immunosuppression. *Transplantation* 68: 701–704

111 Wang ME, Stepkowski SM, Ferraresso M, Kahan BD (1992) Evidence that rapamycin rescue therapy delays rejection of major (MHC) plus minor (non-MHC) histoincompatible heart allografts in rats. *Transplantation* 54: 704–709

Modern Immunosuppressives
ed. by H.-J Schuurman, G. Feutren and J.-F. Bach
© 2001 Birkhäuser Verlag/Switzerland

Inosine monophosphate dehydrogenase inhibition: mycophenolate mofetil

Christophe Legendre and Eric Thervet

Service de Néphrologie, Hôpital Saint-Louis, 1, Avenue C. Vellefaux, 75010, Paris, France

Introduction

Over the past two decades, the development of new immunosuppressive drugs and the prevention of post-transplant infection have substantially improved the survival of transplanted patients and of organ allografts. However, the prevention of acute rejection and consequently of chronic allograft dysfunction, as well as that of long-term metabolic complications and malignancies, are still important issues. In this chapter, we will focus on mycophenolate mofetil, an antiproliferative agent with proven clinical efficacy in human organ transplantation and autoimmune diseases and a satisfactory safety profile.

Pharmacology

Mechanism of action

T-cell activation by alloantigens is a complex process involving an antigenic signal, combined with a costimulatory signal leading to activation of the calcineurin pathway, a process inhibited by cyclosporine A and tacrolimus (Fig. 1). Calcineurin activation allows the activation of the interleukin-2 (IL-2) gene promoters leading to IL-2 production. Subsequently, IL-2 interacts with its receptors, which induces cells to enter cell cycle, and clonal expansion [1]. Antiproliferative agents block DNA replication and therefore clonal expansion by inhibiting either purine synthesis, as observed with azathioprine, mycophenolate mofetil, and mizoribine, or pyrimidine synthesis, as observed with brequinar sodium.

As illustrated in normal mammalian cells (Fig. 2), purine synthesis, i.e., guanine and adenine nucleotide synthesis, involves a *de novo* pathway in which nucleotides are manufactured from small precursors, and a salvage pathway which recycles purine bases. In human lymphocytes, especially proliferating lymphocytes, this pathway plays a preponderant role in purine synthesis [2]. In this pathway, ribose 5-phosphate is phosphorylated to form

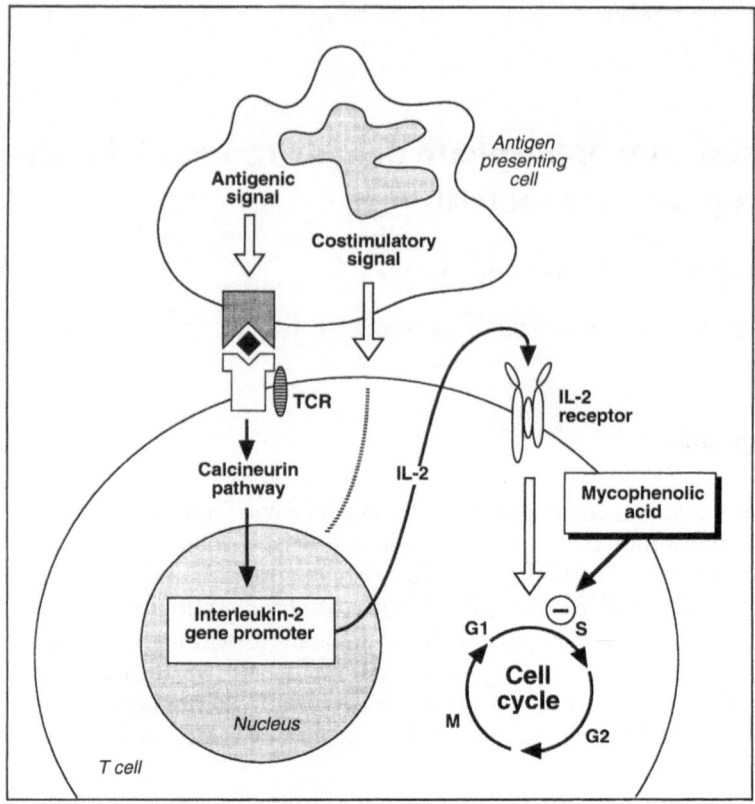

Figure 1. Schematic representation of alloantigen-induced T-cell activation. Mycophenolic acid acts as an antiproliferative drug, fixing cells in the S phase of the cell cycle.

5-phosphoribosyl-1-pyrophosphate (PRPP) by PRPP synthetase, thus leading to the formation of inosine monophosphate (IMP), which may then form either guanosine monophosphate (GMP) through IMPdehydrogenase (IMPDH), or adenosine monophosphate (AMP) through adenosine deaminase (ADA). GMP and AMP are subsequently transformed into RNA and DNA through ribonucleotide reductase. PRPP and ribonucleotide reductase are allosterically regulated by nucleotides. PRPP synthetase and ribonucleotide reductase are both inhibited by adenosine nucleotides and activated by guanosine nucleotides. Hence, depletion of guanosine nucleotides and an excess of adenosine nucleotides reduce the pool of substrates necessary for DNA polymerase.

Mycophenolic acid (MPA, Fig. 3) is a potent, noncompetitive and reversible inhibitor of type II IMPDH, which is of utmost importance in *de novo* purine synthesis of proliferating lymphocytes. Mycophenolic acid indeed inhibits type II IMPDH nearly five times more potently than type I IMPDH, which is predominant in resting cells [3]. MPA therefore induces guanosine nucleotide

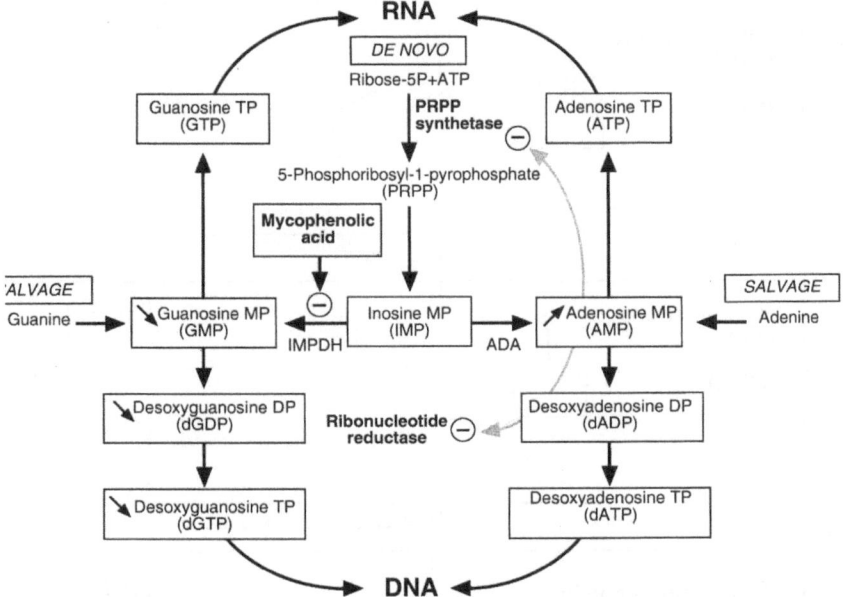

Figure 2. *De novo* and salvage pathways of purine synthesis in human lymphocytes. Mycophenolic acid is a potent, noncompetitive and reversible inhibitor of type II IMPDH (inosine monophosphate dehydrogenase). It induces intracellular depletion of guanosine triphosphate (GTP) and deoxy-GTP without affecting adenosine triphosphate (ATP) or deoxy-ATP.

depletion, which results in somewhat selective inhibition of T- and B-lymphocyte proliferation, as lymphocytes become fixed in the S phase of the cell cycle. As the *de novo* pathway is not of such crucial importance in many other cell types as it is in proliferative lymphocytes, MPA only has a minimal impact on other cell types, and is therefore satisfactorily tolerated. It does not affect the salvage pathway at all.

The mechanism of type II IMPDH inhibition is believed to involve the binding of mycophenolic acid to the nicotinamide site for NAD+, thus preventing the conversion of IMP into xanthine monophosphate and then to GMP [4]. In addition to this mechanism of action, MPA inhibits antibody formation *in vitro*, does not affect production of the cytokines implicated in allograft rejection, inhibits the transfer of fucose and mannose to glycoproteins including adhesion molecules, and inhibits the proliferation of human arterial smooth muscle cells in culture [2]. These properties may be of importance in the prevention of chronic allograft dysfunction in humans.

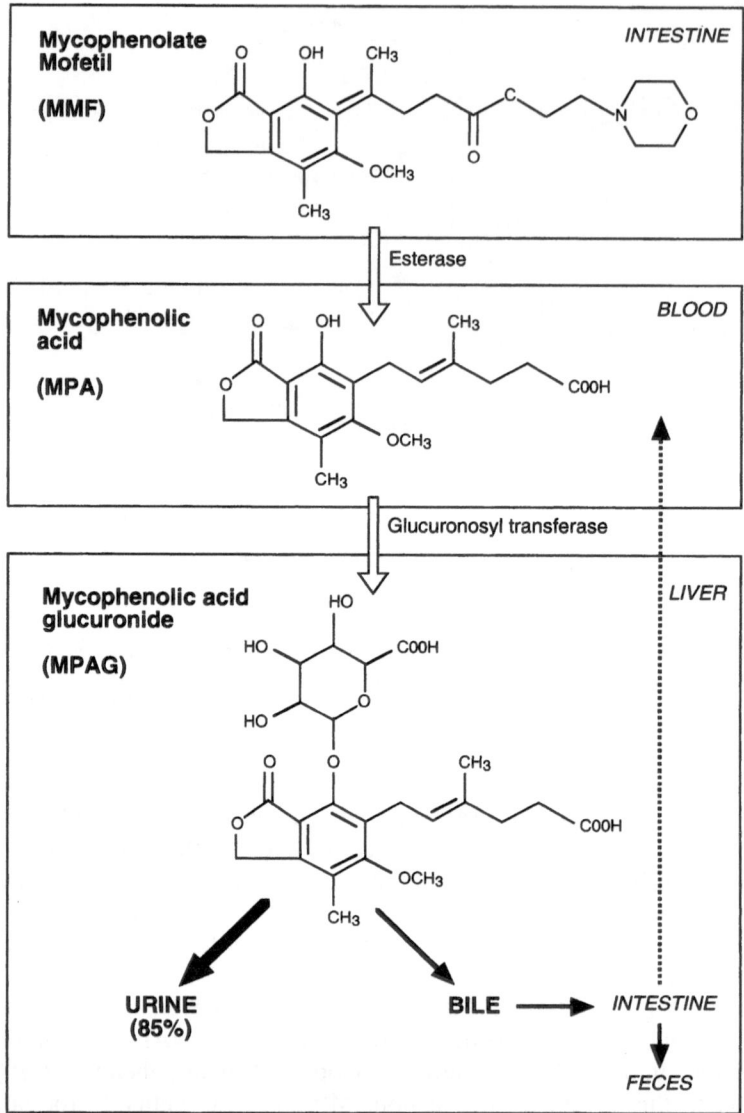

Figure 3. Structure of mycophenolate mofetil (MMF), mycophenolic acid (MPA) and mycophenolic acid glucuronide (MPAG) and sites of interconversion and excretion.

Clinical pharmacology

Pharmacokinetics

Mycophenolate mofetil (MMF, Fig. 3) is rapidly hydrolyzed after absorption and is not measurable at any time after oral administration [5]. The initial concentration peak of MPA occurs 0.80 ± 0.36 h after administration and is followed by secondary concentration peaks 6 to 12 h thereafter. This may be due to the enterohepatic circulatory pathway whose influence varies within and among individuals due to factors such as meal timing in relation to the last MMF dose. Most MPA is bound to human serum albumin (average bound fraction: 97.5%). Free MPA is the pharmacologically active fraction. It is possible that variations in the plasma protein concentration and binding increase the amount of free MPA distributed, as well as its clearance by the liver.

The primary metabolic pathway for MPA is the formation of its glucuronide, i.e., mycophenolic acic glucuronide (MPAG, Fig. 3), *via* a glucuronyltransferase. Since genetic variations of this enzyme have been described, the level of glucuronidation may vary, which might affect individual concentrations, and possibly the efficacy of MPA treatment. The liver is assumed to be the primary site of MPAG production, but its production by other organs such as the kidney and gastrointestinal tract cannot be ruled out. Preliminary results have shown that in patients with severe hepatic oxidative impairment, MPA glucuronidation is gradually impaired in the liver, but is induced in the kidney.

MPAG is mainly eliminated by renal excretion. It is inactive, since inhibitory concentrations (IC_{50}) were found to be up to 1000-fold higher than those for MPA. Lastly, it has been reported that the trough concentration of plasma MPA may diminish in long-term MMF treatment [6], but this preliminary result requires confirmation before any conclusions can be reached about the mechanism and possible potential clinical consequences.

Pharmacodynamics
MPA mediates its effect by inhibiting inosine monophosphate dehydrogenase. An assay to measure IMPDH activity in whole blood as a means of assessing MPA-induced immunosuppression was recently described [7]. This assay is based on the conversion of $[H^3]$ inosine into xanthine, which is measured by the release of tritium. Animal studies have shown an inverse relationship between the activity of IMPDH and its drug concentration. In humans, the peak concentration of MPA, reached 1 h after ingestion, inhibited 40% of IMPDH activity, but there was large inter- and intra-individual variations. IMPDH activity and the MPA concentrations were gradually restored during the intervals between doses. Further studies are needed to evaluate the clinical significance of IMPDH inhibition for the monitoring of MMF treatment efficacy.

Pharmacokinetis-pharmacodynamic (PK/PD) relationships
To date, very few data exist on this topic. In a Japanese trial, the area under the MPA curve from 0 to 12 h postdose (AUC_{0-12}) was obtained in renal transplant recipients. A PK/PD correlation between AUC_{0-12} and the risk of acute rejection was observed, because this risk decreased as the MPA AUC_{0-12} increased [8]. These findings were confirmed in a randomized controlled trial of MMF [9]. No relationship was found between the incidence of adverse events and the AUC during treatment. However, it has not yet been demonstrated that such

monitoring is useful in clinical practice. Interesting data have also been reported for heart transplant recipients, including a good relationship between the MPA trough level and the incidence of acute rejection.

Recommendations

Because of enterohepatic circulatory and the presence of a secondary peak, the MPA trough level measurement does not appear to be a reliable marker. Therapeutic drug monitoring may be useful when drug interaction is suspected or before reducing the dosage of nephrotoxic agents like cyclosporine A or tacrolimus, and for such monitoring, the following measures and findings are important:

- The recommendations and guidelines for the therapeutic drug monitoring of mycophenolic acid, reported in a consensus panel [10], should be implemented;
- A specific method should be used to measure MPA, because it is the active metabolite of MMF;
- Plasma is the preferred matrix;
- Ethylene diaminetetraacetic acid (EDTA) is the recommended anticoagulant;
- Plasma concentrations of MPA remain constant for up to 8 h at room temperature, for at least 96 h at 4 °C, and for 11 months at −20 °C;
- MPAG is the primary metabolite of MPA and is inactive,
- PK/PD studies have demonstrated the predictive relationship between AUC_{0-12} and risk of acute rejection;
- Evaluation of the MPA AUC may be very useful in ensuring that adequate concentrations are present in the early post-transplantation period, and in providing a basis for reducing MMF dosage, to dose reduction of MMF, and to avoid adverse reactions;
- In adult renal transplant recipients, an AUC_{0-12} of 20 μg·h/ml or more is a reasonable choice for the early post-transplant period;

Clinical efficacy

Although most of the clinical experience of MMF accumulated over the past years concerns organ transplantation, there is growing evidence that this drug might be indicated in certain autoimmune diseases as well.

Prevention of acute rejection in solid organ transplantation

MMF has been shown to reduce the incidence of acute rejection significantly more than azathioprine, whatever the organ considered.

Kidney transplantation

Currently, MMF is indicated for the prevention of acute rejection in kidney transplant recipients. Nonblinded, nonrandomized pilot studies by Sollinger et al. [11] indicated an relationship between the MMF dose and the absence of rejection. Subsequently, three large pivotal trials were set up in the USA, Europe, Australia and Canada whose results were reported separately [12–14] and then pooled [15] (Tabs 1 and 2). In the US study [12], first cadaver kidney transplant recipients were given sequential quadruple immunosuppression comprising steroids, cyclosporine A and ATGAM, together with either 2 or 3 g/d MMF, or 1–2 mg/kg/d azathioprine. In the European study [13], first and second cadaver kidney transplant recipients had received triple immunosup-

Table 1. MMF pivotal studies designs

Study sites	USA study [12]	TRI study [14]	EUR study [13]
No. of sites	14	21	20
Allograft type	1st cadaveric	←———— 1st or 2nd cadaveric ————→	
MMF regimens	←———————— 1.0 g b.i.d. (MMF 2 g) ————————→		
	←———————— 1.5 g b.i.d. (MMF 3 g) ————————→		
Control regimen	AZA	AZA	PLA
	1–2 mg/kg/day	100–150 mg/day	
ATG induction	Yes	←———————— No ————————→	
Concomitant immunosuppressive therapy	←———————— CsA and corticosteroids ————————→		

Table 2. First biopsy-proven rejection or treatment failure during first 12 months after transplantation excluding routine biopsies [a] in MMF pivotal studies

	PLA/AZA	MMF 2g	MMF 3g
Patients enrolled	498	505	490
First biopsy-proven rejection (%)	203 (40.8)	100 (19.8)[b]	81 (16.5)[b]
Grade I	84 (16.9)	50 (9.9)	41 (8.4)
Grade II	92 (18.5)	41 (8.1)	30 (6.1)
Grade III	27 (5.4)	9 (1.8)	10 (2.0)
Patients with biopsy-proven rejection or treatment failure (%)	268 (53.8)	186 (36.8)[c]	194 (39.6)[c]

[a] Biopsy-proven rejection was indicated by core biopsy of Banff severity >I. Treatment failure occurred if patient terminated prematurely.
[b] $p < 0.0001$ for pairwise comparisons between MMF 2 g *versus* PLA/AZA and MMF 3 g *versus* PLA/AZA (competing risk analysis using proportional hazards regression, 97.5% confidence intervals).
[c] $p < 0.002$.

pression that included steroids, cyclosporine A and 2 or 3 g/d MMF or place-bo. In the tricontinental study [14], first and second cadaver kidney transplant recipients had received triple immunosuppression comprising steroids, cyclosporine A and 2 or 3 g/d MMF or 100–150 mg/d azathioprine. The authors of all three studies concluded that MMF significantly reduced the incidence of biopsy-proven acute rejection or treatment failure during the 6 months after transplantation (Tab. 2). The time to first biopsy-proven acute rejection or treatment failure was significantly longer for MMF-treated patients than for patients given either placebo or azathioprine [12, 13]. Acute rejections (Banff grade II and III) were more frequent among patients taking azathioprine or placebo than those taking MMF. MMF-treated patients required significantly fewer full courses of anti-rejection therapy and treatment with anti-lymphocyte globulin (ALG) than placebo- or azathioprine-treated patients [12–14]. Six months after transplant, patient and graft survival were similar in all patient subgroups. Note however, that in both the US and Tricontinental trials, the doses of azathioprine were low, at 1–2 mg/kg/d and 100–150 mg/d respectively (100 mg when body weight was below 75 kg). With regard to the MMF safety profile, MMF-treated patients, especially those who took 3 g/d, experienced significantly more adverse gastrointestinal events, neutropenia episodes and tissue-invasive cytomegalovirus (CMV) disease [12–14]. In contrast, the incidence of post-transplant lymphoproliferative disorders was similar in all patient subgroups.

These three trials were sufficiently similar as regards design, patient populations, and timing to allow the statistical analysis of pooled data, in order to obtain a better picture of how MMF performed in renal transplant recipients [15]. The results reported included an extended follow-up at 1 year. Graft survival was 90.4 and 89.2% in the groups given 2 and 3 g/d of MMF respectively, compared to 87.6% in the placebo/azathioprine group, a difference which was not significant. MMF significantly reduced the proportion of rejection episodes, which was 40.8% for placebo/azathioprine patients *versus* 19.8 and 16.5% for the 2 and 3 g/d MMF groups, respectively. Graft function was slightly better in MMF-treated patients.

In the US study, a subgroup analysis was performed in which African-American renal allograft recipients, known to be an immunologically high-risk group, were compared to non-African-American recipients [16]. In the African-American recipients, 3 g/d of MMF significantly reduced the incidence of biopsy-proven acute rejection and delayed its occurrence for significantly longer than in the groups given either azathioprine or 2 g/d MMF, showing a better benefit/risk ratio for this larger MMF dose.

Since the results of these three trials were published, it has been reported that the addition of 2 g/d mycophenolate mofetil to a combination of tacrolimus and prednisone reduced the incidence of acute rejection from 44 to 27% ($p = 0.014$) [17]. However, the optimal dose of MMF when combined with tacrolimus still requires investigation, with regard both to efficacy and the incidence of side-effects.

Kidney-pancreas transplantation

The efficacy of MMF in preventing acute rejection in pancreas kidney transplantation has not been established by perfectly designed studies like in renal transplantation. We will refer to the two major studies reported. At Minneapolis, 120 pancreas transplant recipients were treated with MMF, steroids, tacrolimus and induction with anti-thymocyte globulin (ATG) [18]. Sixty-one underwent a simultaneous pancreas-kidney transplantation, 44 underwent a pancreas transplantation after previous kidney transplantation and 15 underwent a pancreas transplantation alone. A matched-pair analysis was performed using the International Pancreas Transplant Registry database to compare the outcome in MMF *versus* azathioprine recipients. The incidence of acute rejection was significantly lower in the MMF group (15% *versus* 43%). It did not result in significant differences in patient or graft survival. Of note is the high rate of conversion from MMF to azathioprine due to gastrointestinal toxicity, the highest rate being observed in pancreas transplantation alone.

Odorico et al. [19] conducted a retrospective comparison of 358 consecutive primary simultaneous pancreas-kidney transplantations over a 7-year period. Patients received either 3 g MMF ($n = 109$) or 2 mg/kg/d azathioprine ($n = 249$) together with steroids, cyclosporine A and an induction treatment (ATGAM or OKT3). The authors observed a significantly reduced incidence of biopsy-proven kidney rejection, of clinically significant pancreas rejection, and of steroid-refractory rejection. This resulted in a significantly better 2-year graft survival (95 *versus* 86% for the kidney, 95 *versus* 83% for the pancreas). This improvement was not associated with an increased risk of opportunistic infections.

Heart transplantation

The efficacy of MMF in heart transplantation has been studied in a double-blind, active-controlled trial, involving 659 patients at 28 centers [20]. Patients received cyclosporine A, steroids associated with either 3 g MMF or 1.3–3 mg/kg/d azathioprine. Patients were excluded (11%) if they were not able to receive MMF during the first 5 days. In patients that effectively received MMF, mortality at 1 year was significantly reduced compared to that in azathioprine-treated patients, as well as a requirement for rejection treatment. There was a trend for fewer MMF patients to have less than or equal to grade 3A rejection or require poly- or mono-clonal anti-lymphocyte antibodies. Opportunistic infections, mostly herpes virus infections, were more common in the MMF group.

Liver transplantation

Eckhoff et al. [21] compared retrospectively 130 patients who received a primary adult liver transplant with either tacrolimus, 2 g MMF and steroids stopped at 3 months or tacrolimus and steroids. The incidence of acute rejection was significantly reduced in the MMF group (45 *versus* 26%). The incidence of opportunistic infections was similar in both groups. Interestingly,

MMF allowed a significant reduction in tacrolimus dosage and hence a reduced nephrotoxicity. These data were not confirmed by a prospective randomized study [22] comparing the efficacy and toxicity of the association tacrolimus-steroids *versus* tacrolimus-steroids-MMF 2 g. At 1-year, both patient and graft survival were equivalent in both groups as was the incidence of acute rejection. It is interesting to notice that in liver transplantation, MMF was not compared to azathioprine like in other transplanted organs.

Lung transplantation

Ross et al. [23] reported their experience in lung transplantation. They analyzed the incidence of biopsy-proven acute cellular rejection (histology grade ≥ A2) and decrement in pulmonary function in a two-center, nonrandomized concurrent cohort study during the first 12 months following transplantation. Patients received a short induction with ATG, cyclosporine A, steroids associated with either 2 g MMF or 1–2 mg/kg/d azathioprine. The MMF group experienced significantly fewer episodes of acute rejection than the azathioprine group. The change in forced expiratory volume between 3 and 12 months was less pronounced in the MMF group suggesting that MMF may reduce incidence or delay onset of bronchiolitis obliterans syndrome.

Miscellaneous

The experience with MFF in intestinal transplantation is limited [24] and it is difficult to draw definite conclusions. MMF seems to be well tolerated although nausea and diarrhea are difficult to evaluate in this setting. Severe rejections are still observed with a high incidence of severe infections.

Treatment of acute rejection

High doses of MMF can successfully reverse acute renal allograft rejection in a dog model [2]. In humans, the influence of MMF has been studied in cellular acute rejection and in rejection refractory to treatment.

First acute cellular rejection

In a double-blind, double-dummy controlled study, renal allograft recipients experiencing their first biopsy-proven acute cellular rejection in the first 6 months post-transplantation were treated with high-dose steroids associated with either 3 g MMF or 1–2 mg/kg/d azathioprine [25]. The purpose of this study was to compare the efficacy and safety of the addition of MMF or azathioprine to the treatment of a first acute rejection which consisted of intravenous steroids (5 mg/kg/d) for 5 days followed by an oral steroid taper. At 6 months, 16.8% of MMF-treated patients required at least one course of anti-lymphocyte therapy *versus* 41.7% in azathioprine-treated patients ($p < 0.0001$). Also, the number of patients requiring full courses of anti-rejection therapy was significantly lower in the MMF-treated group and there was a trend towards better renal function. However, the incidence of adverse effects was higher in the MMF-group. To determine the long-term influence of treating rejection with MMF, an extended follow-up of these patients has been set-up.

Resistant acute rejection, cellular

In recipients of a first or second cadaver kidney or living-related renal allograft, MMF was compared prospectively to high-dose intravenous steroids in the treatment of biopsy-proven acute cellular rejection refractory to OKT3, ALG or ATG administered for at least 7 days [26]. Intravenous steroids consisted of a 5 mg/kg/d dose for 5 days followed by an oral steroid taper. MMF was given at 3 g/d for 3 months. Patients received steroids and cyclosporine A while those not treated with MMF received azathioprine (up to 2.5 mg/kg/d). The incidence of patients who experienced subsequent biopsy-proven rejection, presumptive rejection or treatment failure (premature termination for any reason including death, graft loss or adverse event) was lower in the MMF group compared to that in the intravenous steroid group, 39% *versus* 64%, respectively ($p < 0.001$). This resulted in a better graft survival at 1 year post-transplantation, i.e., a 42% reduction in graft loss and death incidence. However, the incidence of reported adverse events was higher in the MMF group as well as the incidence of tissue-invasive CMV disease.

Resistant acute rejection, humoral

The treatment of so-called acute humoral rejection is not well standardized and this type of rejection has a bad prognosis. Pascual et al. [27] used a combination of plasma exchange, tacrolimus and MMF to treat acute humoral rejection with development of anti-donor antibodies in five patients. Plasma exchanges first led to a decrease in circulating anti-donor antibodies followed by a subsequent increase. Plasma exchanges together with tacrolimus and MMF led to a sustained result, a good renal function and an excellent 100% graft survival at 1 year post-transplant. Even though it is a small cohort of patients, it constitutes a promising approach to treat this type of rejection.

Prevention and treatment of chronic rejection

Chronic rejection or better chronic allograft dysfunction is a major contributor to declining organ function and graft loss. It is obviously due to immunologic and non-immunologic factors among which acute rejection is probably the most significant. It is often very difficult to make a clear distinction between "true immunologic" chronic rejection and chronic nephrotoxicity due to calcineurin inhibitors.

Kidney transplantation

One possible answer to the preventive role of MMF in chronic allograft nephropathy was to study the long-term results of the tricontinental pivotal study presented above [28], by extending the follow-up to 3 years. Although this study was not initially designed to evaluate long-term issues and was therefore probably biased, it brought some interesting data. One question raised is whether the prevention of acute renal rejection by MMF implies a prevention of chronic rejection. Patients were randomized to receive 100–150 mg of azathioprine ($n = 166$), 2 g MMF ($n = 173$) or 3 g MMF ($n = 164$), in conjunction with cyclosporine A and prednisone from the time of transplantation. At 3 years, both intend-to-treat and on-study analyses of graft and patient survival showed a trend toward advantage for 2–3 g MMF over azathioprine, but this trend did not reach statistical significance. As well, there was no statistical difference regarding graft function, incidence of lymphoproliferative disorders and cancers, and mortality. The deleterious role of acute rejection was again emphasized in this study since patients who experienced a biopsy-proven acute rejection in the first 6 months after transplantation were about five times more likely to lose their graft than those who were free of such rejection. Prevention of acute rejection by MMF was not therefore producing a significant improvement after 3 years of follow-up. Analysis of long-term data from the European study produced similar results [29].

Another approach to study the role of MMF in chronic rejection consists of adding MMF to the current immunosuppression once chronic rejection has been diagnosed. A small retrospective preliminary study was reported by Glicklich et al. [30]. Fourteen patients with clinical and histologic chronic rejection who were receiving cyclosporine or tacrolimus, had MMF added to their immunosuppressive regimen and were compared with patients with chronic rejection but without MMF (patients were matched for serum creatinine levels and transplant duration at time MMF was begun). Over 36 months, including 122 months before MMF and up to 24 months thereafter, there was no significant change in creatinine between the two groups. These data should of course be validated by a randomized controlled trial.

Heart transplantation

Very interestingly, the follow-up of the pivotal heart transplantation study [20] was extended up to 3 years. In the group of patients who received MMF, patient survival was 88.1% *versus* 81.6% in the group of patients who received azathioprine. This results in a 35% decrease in mortality rate. It outlines the close relationship between acute and chronic rejection: the prevention of acute heart rejection is followed by a reduction in mortality due to chronic heart rejection.

Calcineurin inhibitor sparing effect

There is in the literature some evidence that MMF may have a calcineurin inhibitor-sparing effect after transplantation, either early or late. With regard to late calcineurin inhibitor-sparing effect, it is often very difficult to make a clear distinction between chronic nephrotoxicity due to calcineurin inhibitors and "true immunologic" chronic rejection. It is therefore impossible to formally exclude in these studies a potential role of MMF in treating the immunologic part of chronic rejection.

Early effect

Grinyo et al. [31] studied prospectively the results at 6 months of a combination 3 g MMF, ATG and low-dose steroids in 17 immunologic low-risk patients who either received a suboptimal kidney or were at increased risk of delayed graft function. At 6 months post-transplant, all patients were alive with a functioning kidney. Cyclosporine A had to be introduced in 4 patients, one because of gastrointestinal intolerance to MMF, one because of grade I acute rejection, and two because of grade II acute rejection. This preliminary experience suggests that an immunosuppressive regimen including 3 g MMF may safely avoid the use of cyclosporine A in 70% of cases.

Zanker et al. [32] applied a similar immunosuppressive regimen, i.e., 2 g MMF, ATG and steroids, to 12 patients with a median age of 61 years receiving a first cadaver kidney transplant. At 6 months post-transplant, graft function was excellent (creatinine 1.3 mg/dl) and cyclosporine A had to be introduced in two patients, one because of CMV infection and the other because of acute rejection. Again, an immunosuppressive regimen without cyclosporine A was possible and safe (at least within 6 months) in 83% of patients.

As the number of marginal donors is increasing, this approach is potentially very interesting since it avoids cyclosporine nephrotoxicity. However, its efficacy and safety needs to be studied on a larger scale with a valid design.

Late effect

In 1997, Weir et al. [33] evaluated the impact of reduced cyclosporine A dosing and addition of MMF in 28 renal transplant recipients patients who were biopsied because of chronic deterioration of renal function and who demonstrated little or no histologic evidence of acute rejection. Before the change in immunosuppression, the mean loss in renal function as indicated by the least-squares slope of the reciprocal of creatinine *versus* time was 0.006 ± 0.002 mg/dl per month. Following the change in immunosuppression, 21 of the 28 patients improved renal function with a mean slope of 0.007 ± 0.003 mg/dl per month. Interestingly, there was no acute rejection after the immunosuppressive change. In this introductory study, the cyclosporine A-sparing effect of MMF resulted in short-term improvement in renal function in 75% of patients.

A similar experience has been reported by Ducloux et al. [34]. In six patients with cyclosporine A nephrotoxicity, the authors switched the combination cyclosporine-azathioprine for MMF. After a follow-up period of 12 months, serum creatinine decreased from 225 ± 58 to 169 ± 66 µmol/l while hyperlipidemia and hypertension improved. Zanker et al. [32] were even able to switch 13 patients from cyclosporine A monotherapy to MMF monotherapy with a 20% long-lasting improvement in renal function. Hueso et al. [35]

published a similar cyclosporine A-sparing effect of MMF leading to renal function improvement in renal transplant recipients with a suboptimal function. But interestingly, plasma levels of transforming growth factor $\beta1$ decreased in parallel with a good correlation with cyclosporine A trough levels. There again, no acute rejection was observed.

Undoubtedly, the use of MMF is very promising in order to avoid or diminish cyclosporine A nephrotoxicity. But the studies mentioned concern small numbers of patients and should be validated on a larger scale. It is still safest to decrease cyclosporine A dosing when nephrotoxicity is suspected.

The next step is logically to study the conversion from cyclosporine A to MMF in stable patients with good renal function in order to avoid long-term consequences of cyclosporine A nephrotoxicity. In a Dutch study, de Sevaux et al. (oral communication at the American Society Meeting, Chicago, 1999) randomized stable renal transplants recipients at 6 months post-transplantation to stop either cyclosporine A or steroids or to continue a triple combination MMF-CsA-steroids. The withdrawal of cyclosporine A resulted in a rejection incidence of 20%, of which 33% were steroid-resistant. In a French pilot study Legendre et al. (oral communication at the American Society Meeting, Chicago, 1999) switched 20 stable renal transplant recipients from azathioprine to MMF at least 2 years after transplantation. A renal biopsy and a glomerular filtration rate were performed before inclusion in the study and after 40 weeks. Only one patient experienced steroid-responsive acute rejection. However, in 50% of cases, a histologic deterioration was noted. In patients with histologic deterioration, glomerular filtration rate remained stable while it improved in patients without histologic deterioration. Finally, Abramowicz et al. (oral communication at the American Society of Transplantation Meeting, Chicago, 1999) reported preliminary results from a randomized, controlled study investigating the withdrawal of cyclosporine A in stable renal transplant recipients receiving MMF in addition to cyclosporine A and steroids. The incidence of acute rejection was significantly higher in the group of patients who stopped cyclosporine A than in patients who did not. From these preliminary data, it seems therefore very difficult to recommend complete cyclosporine A interruption in stable renal transplant recipients.

Steroid-sparing effect

There is also some evidence that MMF may have a steroid-sparing effect either total or partial. Birkeland et al. [36] reported their experience with 68 kidney transplant recipients who were treated with a 10-day ATG induction together with cyclosporine A and MMF. After a median follow-up of 488 days, 66 patients were alive with a functioning kidney. Fifteen percent of patients developed acute rejection which was not different from historical control patients treated with steroids and cyclosporine A. According to these data, it is therefore possible to completely avoid steroids in a majority of patients.

Another approach was tested in a multicenter French study [37]. Patients were randomized to receive cyclosporine A, MFF and two regimens of steroids: either 30 mg at day 0 tapered until month 3 with a subsequent dose of 10 mg, or 15 mg at day 0 tapered until month 3 and then stopped. With regard to biopsy-proven acute rejection, the incidence was 25% in the low/stop group *versus* 15% in the other group, the difference being explained by more acute rejection episodes in the early period post-transplantation. It was possible to stop steroids at 3 months post-transplant in 75% of patients with excellent function at 1 year post-transplantation.

Bone marrow

Following allogeneic transplantation of bone marrow or peripheral blood stem cells, acute and chronic graft-*versus*-host diseases (GVHD) cause significant morbidity and mortality. There is experimental evidence that MMF combined with cyclosporine A prevents acute GVHD. In humans, Basara et al. [38] reported the use of MMF to treat acute GVHD in combination with cyclosporine A and steroids in 17 patients. In 65% of cases a gradual improvement was noted. Seven patients received MMF for the treatment of the chronic type of GVHD. It led to moderate improvement in half of cases. More recently, Bornhauser et al. [39] studied 14 patients who received 2 g MMF with intravenous cyclosporine A in the prevention of acute GVHD. Patients in the control group received methotrexate instead of MMF. Trilineage engraftment was achieved in all patients. The incidence of acute GVHD in MMF-treated patients was 46.5% *versus* 60% in methotrexate-treated patients. Tolerance was comparable. Interestingly, reduced peak levels of MPA indicated a reduced absorption rate of MMF in the early post-transplant phase.

Other indications

Gout
Hyperuricemia occurs in 30–80% of renal transplant recipients treated with cyclosporine A, with gouty arthritis in 4–10% of these patients. Management of gout is a very difficult therapeutic challenge since allopurinol is dangerous in combination with azathioprine due to myelotoxicity. Also the use of colchicine is limited by its side-effects (diarrhea and rhabdomyolysis). Interestingly, MMF may be substituted for azathioprine to ensure the safe use of allopurinol in kidney transplant recipients, as recently reported by Jacobs et al. [40].

Inhibition of antibody synthesis
Due to its action on B-lymphocytes, MMF has a great potential in situations such as in HLA-immunized patients and the use of xenogeneic therapeutic

antibody. The presencence of anti-HLA antibodies is a source of complications in organ transplantation since is prolongs the waiting time and it has an adverse effect on transplantation results. There is only one report on the use of MMF to decrease anti-HLA antibody production in a patient awaiting heart transplant [41]. After introduction of MMF, panel-reactive antibodies decreased from 50–70% to 5–10% and remained low after MMF was interrupted.

MMF is also able to decrease the production of anti-ATGAM [42] and anti-OKT3 antibodies [43]. With a combination of cyclosporine A (Neoral) and MMF, the immunization rate after a 13-day OKT3 induction therapy went down to 0 out of 11 patients while it was 50% for the combination cyclosporine A (Sandimmun)-azathioprine and 19% for the combination cyclosporine A (Neoral)-azathioprine.

Prevention of pneumocystis carinii infection

It is probably important to note that in virus-free Sprague-Dawley rats induced to get *pneumocystis carinii* pneumonitis, administration of MMF prevented the occurrence of pneumonitis, unlike dexamethazone, tacrolimus and sirolimus, due to possible inhibition of fungal IMPDH [44]. This anti-pneumocystis activity may also be valid in the clinical setting, since no case of *pneumocystis carinii* infection was reported in MMF treated patients in the three pivotal studies presented above [12–14].

Autoimmune diseases

MMF has been extensively tested in various animal models of autoimmune diseases. A beneficial effect has been described in murine lupus (delayed deterioration in renal function and prolonged survival), in experimental autoimmune uveoretinitis, in active Heymann nephritis, in adjuvant-induced arthritis and in experimental allergic encephalomyelitis. In humans to date, only anecdotal reports have been published.

Lupus nephritis

With regard to lupus nephritis [45], clinical observations of 13 patients treated with MMF because of cyclophosphamide-resistant or relapsing lupus nephritis over a mean of 12.8 months showed significant improvement in serum creatinine level and proteinuria.

Glomerulonephritis

Patients with various glomerular diseases [46] including IgA nephropathy, membraneous nephropathy, minimal change disease and focal segmental glomerulosclerosis were also treated successfully with MMF. Like in organ transplant recipients, a steroid or cyclosporine A-sparing effect could be of interest in these patients.

Inflammatory bowel diseases

Another promising field is probably the treatment of inflammatory bowel diseases such as Crohns' disease when azathioprine is either not tolerated or exhibits poor efficacy. Recently, Neurath et al. [47] reported the results of a study in which patients with chronic active Crohn's disease were randomized to receive either azathioprine-steroids or MMF-steroids. Efficacy of the combination MMF-steroids was similar in patients with a moderately active disease, but it was superior in patients with the most active forms.

Dermatology

The use of MMF has been beneficial in patients with erythrodermic psoriasis, bullous pemphigoid, pemphigus vulgaris, dishydrotic eczema and pyoderma gangrenosum. A recent article reports the efficacy of MMF in 11 of 12 patients suffering from pemphigus vulgaris even after tapering the steroid dose [48].

Miscellaneous

Finally, MMF has been used with some success in patients with rheumatoid arthritis, systemic vasculitis associated with anti-neutrophil antibodies, retroperitoneal fibrosis, refractory uveitis or autoimmune haemolytic anemia. Besides these anecdotal reports, prospective controlled trials will be necessary to draw definite conclusions. The challenge resides in the design of such studies, given the infrequency of these individual disorders.

Adverse effects

MMF generally has a satisfying tolerance profile. Gastrointestinal adverse effects such as nausea, abdominal cramping, diarrhea and anorexia are the most commonly observed side-effects at standard doses. Rarely, abdominal bleeding and gastrointestinal ulceration have been described. Thrombocytopenia and anemia may occur, but neutropenia is approximately as frequent as in azathioprine treated patients [12–14]. There is no clear-cut relationship between the frequency and intensity of adverse events and any pharmacologic profile, but this area deserves more attention. The main concern is obviously an increased incidence of invasive CMV infection which was reported in the three pivotal studies in kidney transplantation especially in the 3 g MMF subgroup [12–14]. Sarmiento et al. [49] in a case-controlled study in kidney transplant recipients did not find evidence that 2 g MMF was an independant risk factor for primary CMV viremia or tissue invasion. Of note, MMF markedly potentiates the antiherpesvirus activities of several antiviral agents such as acyclovir, ganciclovir or penciclovir [50]. This issue will probably become of less importance due to the excellent efficacy and safety of anti-CMV prophylaxis either by oral ganciclovir or valacyclovir.

The incidence of EBV-related lymphoproliferative disorders and other malignancies is not increased, at least up to 3 years post-transplantation.

Drug interactions

The number of drug interactions described with MMF is very low [51]. A reduced AUC (33%) has been described in patients receiving antiacids containing aluminum and magnesium hydroxide. It is therefore advisable to give the antacid 2 h after MMF administration. A 40% decrease in the AUC of MMF was observed after a single dose of MMF in healthy volunteers pretreated with 4 g cholestyramine three times a day for 4 days. It is suspected that bile acid sequestrants interfere with enterohepatic circulation. Finally, coadministration of acyclovir and MMF results in higher area under the curve of MPAG.

Concluding remarks

MMF is a potent immunosuppressive agent with an excellent tolerance profile. Its immunosuppressive effect has been proven in comparison with azathioprine. The pharmaco-economic impact of this as well as long-term consequences remain to be precisely defined. The greatest potential of MMF is probably its calcineurin inhibitor-sparing effect to reduce nephrotoxicity either early or late post-transplantation.

References

1 Sayegh MH, Turka LA (1998) The role of T-cell costimulatory activation pathways in transplant rejection. *N Engl J Med* 338: 1813–1821
2 Allison AC, Eugui EM (1993) Immunosuppressive and other effects of mycophenolic acid and an ester prodrug, mycophenolate mofetil. *Immunol Rev* 136: 5–28
3 Natsumeda Y, Carr S (1993) Human type I and II IMP dehydrogenase as targets. *Ann N Y Acad Sci* 696: 88–93
4 Sintchak MD, Fleming MA, Futer O, Raybuck SA, Chambers SP, Caron PR, Murcko MA, Wilson KP (1996) Structure and mechanism of inosine monophosphate dehydrogenase in complex with the immunosuppressant mycophenolic acid. *Cell* 85: 921–930
5 Bullingham RE, Nicholls AJ, Kamm BR (1998) Clinical pharmacokinetics of mycophenolate mofetil. *Clin Pharmacokinet* 34: 429–455
6 Sanquer S, Breil M, Baron C, Dahmane D, Astier A, Lang P (1998) Trough blood concentrations in long-term treatment with mycophenolate mofetil. *Lancet* 351: 1557
7 Yatscoff RW, Aspeslet LJ, Gallant HL (1998) Pharmacodynamic monitoring of immunosuppressive drugs. *Clin Chem* 44: 428–432
8 Takahashi K, Ochiai T, Uchida K, Yasumura T, Ishibashi M, Suzuki S, Otsubo O, Isono K, Takagi H, Oka T et al (1995) Pilot study of mycophenolate mofetil (RS-61443) in the prevention of acute rejection following renal transplantation in Japanese patients. *Transplant Proc* 27: 1421–1424
9 Hale MD, Nicholls AJ, Bullingham RES, Hene R, Hoitsma A, Squifflet JP, Weimar W, Vanrenterghem Y, Van de Woude FJ, Verpooten GA (1998) The pharmacokinetic-pharmacodynamic relationship for mycophenolate mofetil in renal transplantation. *Clin Pharmacol Ther* 64: 672–683
10 Shaw LM, Nicholls A, Hale M, Armstrong VW, Oellerich M, Yatscoff R, Morris RE, Holt DW, Venkataramanan R, Haley J et al (1998) Therapeutic monitoring of mycophenolic acid. A consensus panel report. *Clin Biochem* 31: 317–322
11 Sollinger HW, Deierhoi MH, Belzer FO, Diethelm AG, Kauffman RS (1992) RS-61443: a phase I clinical trial and pilot rescue study. *Transplantation* 53: 428–432

12 Sollinger HW for the USRenal Transplant Mycophenolate Mofetil Study Group (1995) Mycophenolate mofetil for the prevention of acute rejection in primary cadaveric renal allograft recipients. *Transplantation* 60: 225–232

13 European Mycophenolate Mofetil Study Group (1995) Placebo-controlled study of mycophenolate mofetil combined with cyclosporin and corticosteroid for prevention of acute rejection. *Lancet* 345: 1321–1325

14 The Tricontinental Mycophenolate Mofetil Renal Transplantation Study Group (1996) A blinded, randomized clinical trial of mycophenolate mofetil for the prevention of acute rejection in cadaveric renal transplantation. *Transplantation* 61: 1029–1037

15 Halloran P, Mathew T, Tomlanovich S, Groth C, Hooftman L, Barker C (1997) Mycophenolate mofetil in renal allograft recipients. A pooled efficacy analysis of three randomized, double-blind, clinical studies in prevention of rejection. *Transplantation* 63: 39–47

16 Neylan JF for the USRenal Transplant Mycophenolate Mofetil Study Group (1997) Immunosuppressive therapy in high-risk transplant patients. Dose-dependent efficacy of mycophenolate mofetil in African-American renal allograft recipients. *Transplantation* 64: 1277–1282

17 Shapiro R, Jordan ML, Scantlebury VP, Vivas C, Marsh JW, McCauley J, Johnston J, Randhawa P, Irish W, Gritsch HA et al (1999) A prospective, randomized trial of tacrolimus/prednisone *versus* tacrolimus/prednisone/mycophenolate mofetil in renal transplant recipients. *Transplantation* 67: 411–415

18 Gruessner RW, Sutherland DE, Drangstveit MB, Wrenshall L, Humar A, Gruessner AC (1998) Mycophenolate mofetil in pancreas transplantation. *Transplantation* 66: 318–323

19 Odorico JS, Pirsch JD, Knechtle SJ, D'Alessandro AM, Sollinger HW (1998) A study comparing mycophenolate mofetil to azathioprine in simultaneous pancreas-kidney transplantation. *Transplantation* 66: 1751–1759

20 Kobashigawa J, Miller L, Renlund D, Mentzer R, Alderman E, Bourge R, Costanzo M, Eisen H, Dureau G, Ratkovec R et al (1998) A randomized active-controlled trial of mycophenolate mofetil in heart transplant recipients. *Transplantation* 66: 507–515

21 Eckhoff DE, McGuire BM, Frenette JR, Contreras JL, Hudson SL, Bynon JS (1998) Tacrolimus and mycophenolate mofetil combination therapy *versus* tacrolimus in adult liver transplantation. *Transplantation* 65: 180–187

22 Jain AB, Hamad I, Rakela J, Dodson F, Kramer D, Demetris J, McMichael J, Starzl TE, Fung JJ (1998) A prospective randomized trial of tacrolimus and prednisone *versus* tacrolimus, prednisone, and mycophenolate mofetil in primary adult liver transplant recipients: an interim report. *Transplantation* 66: 1395–1398

23 Ross DJ, Waters PF, Levine M, Kramer M, Ruzevich S, Kass RM (1998) Mycophenolate mofetil *versus* azathioprine immunosuppressive regimens after lung transplantation: preliminary experience. *J Heart Lung Transplant* 17: 768–774

24 Tsakis AG, Weppler D, Khan MF, Koutouby R, Romero R, Viciana AL, Raskin J, Nery JR, Thompson J (1998) Mycophenolate mofetil as primary and rescue therapy in intestinal transplantation. *Transplant Proc* 30: 2677–2679

25 The Mycophenolate Mofetil Acute Renal Rejection Study Group (1998) Mycophenolate mofetil for the treatment of a first acute renal allograft rejection. *Transplantation* 65: 235–241

26 The Mycophenolate Mofetil Renal Refractory Rejection Study Group (1996) Mycophenolate mofetil for the treatment of refractory, acute, cellular renal transplant rejection. *Transplantation* 61: 722–729

27 Pascual M, Saidman S, Tolkoff-Rubin N, Williams WW, Mauiyyedi S, Duan JM, Farrell ML, Colvin RB, Cosimi AB, Delmonico FL (1998) Plasma exchange and tacrolimus-mycophenolate rescue for acute humoral rejection in kidney transplantation. *Transplantation* 66: 1460–1464

28 Mathew TH for the Tricontinental Mycophenolate Mofetil Renal Transplantation Study Group (1998) A blinded, long-term, randomized multicenter study of mycophenolate mofetil in cadaveric renal transplantation. *Transplantation* 65: 1450–1454

29 USRenal Transplant Mycophenolate Mofetil Study Group (1999) Mycophenolate Mofetil in cadaveric renal transplantation. *Amer J Kidney Dis* 34: 296–303

30 Glicklich D, Gupta B, Schurter-Frey G, Greenstein SM, Schechner RS, Tellis VA (1998) Chronic renal allograft rejection: no response to mycophenolate mofetil. *Transplantation* 66: 398–399

31 Grinyo JM, Gil-Vernet S, Seron D, Hueso M, Fulladosa X, Cruzado JM, Moreso F, Fernandez A, Torras J, Riera L et al (1998) Primary immunosuppression with mycophenolate mofetil and

antithymocyte globulin for kidney transplant recipients of a suboptimal kidney. *Nephrol Dialysis Transplant* 13: 2601–2604

32 Zanker B, Schneeberger H, Rothenpieler U, Hillebrand G, Illner WD, Theodorakis I, Stangl M, Land W (1998) Mycophenolate mofetil-based, cyclosporine-free induction and maintenance immunosuppression: first-3-months analysis of efficacy and safety in two cohorts of renal allograft recipients. *Transplantation* 66: 44–49

33 Weir MR, Anderson L, Fink JC, Gabregiorgish K, Schweitzer EJ, Hoehn-Saric E, Klassen DK, Cangro CB, Johnson LB, Kuo PC et al (1997) A novel approach to the treatment of chronic allograft nephropathy. *Transplantation* 64: 1706–1710

34 Ducloux D, Fournier V, Bresson-Vautrin C, Rebibou JM, Billerey C, Saint-Hillier Y, Chalopin JM (1998) Mycophenolate mofetil in renal transplant recipients with cyclosporine-associated nephrotoxicity: a preliminary report. *Transplantation* 65: 1504–1506

35 Hueso M, Bover J, Seron D, Gil-Vernet S, Sabate I, Fulladosa X, Ramos R, Coll O, Alsina J, Grinyo JM (1998) Low-dose cyclosporine and mycophenolate mofetil in renal allograft recipients with suboptimal function. *Transplantation* 66: 1727–1731

36 Birkeland SA (1998) Steroid-free immunosuppression after kidney transplantation with antithymocyte globulin induction and cyclosporine and mycophenolate mofetil maintenance therapy. *Transplantation* 66: 1207–1210

37 Lebranchu Y for the M 55002 Study Group (1999) Comparison of 2 corticosteroid regimens in combination with MMF and cyclosporine for prevention of acute allograft rejection: 12 month results of a double-blind, randomized, multi-center study. *Transplant Proc* 31: 249–250

38 Basara N, Blau WI, Romer E, Rudolphi M, Bischoff M, Kirsten D, Sanchez H, Gunzelmann S, Fauser AA (1998) Mycophenolate mofetil for the treatment of acute and chronic GVHD in bone marrow transplant patients. *Bone Marrow Transplant* 22: 61–65

39 Bornhauser M, Schuler U, Porksen G, Naumann R, Geissler G, Thiede C, Schwerdtfeger R, Ehninger G, Thiede HM (1999) Mycophenolate mofetil and cyclosporine as graft-*versus*-host disease prophylaxis after allogeneic blood stem cell transplantation. *Transplantation* 67: 499–504

40 Jacobs F, Mamzer-Bruneel MF, Skhiri H, Thervet E, Legendre C, Kreis H (1997) Safety of the mycophenolate mofetil-allopurinol combination in kidney transplant recipients with gout. *Transplantation* 64: 1087–1088

41 Schmid C, Garritsen HS, Kelsch R, Cassens U, Baba HA, Sibrowski W, Scheld HH (1998) Suppression of panel-reactive antibodies by treatment with mycophenolate mofetil. *Thorac Cardiovasc Surg* 46: 161–162

42 Kimball JA, Pescovitz MD, Book BK, Norman DJ (1995) Reduced human IgG anti-ATGAM antibody formation in renal transplant recipients receiving mycophenolate mofetil. *Transplantation* 60: 1379–1383

43 Broeders N, Wissing M, Crusiaux A, Kinnaert P, Vereerstraeten P, Abramowicz D (1998) Mycophenolate mofetil together with cyclosporin A prevents anti-OKT3 antibody response in kidney transplant recipients. *J Amer Soc Nephrol* 9: 1521–1525

44 Oz HS, Hughes WT (1997) Novel anti-pneumocystis carinii effects of the immunosuppressant mycophenolate mofetil in contrast to provocative effects of tacrolimus, sirolimus, and dexamethasone. *J Infect Dis* 175: 901–904

45 Glicklich D, Acharya A (1998) Mycophenolate mofetil therapy for lupus nephritis refractory to intravenous cyclophosphamide. *Amer J Kidney Dis* 32: 318–322

46 Briggs WA, Choi MJ, Scheel PJ (1998) Successful mycophenolate mofetil treatment of glomerular disease. *Amer J Kidney Dis* 31: 213–217

47 Neurath MF, Wanitschke R, Peters M, Krummenauer F, Meyer zum Buschenfelde KH, Schlaak JF (1999) Randomised trial of mycophenolate mofetil *versus* azathioprine for treatment of chronic active Crohn's disease. *Gut* 44: 625–628

48 Enk AH, Knop J (1999) Mycophenolate is effective in the treatment of pemphigus vulgaris. *Arch Dermatol* 135: 54–56

49 Sarmiento JM, Munn SR, Paya CV, Velosa JA, Nguyen JH (1998) Is cytomegalovirus infection related to mycophenolate mofetil after kidney transplantation? *Clin Transplant* 12: 371–374

50 Neyts J, Andrei G, De Clercq E (1998) The novel immunosuppressive agent mycophenolate mofetil markedly potentiates the antiherpesvirus activities of acyclovir, ganciclovir, penciclovir *in vitro* and *in vivo*. *Antimicrob Agents Chemother* 42: 216–222

51 Mignat C (1997) Clinically significant drug interactions with new immunosuppressive agents. *Drug Safety* 16: 267–278

Biologicals

Modern Immunosuppressives
ed. by H.-J Schuurman, G. Feutren and J.-F. Bach
© 2001 Birkhäuser Verlag/Switzerland

Therapeutic anti-T-cell monoclonal antibodies

Lucienne Chatenoud and Jean-François Bach

INSERM U25, Hôpital Necker, 161 Rue de Sèvres, F-75015 Paris, France

Introduction

In its first three decades of existence, clinical immunosuppression had essentially been based on chemical drugs that inhibit various lymphocyte functions, notably proliferation and cytokine production. In the early 1960s major successes were obtained with azathioprine and corticosteroids and then, in the 1980s, with cyclosporine A which represented an important breakthrough due to its high T-cell selectivity. More recently new chemicals were proposed namely, FK506 and mycophenolic acid, but there is not strong evidence suggesting that, when compared to cyclosporine A, these drugs are more selective, less toxic (for an equal therapeutic activity) or have an increased capacity to prevent chronic rejection or to induce tolerance.

At variance, both experimental and more recent clinical data [1–11] have suggested that a real bonus could be derived from the usage of monoclonal antibodies (MoAbs) to T-cell receptors. The degree of immunosuppression induced by these biologicals is stronger than that observed with chemical agents. More importantly, presently available data, predominantly in transplantation, but also in autoimmunity, clearly suggest their capacity to promote immune tolerance, which has not been clearly proven to be the case with most of the drugs previously mentioned.

Available specificities

One could in theory produce MoAbs against any T-cell membrane antigen and expect a favorable therapeutic effect. It was, in fact, initially thought that cell depletion was one pivotal mode of action of MoAbs and that any surface protein could serve as a target for depleting antibodies. However, the results obtained do not support this contention since mechanisms other than mere depletion, such as the inhibition or blockade of the functional capacity of the target cells and/or the unique capacity of some anti-T-cell MoAbs to establish immunoregulatory pathways that redirect a "destructive" alloreactive or autoreactive effector response towards a "non-destructive type" one, are of importance in explaining their *in vivo* effects.

We shall focus here on lymphocyte surface molecules involved in the transduction of signals derived from the T-cell antigen receptor, such as CD3 and CD4, that appear among the relevant targets that have been characterized. Recent data also pointed to the importance of receptors involved in the transduction of costimulatory signals, such as CD28 and CD40-Ligand or CD154, that are reviewed by Knechtle elsewhere in this volume. The topic of antibodies that are specific for receptors selectively expressed at the surface of activated T-cells, such as the receptor for interleukin-2 (IL-2), which also constitute relevant therapeutic tools, is also covered in the chapter by Strom.

CD3 is a multichain protein complex, including the γ, δ, ε, ζ and η invariant polypeptides, that is tightly although noncovalently associated with the αβ-heterodimer that is the T-cell antigen receptor (TCR) [12–14]. CD3 is present on both CD4 and CD8 cells, i.e., on the totality of peripheral blood T-lymphocytes, and is absent from NK cells. CD3 constitutes the transduction element of signals delivered through the TCR upon recognition of peptide antigens presented by major histocompatibility complex (MHC) molecules which explains its major functional relevance. Over the years, several MoAbs have been raised against the mouse, rat, monkey and human ε chains of the CD3 complex that were all endowed with very interesting therapeutic properties. Most studies in the mouse have used the 145 2C11 hamster MoAb produced Leo et al. [15]. In humans, OKT3, a murine IgG2a MoAb, initially developed by Kung and Goldstein [16], has been the first widely used MoAb which was introduced in clinical transplantation in 1981 [17, 18].

CD4 is a single-chain molecule including different domains expressed at the surface of one major subset of T-lymphocytes mainly expressing helper properties. CD4 binds MHC class II molecules and was initially considered as a simple adhesion molecule. However, it soon became apparent that the expression of CD4 significantly improved the effectiveness of signal transduction through CD3/TCR, an effect which was linked to its intracytoplasmic noncovalent association to the lymphocyte-specific tyrosine kinases p56[lck] [19, 20]. CD4 is in functional terms a CD3-TRC "co-receptor" that, according to the data by Tome et al. [21] through p56[lck] associates to the "activated" form of the tyrosine phosphorylated CD3 ζ-ζ/ZAP-70 intracytoplasmic complex thus amplifying CD3/TCR-mediated signaling. A multitude of MoAbs have been produced against CD4 molecules in various species. Various antibodies have been used in man, but none has yet been granted approval by regulatory authorities.

Mode of action of anti-T-cell monoclonal antibodies

A large number of studies since the early 1960s had been devoted to the mode of action of polyclonal anti-lymphocyte antibodies. Three major modes of actions have been delineated, including cell depletion, receptor blockade through lymphocyte coating and/or antigenic modulation and lymphocyte activation, intended as the capacity to trigger T-cell-mediated immunoregulatory circuits. Not surprisingly, these mechanisms are also the ones invoked to explain the therapeutic activity of anti-T-cell MoAbs. Importantly, however, each of these mechanisms contributes to the immunosuppressive activity in quite different proportions according to the fine specificity of the monoclonal antibody considered.

Depletion

Some MoAbs promote a very efficient T-cell depletion which, depending on the antibody specificity, will involve all T-cells, as in the case of CD52 antibodies [22], or only certain subsets, as with depleting CD4 antibodies [23]. Depending on the isotype probably linked to complement fixation, but also on other less defined properties such as affinity for the target antigen, the depletion may be nearly complete or very partial, durable or short lived.

The molecular mechanisms involved in monoclonal antibody-mediated cell destruction *in vivo* are variable and complex and, at variance with what was initially expected, do not only rely on the capacity of the constant Fc antibody portion, bearing the antibody isotypes, to interact with Fc receptors on monocyte/macrophages and/or to activate the complement cascade. When injected into humans, most mouse and rat monoclonal anti-T-cell antibodies showed, upon *in vivo* injection into humans, a poor lytic capacity due to the membrane-bound factors that inhibit complement activation in a species-restricted manner. Despite this, some antibody specificities such as CD52 (CAMPATH-1) were highly depleting [22]. Important conclusions came from the study of molecularly-engineered sets of recombinant antibodies, sharing identical specificities but different constant regions [24]. Thus, the potential lytic or nonlytic capacity of a given antibody depends on both its fine specificity and on the density and the distribution of the target cell antigen. In addition, among a given set of MoAbs sharing the same fine specificity, the isotype will also impact on the potential lytic capacity so that a hierarchy can be established, for instance in the case of human immunoglobulins this reads as follows: IgG1 > IgG2 > IgG3 >> IgG4 [24].

An antigen will be a poor target for profound cell lysis if it easily undergoes antigenic modulation, as is the case with molecules such as CD3.

Other mechanisms involved in antibody-mediated depletion are redirected T-cell lysis upon bridging cytotoxic T-cells to the target [25] and, in particular for antibodies to CD3 and CD4, the induction of apoptosis or programmed cell death. Apoptosis mediated *via* CD3/TCR signaling was initially demonstrated in immature thymocytes, but accumulating evidence indicates that it can also be triggered in activated mature peripheral T-cells [26–28]. There is also evidence that antibodies to CD4 may trigger apoptosis especially of activated T-cells.

In order to increase their lytic potential, some antibodies have been coupled with toxins (diphtheria toxin or ricin) [29, 30]. Such immunotoxins specifically bind to the target cells through the antibody portion and kill them after internalization. It has been recently shown in monkeys using CD3-immunotoxins [31, 32], and in humans using CAMPATH-1H [33], that the induction of a profound though transient lymphocyte depletion at the time of implanting a fully mismatched organ allograft is of great benefit to promote long-term engraftment and immune tolerance. However, some concern is raised on the capacity of the immune system to fully reconstitute after such treatments. In fact, large differences exist between the reconstitution capacity of the different lymphocyte subsets, the CD4$^+$ T-cell subset being, for unknown reasons, in all the species studied (mice, monkeys and humans) much more sensitive than the CD8$^+$ T-cell subset. In fact, the general experience has been that transplant patients treated with polyclonal anti-lymphocyte antibodies will very frequently keep for several months low circulating CD4$^+$ T-cell counts and an inversed CD4/CD8 ratio. This was further stressed by the case of the chimeric (human IgG1) CD4 antibody MT-512. Especially at high doses (700 mg of cumulated dosage) the CD4 lymphocytopenia lasted for several consecutive months [23]. Importantly, only a modest increase in the predisposition to infections was reported, which essentially appeared in patients who received high doses of additional immunosuppressants (i.e., methotrexate in rheumatoid arthritis patients).

Because of this risk, particular interest was focused on nondepleting CD4 antibodies that possess many properties of the depleting ones [7, 34–38].

Receptor blockade

There are essentially two non-mutually exclusive mechanisms that may account for an antibody-mediated physical blockade of the cell receptor function, by hampering the interactions with the physiological ligand, and that include the antigenic modulation of the target cell receptor and the MoAb-mediated cell coating (also termed blindfolding). Cell-directed antibodies, and in particular monoclonal antibodies to CD3, can also promote an active phenomenon termed antigenic modulation that is widely observed in the context of various receptor-ligand interactions. In practice it implies that upon binding to its ligand, or to the specific MoAb, the so-formed receptor-antibody (or receptor ligand) complexes will form microaggregates that redistribute at one pole of the cell surface (a phenomenon also known as "capping") and ultimately disappear upon internalization or shedding [39]. Antigenic modulation was shown to be one major mode of action explaining the immunosuppressive capacity of monoclonal antibodies to CD3. In fact, CD3-modulated cells that lose the expression of both CD3 and TCR, while keeping a normal expression of other differentiation antigens such as CD4 or CD8, are fully unresponsive to antigen-specific or mitogen stimulation [39, 40]. This is consistent with the clinical data showing that in CD3-treated transplant patients no allograft rejection is observed while T-cells in the circulation do not express CD3 [17, 41].

Several MoAbs to human, mouse and rat CD4 have been described that are nondepleting and still express potent immunosuppressive and tolerogenic properties. *In vivo* these antibodies essentially act by coating target cells and in most cases, at variance with CD3 MoAbs, do not modulate the CD4 receptor [7, 34–38]. This particular "lack of mobility" of the CD4 molecule at the cell membrane is due to its intracytoplasmic association to $p56^{lck}$ that plays the role of a physical "anchor". Cell transfection experiments using mutant CD4 molecules lacking the intracytoplasmic domain that associate to $p56^{lck}$ have confirmed their ability to undergo antigenic modulation upon CD4 antibody binding.

Lymphocyte signaling

Anti-T-cell MoAbs do not only interfere with physiological receptor/ligand interactions, but may be endowed with agonistic or antagonistic properties thus triggering signal transduction pathways. Importantly, evidence is now accumulating to show that this "activation" may play an essential role in the imunosuppressive and/or tolerogenic capacity of these antibodies.

Most CD3 antibodies are very potent lymphocyte mitogens both *in vitro* and *in vivo*. This mitogenicity is the basis for the massive, though transient, release of several cytokines, both of the T-helper 1 and T-helper 2 type, that follows the first administration of the antibody and is responsible for the well known "flu-like syndrome" [42]. This mitogenic capacity relies on the capacity of the CD3 antibody Fc portion to interact with monocyte Fc receptors. Thus, CD3 F(ab')$_2$ fragments, which lack the Fc portion, or CD3 antibodies which Fc regions have been engineered to prevent them binding to specific receptors completely lose their mitogenic potential [43–46]. Both the experimental and clinical data stress that the therapeutic activity of these nonmitogenic CD3 antibodies is identical to that of the mitogenic ones [44, 47–51]. However, one major finding is that although devoid of mitogenic activity, CD3 F(ab')$_2$ fragments do still trigger T-cell "activation". Thus, using PCR on spleen cell samples from anti-CD3 F(ab')$_2$-treated mice, specific mRNA for different cytokine genes including IL-2, IL-4, IL-10 and interferon-γ may clearly be identified [47]. Moreover, this T-cell "activation" is indispensable for the therapeutic effectiveness of nonmitogenic CD3 antibodies since cyclosporine A, which selectively prevents T-cell cytokine gene transcription amongst which IL-2, interferon-γ and IL-4 [52–54], completely blocks the tolerogenic capacity of nonmitogenic CD3 antibodies when applied concomitantly [47].

Antibodies to CD4 may also promote T-cell signaling. Given the previously discussed contribution of CD4 to TCR/CD3-mediated signaling, some authors have proposed that effective CD4 coating could trigger therapeutically relevant negative "signals" [55]. This is supported by the observations that the proliferative response and lymphokine production in response to various stimuli of resting T-cells is significantly inhibited upon independent *in vitro* ligation of CD3 and CD4, as one may observe after the injection of mono-clonal antibodies to CD4 [56].

In vivo functional properties of therapeutic anti-T-cell monoclonal antibodies

A clear distinction between non-antigen specific immunosuppression and immune tolerance has to be made. In the first case, immune responses are globally depressed, especially for most primary responses, but less common-ly for secondary responses, and this effect does not last more than a few days after clearance of the therapeutic antibody or, in the case of depleting anti-bodies, after reconstitution of the target cell population. In contrast, opera-tional immune tolerance is intended as the establishment of a durable antigen-specific unresponsiveness (prolonged survival of an allograft, prevention of an autoimmune disease relapse) which persists in the absence of generalised immunosuppression. Such quite broad definition does not take into account the underlying immune mechanisms which at present are only partially under-stood.

The degree of non-specific immunosuppression that one may achieve tight-ly correlates with the cumulative drug dosage applied. At least in transplanta-tion, therapeutic anti-T-cell antibodies are given in association with several chemical immunosuppressants, making it difficult to appreciate the contribu-tion of each individual therapeutic agent. One major drawback of this strategy is of course the infectious and tumorigenic risks as well as its incomplete effectiveness. In fact, in clinical transplantation the substantial increase over the last 15 years in the potency of the nonspecific immunosuppression strate-gies applied allowed to almost completely solve the problem of acute rejec-tion. However, chronic vascular rejection remains a major cause of long-term graft failure for which no effective therapy is available yet.

The first observation of the unique tolerogenic capacity of antibodies to CD4 derived from studies showing that rat MoAbs to CD4 injected to mice, in contrast to other rat anti-T-cell MoAbs, did not trigger an anti-globulin response [1, 2]. It was further demonstrated that specific tolerance to soluble antigens and tissue alloantigens could be induced by delivering these antigens into normal adult animals under the cover of depleting or nondepleting anti-bodies to CD4 [1, 3, 7]. Importantly, the continuous presence of the tolerogen is essential to maintain this antigen-specific unresponsiveness.

In adult euthymic mice combinations of antibodies to CD4 and CD8, even if nondepleting, can induce classical transplantation tolerance to skin grafts in partial and fully mismatched combinations [58]. This antibody-induced toler-ance can also be induced and maintained in thymectomized animals, clearly showing that it is a peripheral event; no evidence for clonal deletion of specif-ic alloreactive T-cells was found [4, 34].

Despite the fact that most studies on tolerance induction to organ allografts have focused on antibodies to CD4, other specificities also deserve interest. For instance, antibodies to CD3 can be mentioned, as well as the combination of antibodies to LFA-1 and ICAM-1 and antibodies to CD25 (especially in rat transplant models). Combined administration of MoAbs to LFA-1 and ICAM-1 into mice resulted in permanent engraftment of fully mismatched vascularized heart allografts, but also specific tolerance to donor-type skin allografts [5]. In a mouse heart and skin allograft model the simultaneous blockade of the CD28 and CD40 costimulatory pathways promoted long-term, although not indefinite, allograft survival, whereas the independent blockade of the CD28 and CD40 costimulatory pathways was not effective. More importantly, the simultaneous blockade also inhibited the development of chronic vascular rejection in the grafted hearts [59]. More recent data have shown long-term survival of renal allografts in nonhuman primates treated with MoAbs to CD40 Ligand (CD154) [60].

MoAbs to CD3 can also promote long-term specific unresponsiveness to both alloantigens and autoantigens. In the rat, CD3 antibody induces permanent engraftment of histoincompatible vascularized heart grafts and permanent tolerance (i.e., skin graft acceptance) [61]. Moreover, in NOD mice, who develop a spontaneous form of T-cell mediated autoimmune insulin-dependent diabetes mellitus, a low-dose CD3 treatment applied at the stage of overt disease induces permanent remission and restores self tolerance [11, 47]. Recent results have extended these results to nonhuman primates showing that the use of a CD3-immunotoxin associated either with donor bone marrow cells or with 15-deoxyspergualin induced long-term survival of completely mismatched renal allografts [31, 32].

The major feature characterising most of these models is the strict antigen-dependence and the active or dominant nature of the peripheral immune tolerance achieved. Thus tolerant hosts resist the transfer of immunocompetent naïve and sensitized effectors and one may reverse or "break" the tolerant state upon elimination or functional blockade of defined immune cell subsets i.e., mainly regulatory CD4$^+$ cells that mediate suppression upon adoptive transfer into naïve recipients [34, 62]. In the NOD mouse model, the CD3 antibody-mediated permanent remission of diabetes also associates with the presence of a subset of regulatory T-cells (CD4$^+$CD62L$^+$) that do transfer the protection to naïve recipients (Chatenoud et al., unpublished results).

The molecular basis for these effects is still elusive. In some models of CD4 antibody-induced tolerance to cardiac and renal allografts, the presence of a dominant T-helper 2 response was reported [63]. However, when it comes to the phenomenon of transferable suppression, the available data show only a partial blockade upon treatment with anti-IL-4 MoAb [34]. Another important unresolved question concerns the cellular source of IL-4. Although the assumption is that tolerant or suppressor cells would produce it, there is no firm evidence to show their T-helper 2 subtype nature. It is important to mention at this point that in models of tolerance applied to autoimmunity, other forms of immune deviation were found to correlate with active or transferable suppression phenomena. Thus, T-helper 3 and T-regulatory type 1 CD4$^+$ T-cells, producing transforming growth factor-β and IL-10, respectively, have been shown to play a major immunoregulatory role in models of experimental allergic encephalomyelitis and inflammatory bowel disease [64, 65].

Finally, it has also been proposed that tolerant cells would in fact be to some extent anergic, that is, providing no help, and compete with potentially reactive effectors for binding to antigen-presenting cells. *In vitro*, anergic human T-cell clones could suppress the proliferation of potentially reactive nonanergic cells provided the same antigen-presenting cell was presenting the peptides specific for both partners [66, 67].

Clinical considerations

It is clear that anti-T-cell MoAb therapy represent a very useful complement to chemical immunosuppression in the management of allograft recipients. This applies both for induction treatments and for the reversal of established acute rejection. In a context of non-specific immunosuppression, antibodies have the main merit to reduce the dosage of associated chemical immunosuppressants thus limiting their toxicity. In fact, they probably achieve more than a simple synergistic effect if they can also contribute to tolerance induction.

However, chemical immunosuppressants can also antagonize the tolerogenic properties of anti-T-cell MoAbs. Thus, there is good experimental evidence suggesting that cyclosporine A can inhibit tolerance induction by anti-T-cell MoAbs. This has been shown for the combination of CTLA4-Ig and CD40 Ligand (CD154) antibodies in heart allograft recipients [59] and for CD3 antibodies in the treatment of diabetic NOD mice [47]. As previously discussed, one explanation for these results is that cyclosporine A interferes with some T-lymphocyte activation pathways and cytokine gene transcription [52, 68] that are indispensable for the establishment of immunoregulatory pathways. The clinical relevance of these findings is suggested by the report from the Collaborative Transplant Study Group showing that the kidney allograft survival of patients who received OKT3 as part of their prophylactic regimen was significantly lower if cyclosporine A was associated since the begining of OKT3 treatment as compared to patients in whom the association was protracted [69].

The problem of sensitization

Historically, MoAbs that were initially used therapeutically were of xenogeneic origin, mainly mouse or rat anti-human antibodies. Even in rodents, antibodies were also most often xenogeneic, i.e., hamster and rat anti-mouse antibodies. Administration of such xenogeneic antibodies regularly lead to the appearance of an anti-monoclonal globulin response often endowed with a potent neutralizing activity. Extensive studies, initially performed with the human antibodies and subsequently with the rodent ones, have allowed a better definition of the pattern of the anti-globulin response. Ultimately, various methods have been proposed to circumvent the problem.

Anti-monoclonal globulins express two major specificities that are anti-isotypic and anti-idiotypic [70, 71]. Anti-idiotypic antibodies represent the majority if not the total of neutralizing antibodies. Their detection is based on ELISA and by the inhibition of the binding of the MoAb to the target cell. Studies performed on immunized patients and monkey sera using affinity purified anti-idiotypic antibodies showed that the response is oligoclonal [72]. Anti-isotypic antibodies appear for the majority to be essentially non-neutralizing [73].

It thus appears that the neutralizing potential of the humoral response to monoclonal antibodies is more dependent on its specificity than on the overall amount of antibodies produced, since only a few specific clones are recruited. This explains why serum sickness does not occur, as the amount of immune complexes formed is insufficient to elicit a generalized reaction. The anti-monoclonal globulin response may also include IgE antibodies, associated with the potential risk of anaphylaxis, but in practice this has appeared to be an extremely rare observation [74]. Thus, from the clinical point of view sensitization essentially poses the problem of the abrogation of the therapeutic efficacy of the MoAb.

In practice, the adjunct of appropriate dosages of chemical immunosuppressants to the monoclonal antibody significantly decreased the frequency and intensity of sensitization In the case of OKT3, adding corticosteroids and azathioprine and cyclosporine A at adequate doses decreased the frequency of sensitization from 90–95% to 15–25% [75]. In most cases antibodies appeared only at or after the end of OKT3 treatment and did not affect efficacy. Although this approach has been quite useful, to get a more complete protection from sensitization, a common trend has been to generate "humanized" antibodies or more recently human MoAbs.

Humanized antibodies

Humanized chimeric or complementarity-determining region (CDR)-grafted MoAbs were produced in the attempt to reduce as much as possible the amount of xenogeneic sequences expressed [76]. Chimeric antibodies present with intact variable regions (F_{ab}) from the parental rodent antibody coupled to a human immunoglobulin constant portion. Such chimeric immunoglobulins were initially derived by chemical procedures and subsequently by molecular engineering. In the case of recombinant CDR-grafted antibodies, the rodent CDRs carrying the hypervariable regions that specifically interact with the antigen are inserted into human heavy- and light-chain immunoglobulin frameworks. These two approches allow to select for the desired human Fc fragment that will impact on the final antibody effector capacities (complement fixation, opsonisation, antibody-dependent cellular cytotoxicity (ADCC) and, as previously discussed, potential mitogenic capacity).

The risk of a deleterious anti-idiotypic response still occurring with these humanized antibodies is a valid concern. In fact the clinical data available so far show that chimeric and reshaped humanized antibodies are immunogenic in some patients, but only when the monoclonal is administered alone (in the absence of associated immunosuppressants) and after more than two to three repeated antibody courses [77]. Thus, several centers have now reported on the use of humanized MoAbs in clinical transplantation, where single antibody courses in association with other immunosuppressants is mostly the rule, in the absence of sensitization. From a fundamental point of view, these data are the first indication of the crucial role of the monoclonal antibody constant portions in the induction of the anti-idiotypic response.

In the particular case of CD3 antibodies, as previously discussed, the humanization has offered the double advantage of circumventing the problems linked to the sensitization and the mitogenicity that is responsible for the cytokine-related "flu-like" syndrome which is a major side-effect. Thus, within the first few hours after CD3 MoAb administration a massive but transient systemic release of several cytokines is observed (tumor necrosis factor, interferon-γ, IL-2, IL-3, IL-4, IL-6, IL-10, granulocyte-macrophage colony-stimulating factor) which induces high fever, chills and headache, together with repeated episodes of vomiting and diarrhea; patients become prostrated through massive fluid and electrolyte loss. A minor proportion of patients may develop more severe and potentially life-threatening conditions, such as severe respiratory distress (related to pulmonary edema in patients with significant fluid overload), neurotoxicity and hypotension, but only after the first injection. As we already mentioned, this mitogenic capacity is due to the ability of the Fc portion of CD3 antibodies to interact with monocyte Fc receptors. Thus, by mutating or aglycosylating [45, 46] the Fc portion engineered humanized nonmitogenic CD3 MoAbs have been obtained. Results from pilot trials are very encouraging since they confirmed the good tolerance as well as the capacity of these humanized CD3 antibodies to reverse ongoing kidney allograft rejection.

Human antibodies

Three approaches have recently been made available to produce human therapeutic monoclonal antibodies. The first one consists of the use of mice whose endogenous immunoglobulin genes have been knocked-out and that have been made transgenic for human constant and variable regions of immunoglobulin-encoding genes. Almost all the B-cells in these animals express human immunoglobulin chains and produce human antibodies. The number of human immunoglobulin-encoding sequences introduced proved sufficient to allow the generation of a sufficient diversity. This method has the advantage of simplicity (once the transgenic mice are available) and of the production of high-affinity antibodies using an *in vivo* antigen-driven selection of high-affinity antibody-forming clones upon immunization.

An alternative is the phage-display technique using cDNA libraries expressed on filamentous phages allowing a rapid, fully *in vitro* selection of antibodies with high specificity [78].

The third approach consists in establishing human-mouse chimeras. Irradiated mice are reconstituted with bone marrow cells from scid mice. Human lymphocytes from presensitized donors are then injected into the reconstituted mice that are boosted with defined antigens and used for fusion with myeloma cells [79].

Concluding remarks

All the experience that has been gained in using immunosuppressive MoAbs in transplantation and autoimmunity has clearly demonstrated the existence of therapeutic activities not shared by conventional chemical immunosuppressants, in that MoAbs can promote immune tolerance. Thus, despite the different problems surrounding their preclinical/clinical development, continued effort in pursuing the study of therapeutic humanized and human monoclonals appears worthwhile.

The very stimulating results that have been recently obtained in nonhuman primates (with CD3-immunotoxins and CD40 Ligand (CD154) antibodies) as well as in the clinics (with the CAMPATH-1H antibody) should encourage the design of protocols more directly aimed at inducing "operational" tolerance. These should take into account the potentially deleterious effect of some drug combinations. This is in fact the only way to avoid the two major hazards of chronic immunosuppressive therapy namely, its relative long-term ineffectiveness with consequent recurrence of the destructive immunopathologic processes, and the well-documented infectious and tumorigenic risks. Moreover, from a more fundamental point of view, an understanding of the molecular basis of the tolerogenic properties of monoclonal antibodies would clear the way for development of more easily accessible therapeutic strategies i.e., simple chemicals or recombinant receptor agonist and/or antagonist ligands that would mimic the desired therapeutic effect.

References

1 Benjamin RJ, Waldmann H (1986) Induction of tolerance by monoclonal antibody therapy. *Nature* 320: 449–451
2 Gutstein NL, Seaman WE, Scott JH, Wofsy D (1986) Induction of immune tolerance by administration of monoclonal antibody to L3T4. *J Immunol* 137: 1127–1132
3 Cobbold SP, Qin S, Leong LY, Martin G, Waldmann H (1992) Reprogramming the immune sys-

tem for peripheral tolerance with CD4 and CD8 monoclonal antibodies. *Immunol Rev* 129: 165–201

4 Qin S, Cobbold SP, Pope H, Elliott J, Kioussis D, Davies J, Waldmann H (1993) "Infectious" transplantation tolerance. *Science* 259: 974–977

5 Isobe M, Yagita H, Okumura K, Ihara A (1992) Specific acceptance of cardiac allograft after treatment with antibodies to ICAM-1 and LFA-1. *Science* 255: 1125–1127

6 Lin H, Bolling SF, Linsley PS, Wei RQ, Gordon D, Thompson CB, Turka LA (1993) Long-term acceptance of major histocompatibility complex mismatched cardiac allografts induced by CTLA4Ig plus donor-specific transfusion. *J Exp Med* 178: 1801–1806

7 Pearson TC, Madsen JC, Larsen CP, Morris PJ, Wood KJ (1992) Induction of transplantation tolerance in adults using donor antigen and anti-CD4 monoclonal antibody. *Transplantation* 54: 475–483

8 Wofsy D, Seaman WE (1987) Reversal of advanced murine lupus in NZB/NZW F1 mice by treatment with monoclonal antibody to L3T4. *J Immunol* 138: 3247–3253

9 Wood KJ (1990) Transplantation tolerance with monoclonal antibodies. *Semin Immunol* 2: 389–399

10 Shizuru JA, Taylor-Edwards C, Banks BA, Gregory AK, Fathman CG (1988) Immunotherapy of the nonobese diabetic mouse: treatment with an antibody to T-helper lymphocytes. *Science* 240: 659–662

11 Chatenoud L, Thervet E, Primo J, Bach JF (1994) Anti-CD3 antibody induces long-term remission of overt autoimmunity in nonobese diabetic mice. *Proc Natl Acad Sci USA* 91: 123–127

12 Clevers H, Alarcon B, Wileman T, Terhorst C (1988) The T-cell receptor/CD3 complex: a dynamic protein ensemble. *Annu Rev Immunol* 6: 629–662

13 Weiss A (1991) Molecular and genetic insights into T cell antigen receptor structure and function. *Annu Rev Genet* 25: 487–510

14 Rudd CE (1990) CD4, CD8 and the TCR-CD3 complex: a novel class of protein-tyrosine kinase receptor. *Immunol Today* 11: 400–406

15 Leo O, Foo M, Sachs DH, Samelson LE, Bluestone JA (1987) Identification of a monoclonal antibody specific for a murine T3 polypeptide. *Proc Natl Acad Sci USA* 84: 1374–1378

16 Kung P, Goldstein G, Reinherz EL, Schlossman SF (1979) Monoclonal antibodies defining distinctive human T cell surface antigens. *Science* 206: 347–349

17 Cosimi AB, Colvin RB, Burton RC, Rubin RH, Goldstein G, Kung PC, Hansen WP, Delmonico FL, Russell PS (1981) Use of monoclonal antibodies to T-cell subsets for immunologic monitoring and treatment in recipients of renal allografts. *N Engl J Med* 305: 308–314

18 Cosimi AB, Burton RC, Colvin RB, Goldstein G, Delmonico FL, Laquaglia MP, Tolkoff-Rubin N, Rubin RH, Herrin JT, Russell PS (1981) Treatment of acute renal allograft rejection with OKT3 monoclonal antibody. *Transplantation* 32: 535–539

19 Emmrich F, Rieber P, Kurrle R, Eichmann K (1988) Selective stimulation of human T lymphocyte subsets by heteroconjugates of antibodies to the T cell receptor and to subset-specific differentiation antigens. *Eur J Immunol* 18: 645–648

20 Julius M, Maroun CR, Haughn L (1993) Distinct roles for CD4 and CD8 as co-receptors in antigen receptor signaling. *Immunol Today* 14: 177–183

21 Thome M, Duplay P, Guttinger M, Acuto O (1995) Syk and ZAP-70 mediate recruitment of p56lck/CD4 to the activated T cell receptor/CD3/zeta complex. *J Exp Med* 181: 1997–2006

22 Bindon CI, Hale G, Waldmann H (1988) Importance of antigen specificity for complement-mediated lysis by monoclonal antibodies. *Eur J Immunol* 18: 1507–1514

23 Moreland LW, Pratt PW, Bucy RP, Jackson BS, Feldman JW, Koopman WJ (1994) Treatment of refractory rheumatoid arthritis with a chimeric anti-CD4 monoclonal antibody. Long-term followup of CD4+ T cell counts. *Arthritis Rheum* 37: 834–838

24 Isaacs JD, Clark MR, Greenwood J, Waldmann H (1992) Therapy with monoclonal antibodies. An *in vivo* model for the assessment of therapeutic potential. *J Immunol* 148: 3062–3071

25 Wong JT, Colvin RB (1991) Selective reduction and proliferation of the CD4+ and CD8+ T cell subsets with bispecific monoclonal antibodies: evidence for inter-T cell-mediated cytolysis. *Clin Immunol Immunopathol* 58: 236–250

26 Smith CA, Williams GT, Kingston R, Jenkinson EJ, Owen JJ (1989) Antibodies to CD3/T-cell receptor complex induce death by apoptosis in immature T cells in thymic cultures. *Nature* 337: 181–184

27 Wesselborg S, Janssen O, Kabelitz D (1993) Induction of activation-driven death (apoptosis) in

activated but not resting peripheral blood T cells. *J Immunol* 150: 4338–4345

28 Choy EH, Adjaye J, Forrest L, Kingsley GH, Panayi GS (1993) Chimaeric anti-CD4 monoclonal antibody cross-linked by monocyte Fc gamma receptor mediates apoptosis of human CD4 lymphocytes. *Eur J Immunol* 23: 2676–2681

29 Kronke M, Schlick E, Waldmann TA, Vitetta ES, Greene WC (1986) Selective killing of human T-lymphotropic virus-I infected leukemic T-cells by monoclonal anti-interleukin 2 receptor antibody-ricin A chain conjugates: potentiation by ammonium chloride and monensin. *Cancer Res* 46: 3295–3298

30 Waldmann TA, O'Shea J (1998) The use of antibodies against the IL-2 receptor in transplantation. *Curr Opin Immunol* 10: 507–512

31 Thomas JM, Neville DM, Contreras JL, Eckhoff DE, Meng G, Lobashevsky AL, Wang PX, Huang ZQ, Verbanac KM, Haisch CE et al (1997) Preclinical studies of allograft tolerance in rhesus monkeys: a novel anti-CD3-immunotoxin given peritransplant with donor bone marrow induces operational tolerance to kidney allografts. *Transplantation* 64: 124–135

32 Hamawy MM, Knechtle SJ (1998) Strategies for tolerance induction in nonhuman primates. *Curr Opin Immunol* 10: 513–517

33 Calne R, Friend P, Moffatt S, Bradley A, Hale G, Firth J, Bradley J, Smith K, Waldmann H (1998) Prope tolerance, perioperative campath 1H, and low-dose cyclosporin monotherapy in renal allograft recipients. *Lancet* 351: 1701–1702

34 Cobbold SP, Adams E, Marshall SE, Davies JD, Waldmann H (1996) Mechanisms of peripheral tolerance and suppression induced by monoclonal antibodies to CD4 and CD8. *Immunol Rev* 149: 5–33

35 Cosimi AB, Burton RC, Kung PC, Colvin R, Goldstein G, Lifter J, Rhodes W, Russell PS (1981) Evaluation in primate renal allograft recipients of monoclonal antibody to human T-cell subclasses. *Transplant Proc* 13: 499–503

36 Jonker M, Neuhaus P, Zurcher C, Fucello A, Goldstein G (1985) OKT4 and OKT4A antibody treatment as immunosuppression for kidney transplantation in rhesus monkeys. *Transplantation* 39: 247–253

37 Goldberg D, Morel P, Chatenoud L, Boitard C, Menkes CJ, Bertoye PH, Revillard JP, Bach JF (1991) Immunological effects of high dose administration of anti-CD4 antibody in rheumatoid arthritis patients. *J Autoimmun* 4: 617–630

38 Mathieson PW, Cobbold SP, Hale G, Clark MR, Oliveira DB, Lockwood CM, Waldmann H (1990) Monoclonal-antibody therapy in systemic vasculitis. *N Engl J Med* 323: 250–254

39 Chatenoud L, Bach JF (1984) Antigenic modulation: a major mechanism of antibody action. *Immunol Today* 5: 20–25

40 Chatenoud L, Baudrihaye MF, Kreis H, Goldstein G, Schindler J, Bach JF (1982) Human *in vivo* antigenic modulation induced by the anti-T cell OKT3 monoclonal antibody. *Eur J Immunol* 12: 979–982

41 Vigeral P, Chkoff N, Chatenoud L, Campos H, Lacombe M, Droz D, Goldstein G, Bach JF, Kreis H (1986) Prophylactic use of OKT3 monoclonal antibody in cadaver kidney recipients: utilization of OKT3 as the sole immunosuppressive agent. *Transplantation* 41: 730–733

42 Chatenoud L, Legendre C, Ferran C, Bach JF, Kreis H (1991) Corticosteroid inhibition of the OKT3-induced cytokine-related syndrome – dosage and kinetics prerequisites. *Transplantation* 51: 334–338

43 Van Lier RA, Boot JH, de Groot ER, Aarden LA (1987) Induction of T cell proliferation with anti-CD3 switch-variant monoclonal antibodies: effects of heavy chain isotype in monocyte-dependent systems. *Eur J Immunol* 17: 1599–1604

44 Hirsch R, Bluestone JA, de Nenno L, Gress RE (1990) Anti-CD3 F(ab')2 fragments are immunosuppressive *in vivo* without evoking either the strong humoral response or morbidity associated with whole mAb. *Transplantation* 49: 1117–1123

45 Bolt S, Routledge E, Lloyd I, Chatenoud L, Pope H, Gorman SD, Clark M, Waldmann H (1993) The generation of a humanized, non-mitogenic CD3 monoclonal antibody which retains *in vitro* immunosuppressive properties. *Eur J Immunol* 23: 403–411

46 Alegre ML, Peterson LJ, Xu D, Sattar HA, Jeyarajah DR, Kowalkowski K, Thistlethwaite JR, Zivin RA, Jolliffe L, Bluestone JA (1994) A non-activating "humanized" anti-CD3 monoclonal antibody retains immunosuppressive properties *in vivo. Transplantation* 57: 1537–1543

47 Chatenoud L, Primo J, Bach JF (1997) CD3 antibody-induced dominant self tolerance in overtly diabetic NOD mice. *J Immunol* 158: 2947–2954

48 Hirsch R, Archibald J, Gress RE (1991) Differential T cell hyporesponsiveness induced by *in vivo* administration of intact or F(ab')2 fragments of anti-CD3 monoclonal antibody. F(ab')2 fragments induce a selective T helper dysfunction. *J Immunol* 147: 2088–2093

49 Hughes C, Wolos JA, Giannini EH, Hirsch R (1994) Induction of T helper cell hyporesponsiveness in an experimental model of autoimmunity by using nonmitogenic anti-CD3 monoclonal antibody. *J Immunol* 153: 3319–3325

50 Herold KC, Bluestone JA, Montag AG, Parihar A, Wiegner A, Gress RE, Hirsch R (1992) Prevention of autoimmune diabetes with nonactivating anti-CD3 monoclonal antibody. *Diabetes* 41: 385–391

51 Johnson BD, McCabe C, Hanke CA, Truitt RL (1995) Use of anti-CD3 epsilon F(ab')2 fragments *in vivo* to modulate graft-*versus*-host disease without loss of graft-*versus*-leukemia reactivity after MHC-matched bone marrow transplantation. *J Immunol* 154: 5542–5554

52 Granelli-Piperno A, Keane M, Steinman RM (1988) Evidence that cyclosporine inhibits cell-mediated immunity primarily at the level of the T lymphocyte rather than the accessory. *Cell Transplant* 46: 53S-60S

53 Granelli-Piperno A, Andrus L, Steinman RM (1986) Lymphokine and nonlymphokine mRNA levels in stimulated human T cells. Kinetics, mitogen requirements, and effects of cyclosporin A. *J Exp Med* 163: 922–937

54 Sigal NH, Dumont FJ (1992) Cyclosporin A, FK-506, and rapamyc*In*: pharmacologic probes of lymphocyte signal transduction. *Annu Rev Immunol* 10: 519–560

55 Bank I, Chess L (1985) Perturbation of the T4 molecule transmits a negative signal to T cells. *J Exp Med* 162: 1294–1303

56 Emmrich F, Kanz L, Eichmann K (1987) Cross-linking of the T cell receptor complex with the subset-specific differentiation antigen stimulates interleukin 2 receptor expression in human CD4 and CD8 T cells. *Eur J Immunol* 17: 529–534

57 Wofsy D, Mayes DC, Woodcock J, Seaman WE (1985) Inhibition of humoral immunity *in vivo* by monoclonal antibody to L3T4: studies with soluble antigens in intact mice. *J Immunol* 135: 1698–1701

58 Qin SX, Cobbold S, Benjamin R, Waldmann H (1989) Induction of classical transplantation tolerance in the adult. *J Exp Med* 169: 779–794

59 Larsen CP, Elwood ET, Alexander DZ, Ritchie SC, Hendrix R, Tuckerburden C, Cho HR, Aruffo A, Hollenbaugh D, Linsley PS et al (1996) Long-term acceptance of skin and cardiac allografts after blocking CD40 and CD28 pathways. *Nature* 381: 434–438

60 Kirk AD, Burkly LC, Batty DS, Baumgartner RE, Berning JD, Buchanan K, Fechner JR Jr, Germond RL, Kampen RL, Patterson NB et al (1999) Treatment with humanized monoclonal antibody against CD154 prevents acute renal allograft rejection in nonhuman primates. *Nat Med* 5: 686–693

61 Nicolls MR, Aversa GG, Pearce NW, Pospinelli A, Berger MF, Gurley KE, Hall BM (1993) Induction of long-term specific tolerance to allografts in rats by therapy with an anti-CD3-like monoclonal antibody. *Transplantation* 55: 459–468

62 Cobbold S, Waldmann H (1998) Infectious tolerance. *Curr Opin Immunol* 10: 518–524

63 Nickerson P, Steurer W, Steiger J, Zheng X, Steele AW, Strom TB (1994) Cytokines and the Th1/Th2 paradigm in transplantation. *Curr Opin Immunol* 6: 757–764

64 Miller A, Lider O, Roberts AB, Sporn MB, Weiner HL (1992) Suppressor T cells generated by oral tolerization to myelin basic protein suppress both *in vitro* and *in vivo* immune responses by the release of transforming growth factor beta after antigen-specific triggering. *Proc Natl Acad Sci USA* 89: 421–425

65 Groux H, O'Garra A, Bigler M, Rouleau M, Antonenko S, de Vries JE, Roncarolo MG (1997) A CD4+ T-cell subset inhibits antigen-specific T-cell responses and prevents colitis. *Nature* 389: 737–742

66 Lombardi G, Sidhu S, Batchelor R, Lechler R (1994) Anergic T cells as suppressor cells *in vitro*. *Science* 264: 1587–1589

67 Van Eden W, Anderton SM, van der Zee R, Prakken BJ, Broeren CP, Wauben MH (1996) Altered self peptides and the regulation of self reactivity in the peripheral T cell pool. *Immunol Rev* 149: 55–73

68 Durez P, Abramowicz D, Gerard C, van Mechelen M, Amraoui Z, Dubois C, Leo O, Velu T, Goldman M (1993) *In vivo* induction of interleukin 10 by anti-CD3 monoclonal antibody or bacterial lipopolysaccharide: differential modulation by cyclosporin A. *J Exp Med* 177: 551–555

69 Opelz G (1995) Efficacy of rejection prophylaxis with OKT3 in renal transplantation. Collaborative Transplant Study. *Transplantation* 60: 1220–1224

70 Chatenoud L, Baudrihaye MF, Chkoff N, Kreis H, Goldstein G, Bach JF (1986) Restriction of the human *in vivo* immune response against the mouse monoclonal antibody OKT3. *J Immunol* 137: 830–838

71 Benjamin RJ, Cobbold SP, Clark MR, Waldmann H (1986) Tolerance to rat monoclonal antibodies. Implications for serotherapy. *J Exp Med* 163: 1539–1552

72 Chatenoud L, Jonker M, Villemain F, Goldstein G, Bach JF (1986) The human immune response to the OKT3 monoclonal antibody is oligoclonal. *Science* 232: 1406–1408

73 Baudrihaye MF, Chatenoud L, Kreis H, Goldstein G, Bach JF (1984) Unusually restricted anti-isotype human immune response to OKT3 monoclonal antibody. *Eur J Immunol* 14: 686–691

74 Abramowicz D, Crusiaux A, Goldman M (1992) Anaphylactic shock after retreatment with OKT3 monoclonal antibody. *N Engl J Med* 327: 736

75 Hricik DE, Mayes JT, Schulak JA (1990) Inhibition of anti-OKT3 antibody generation by cyclosporine – results of a prospective randomized trial. *Transplantation* 50: 237–240

76 Riechmann L, Clark M, Waldmann H, Winter G (1988) Reshaping human antibodies for therapy. *Nature* 332: 323–327

77 Elliott MJ, Maini RN, Feldmann M, Long-Fox A, Charles P, Bijl H, Woody JN (1994) Repeated therapy with monoclonal antibody to tumour necrosis factor alpha (cA2) in patients with rheumatoid arthritis. *Lancet* 344: 1125–1127

78 Marks JD, Hoogenboom HR, Bonnert TP, McCafferty J, Griffiths AD, Winter G (1991) By-passing immunization. Human antibodies from V-gene libraries displayed on phage. *J Mol Biol* 222: 581–597

79 Lubin I, Segall H, Marcus H, David M, Kulova L, Steinitz M, Erlich P, Gan J, Reisner Y (1994) Engraftment of human peripheral blood lymphocytes in normal strains of mice. *Blood* 83: 2368–2381

Modern Immunosuppressives
ed. by H.-J Schuurman, G. Feutren and J.-F. Bach
© 2001 Birkhäuser Verlag/Switzerland

Targeting the IL-2 receptor with antibodies or chimeric toxins

Terry B. Strom

Department of Medicine, Harvard Medical School, Division of Immunology, Beth Israel Deaconess Medical Center, Research North, Room 380, P.O. Box 15707, Boston, MA 02215, USA

Introduction

Although various mouse anti-rat and rat anti-mouse monoclonal antibodies (mAbs) produce profound immunosuppressive effects, the experience with rodent anti-human mAb has been somewhat disappointing. The impetus for creating chimeric or humanized mAbs or fusion proteins to be used as immunosuppressive agents in allograft recipients stems directly from the clinical experience with rodent antihuman mAbs. With the exception of antibodies directed against proteins of the TCR/CD3 complex, murine mAbs have failed to deliver on their many potential advantages for treating or preventing rejection. The favorable attributes of chimeric or humanized mAbs include: (i) high specificity and affinity; (ii) long circulating half-lives; and (iii) a variety of mechanisms by which they can mediate an immunosuppressive effect. Cytolytic immune effector mechanisms of the host, antibody-mediated cell-mediated cytotoxicity (ADCC), and complement-mediated cytotoxicity (CDC) can theoretically be recruited directed against antibody coated target cells. Moreover, mAbs can interrupt signaling at the cell surface by blocking key receptor sites.

The discrepancy between the high promise and poor delivery of therapeutic benefit through use of rodent mAbs in the clinic is explained at least in part by (i) the limiting effect of the ubiquitous human anti-xenoantibody response; and (ii) the failure of most murine mAb to activate human complement or Fc-receptor-positive cytolytic cells and thereby trigger target cell lysis. In the case of murine mAbs, this host antibody response is denoted as the human anti-murine antibody (HAMA) response [1–3]. The HAMA response entails both anti-idiotypic and anti-isotypic antibody responses, often within the first 14–20 days following initiation of treatment. Anti-idiotypic antibodies block the capacity of the mAb to bind antigen and are therefore neutralizing. Anti-isotypic antibodies, although not neutralizing, adversely affect the circulating half-life and volume of distribution [1]. The circulating half-lives of murine mAbs are considerably shorter in humans (about 20 h) than those of human antibodies of the same class (about 20 days), and the development of HAMA acts to further increase clearance.

Chimeric and humanized monoclonal antibodies

The majority of xenoantibodies are, at best, only poorly able to recruit ADCC or CDC human immune effector mechanisms. This means that the majority of conventional rodent anti-human mAbs will be restricted to non-cytolytic mechanisms of immunosuppression, e.g., OKT3. In order to improve the clinical utility of rodent anti-human mAbs, human sequences are introduced, generating either chimeric or humanized antibody

Chimeric antibodies are produced through a gene fusion strategy in which codons for the entire antigen-binding Fv region ($V_L + V_H$) from an existing murine mAb are joined to codons for human constant region sequences [4]. This simple approach has been extended and refined to create hyperchimeric, humanized antibodies [4, 5]. This strategy incorporates the basic concept that led to production of chimeric antibodies in which the antigen-binding portions of a rodent mAb are genetically fused to human Fc sequences, but an additional step is added. This scheme, which seeks to introduce as little of the xenogeneic rodent V region sequences as possible while retaining antigen specificity and affinity of a rodent mAb, is accomplished by splicing any of the appropriately spaced codons for the six murine antigen-binding complementarity-determining regions (CDRs) of a rodent mAb into a human V region framework and Fc region cDNA. In practice, this approach creates a totally synthesized V region cDNA to achieve CDR plus framework grafting. Amino acid residues outside of the CDRs, but in spatial proximity or "contact" with them, are also often grafted because they may be necessary to retain proper conformation of the antigen-binding CDR. The goals of these engineering efforts are to reduce immunogenicity and to gain human ADCC and CDC effector functions.

The IL-2 receptor as a therapeutic target

Only certain leukemic or lymphoma cells, or recently activated immune cells, especially T-cells, bear the trimolecular high-affinity interleukin-2 receptor (IL-2R). The high affinity IL-2R is absent from the surface of resting T-cells and nonlymphoid tissues [6]. The *de novo* acquisition of high-affinity IL-2Rs is a critical event in the course of T-cell activation [6–9]. The IL-2R can be expressed as high-, intermediate-, or low-affinity binding sites. The high-affinity site is a multimeric complex containing at least three peptides: the 55-kDa α-chain and the 70-kDa β- and 64-kDa γ-chains that participate in signal transduction. The β- and γ-chains, but not the α-chain, are sparsely expressed on resting T-cells and NK cells. With T-cell activation marked amplification of expression of the β- and γ-chains and *de novo* expression of the α-chain ensues [6–9]. The IL-2R β/γ heterodimer possesses intermediate binding affinity, whereas the isolated 55-kDa α-chain (CD25) is a low-affinity binding site [6–11].

Because the high-affinity receptor is only transiently expressed during the brief antigen-triggered proliferative burst of lymphocytes, we wondered whether administration of anti-IL-2R mAb, e.g., anti-CD25 or chimeric IL-2 toxins would provide a utilitarian approach to achieve selective immunosuppression aimed directly at activated lymphocytes [12]. In theory, agents directed against the IL-2R can be used in every situation of unwanted T-cell-dependent immunity to achieve selective immunosuppression.

Based on extensive and highly successful experimentation in rodent transplant and autoimmune models [12, 13], several murine anti-human-CD25 mAbs have been tested in human renal transplant recipients as an adjunct to traditional therapy. Modest beneficial effects were obtained [14–20]. Nonetheless, the number of early rejection episodes were reduced and/or delayed. The HAMA response severely limited effectiveness. The modest beneficial effects produced by the conventional mAbs spurred efforts to develop refined mAbs bearing human sequences to increase potency [21, 22].

As the HAMA response was an obvious barrier to successful employment of anti-CD25 mAbs, both the chimeric basiliximab (Simulect) [21] and the hyperchimeric daclizumab (Zenapax) [22] have been produced and tested for therapeutic efficacy as an adjunct to conventional treatment in human renal allograft recipients [23–25]. Zenepax and Simulect are first administered in the immediate peritransplant period. Only one additional dose of Simulect is given 4 to 5 days later [21], while five additional doses of Zenapax are given at 2-week intervals [25]. The individual doses of Simulect are greater than those used for Zenapax. Structural differences in antibodies are considerable. While daclizumab (Zenapax) is a humanized mAb and should be less inherently immunogenic, Simulect exerts a superior affinity for the IL-2 receptor. Thus it is difficult to assess the relative value of these in Abs using either clinical trial results or perceived superior biologic attributes.

Although intuition would suggest clear therapeutic superiority for the humanized mAb, it is not certain that this will prove to be true. Direct comparison of Simulect and Zenapax through therapeutic trials has not been conducted. The treatment protocols are quite different in terms of the number of injections and the dose/injection. The data from double-blind placebo-controlled phase III trials in kidney transplantation are summarized in Table 1. Both the chimeric mouse-human Simulect and hyperchimeric ("humanized") Zenapax anti-CD25 mAbs have been approved by the Food and Drug Administration for use in renal allograft recipients. As anticipated, a single infection of mAb leads to sustained blood levels. Treatment with either mAb diminishes the incidence of acute rejection episodes by 33–50%. In treated patients the rejection episodes that do occur are delayed and less virulent than those observed in control patients. The incidence of neutralizing HAMA

Table 1. Results of randomized double-blind placebo-controlled phase III trials using anti-CD25 in induction immunosuppression after kidney transplantation

	Placebo group	Treatment group	p
Daclizumab (Zenapax): US/CAN/Sweden trial [25][1]			
Number of patients	134	126	
Number of patients with biopsy-proven acute rejection episodes in first half-year	47	28	0.03
Number of patients with biopsy-proven or presumed acute rejection episodes in first half-year	52	32	0.04
Number of rejection episodes per patient	0.6	0.3	0.01
Time to first rejection (days)	30 ± 27	73 ± 59	0.008
Basiliximab (Simulect): US trial [23][2]			
Number of patients	173	173	
Number of patients with biopsy-proven acute rejection episodes in first year	85	61	0.009
Number of patients with biopsy-proven or presumed acute rejection episodes in first year	95	65	0.001
Number of rejection-free patients after first year	79	104	0.009
Basiliximab (Simulect): Canadian/European trial [24][2]			
Number of patients	186	190	
Number of patients with biopsy-proven acute rejection episodes in first half-year	73	51	0.012
Number of patients with biopsy-proven or presumed acute rejection episodes in first half-year	97	65	0.001
Number of rejection-free patients after first year	73	95	0.002

[1] In this trial daclizumab or placebo was given in five doses each or 1 mg/kg, one within 24 h before transplantation, and one at 2, 4, 6, and 8 weeks after transplantation, respectively. This was given in addition to standard triple-immunosuppression comprising cyclosporine, azathioprine and steroids
[2] In this trial basiliximab or placebo was given twice, 20 mg just before transplantation and 20 mg on day 4 post-transplantation. This was given in addition to standard double-immunosuppression comprising cyclosporine and steroids

responses formed in patients treated with either mAb is very low. The overall incidence of adverse events including lymphoma, other malignancies, and opportunistic infections are very low and similar to the incidence noted with placebo adjustive treatment. Similar data are evolving in studies on liver and cardiac allograft recipients.

Thus, it is difficult to assess the relative value of these mAbs. Because of the extreme safety and relative effectiveness of the anti-CD25 antibodies, many transplantation units now use these antibodies as adjuncts to conventional immunosuppressive agents. The anti-CD25 compete with polyclonal antilymphocyte for this application. There is little question that anti-CD25 mAbs are safer than polyclonal antilymphocyte antibodies in terms of the selective targeting of activated lymphocytes, freedom from anaphylactoid reactions and the low risk for opportunistic infection. At this early date in the clinical application of anti-CD25 mAbs, it is uncertain as to whether the polyclonal antibodies or anti-CD25 mAbs exert similar potency in the patient populations at high risk for immunologic graft failure.

IL-2 toxin fusion protein

The great German scientist Paul Ehrlich first suggested *"Zauberkugeln"* (i.e., "magic bullet") hybrid molecules, consisting of cell-specific antibodies linked to a toxin (immunotoxin), to be constructed for various therapeutic purposes. He envisioned that immunotoxins could be used as magic bullets to destroy a highly selective population of target cells. By genetically linking cytokines to select portions of toxins, we and others have pursued a strategy closely related to that proposed by Ehrlich many years ago. Naturally occurring bacterial and plant toxins possess domain-specific structure-function activity; therefore, the structure can be manipulated to create biological agents that specifically target and kill disease-causing cells [26–28].

Functional domains of diphtheria toxin and Pseudomonas exotoxin

The holotoxins used in construction of hybrid toxins possess three functionally specialized domains that bind to specific target cell surface receptors; translocate the toxin into the appropriate subcellular compartment; and enzymatically intoxicate the target cell [26–28]. The three functional domains of diphtheria toxin (DT) are segregated into three separate structural domains [26]. In both diphtheria toxin (DT) and *Pseudomonas* exotoxin A (PEA) [27], the enzymatically active core is an adenosine diphosphate-ribosyltransferase that targets elongation factor-2. This factor is an essential element in the translational apparatus of the cell. Following adenosine diphosphate-ribosylation, elongation factor-2 is inactivated and the intoxicated cell dies because it does not manufacture new cellular proteins. The extreme carboxy terminus of DT and the amino terminus of PEA function as receptor-binding elements and are responsible for the binding of the toxin to specific eukaryotic cell surface receptors. The third centrally located domain of both toxins serves as a translocating element and enables the intact toxin to traverse the target cell membrane, thereby permitting the toxin to enter the endosome and ensuring subsequent delivery of the toxophore to the cytosol [26–28].

IL-2 fusion toxins – DAB₄₈₆ IL-2 and DAB₃₉₈ IL-2

The genetic replacement of the receptor-binding domain of native DT or PEA with a cytokine (e.g., IL-2) or other growth factors has resulted in the development of a new class of biological response modifiers, the fusion toxins [29–37]. IL-2 fusion toxins (DAB₄₈₆ IL-2 and DAB₃₉₈ IL-2), the first of this new class of targeted biologicals to be tested in the clinic, are specifically cytotoxic for IL-2R-expressing cells [31–33, 37]. The receptor binding domain of DT has been replaced by a specific targeting ligand, human interleukin-2, creating a recombinant protein that kills activated IL-2R-expressing lymphocytes at 10^{-10}–10^{-11} M concentrations [31–33, 37]. DAB₄₈₆ IL-2 (67 kDa) was the first fusion toxin to be evaluated clinically; DAB₃₉₈ IL-2, which possesses a higher affinity for the IL-2R than DAB₃₉₈ IL-2, is approximately 10 times more potent than DAB₄₈₆ IL-2.

IL-2 fusion toxins, once bound to the cell membrane IL-2R, are rapidly internalized into an acidic endocytic vesicle. The toxic fragment then reaches the cell cytosol, initiating a cytotoxic event within 5–15 min. Protein synthesis is irreversibly inhibited as a result of adenosine diphosphate ribosylation of elongation factor-2, and cell death occurs over 36–72 h [31, 32, 37].

This early clinical experience provides a basis for evaluation of DAB₃₉₈ IL-2 in randomized, placebo-controlled clinical trials in patients with lymphoma [38] or psoriasis [39]. DAB₃₉₈ IL-2 produced five complete remissions and eight partial responses involving 35 patients with cutaneous T-cell lymphoma. In 17 patients with non-Hodgkin's lymphoma DAB₃₉₈ IL-2 treatment resulted in one complete remission and two partial responses. This biological has now been approved by the FDA for use in instantaneous T-cell lymphoma.

DAB₃₉₈ IL-2 represents a specific immunoregulatory agent with a targeted mechanism of action, offering an opportunity to assess the immunopathogenesis of rejection. Generalized or persistent immunosuppression has not been evident in IL-2 fusion toxin clinical trials.

References

1 Chatenoud L, Baudrihay MF, Chkoff N, Kreis H, Goldstein G, Bach J-F (1986) Restriction of the human *in vivo* immune response against the mouse monoclonal antibody OKT3. *J Immunol* 137: 830–838

2 Jaffers GJ, Fuller TC, Cosimi AB, Russell PS, Winn HJ, Colvin RB (1986) Monoclonal antibody therapy anti-idiotypic and non-anti-idiotypic antibodies to OKT3 arising despite intense immunosuppression. *Transplantation* 41: 572–578

3 Thistlethwaite JR, Stuart JK, Mayes JT, Gaber AO, Woodle S, Buckingham MR, Stuart FP (1988) Monitoring and complications of monoclonal therapy: complications and monitoring of OKT3 therapy. *Amer J Kidney Dis* 11: 112–119

4 Morrison SL, Johnson MJ, Herzenberg LA, Oi VT (1984) Chimeric human antibody molecules: mouse antigen-binding domains with human constant region domains. *Proc Natl Acad Sci USA* 81: 6851–6855

5 Jones PT, Dear PH, Foote J, Neuberger MS, Winter G (1986) Replacing the complementarity-determining regions in a human antibody with those from a mouse. *Nature* 321: 522–525

6 Smith KA (1987) The two chain structure of high-affinity IL-2 receptors. *Immunol Today* 8: 11–13
7 Cantrell PA, Smith KA (1984) The interleukin-2 T-cell system: a new cell growth model. *Science* 224: 1312–1316
8 Leonard WJ, Depper JM, Uchiyama T, Smith KA, Waldmann TA, Greene WC (1982) A monoclonal antibody that appears to recognize the receptor for human T-cell growth factor; partial characterization of the receptor. *Nature* 300: 267–269
9 Maddock EO, Maddock SW, Kelley VE, Strom TB (1985) Rapid stereospecific stimulation of lymphocytic metabolism by interleukin-2. *J Immunol* 135: 4004–4008
10 Tsudo M, Kozak RW, Goldman CK, Waldmann TA (1986) Demonstration of a non-Tac peptide that binds interleukin 2: a potential participant in a multichain interleukin 2 receptor complex. *Proc Natl Acad Sci USA* 83: 9694–9698
11 Takeshita T, Asao H, Ohtani K, Ishii N, Kumaki S, Tanaka N, Munakata H, Nakamura M, Sugamura K (1992) Cloning of the gamma chain of the human IL-2 receptor. *Science* 257: 379–382
12 Strom TB, Kelley VR, Murphy JR, Nichols N, Woodworth TG (1993) Interleukin-2 receptor-directed therapies: antibody- or cytokine-based targeting molecules. *Annu Rev Med* 44: 343–353
13 Waldmann TA, O'Shea J (1998) The use of antibodies against the IL-2 receptor in transplantation. *Curr Opin Immunol* 10: 507–512
14 Kirkman RL, Shapiro ME, Carpenter CB, Milford EL, Ramos EL, Tilney NL, Waldmann TA, Zimmerman CE, Strom TB (1989) Early experience with anti-Tac, an antihuman IL-2 receptor mAb. *Transplantation* 21: 1766–1768
15 Soulillou JP, Peyronnet P, Le Mauff B, Hourmant M, Olive D, Mawas C, Delaage M, Hirn M, Jacques Y (1987) Prevention of rejection of kidney transplants by mAb directed against interleukin 2. *Lancet* 1: 1339–1342
16 Soulillou JP, Cantarovich D, Le Mauff B, Giral M, Robillard N, Hourmant M, Hirn M, Jacques Y (1990) Randomized controlled trial of a monoclonal antibody against the interleukin-2 receptor (33B3.1) as compared with rabbit antithymocyte globulin for prophylaxis against rejection of renal allografts. *N Engl J Med* 322: 1175–1182
17 Kirkman RL, Shapiro ME, Carpenter CB, McKay DB, Milford EL, Ramos EL, Tilney NL, Waldmann TA, Zimmerman CE, Strom TB (1991) A randomized prospective trial of anti-Tac monoclonal antibody in human renal transplantation. *Transplantation* 51: 107–113
18 Van Gelder T, Zietse R, Mulder AH, Yzermans JN, Hesse CJ, Vaessen LM, Weimar W (1995) A variable blind study of uroclonal anti-interleukin-2 receptor antibody (BT563) administration to prevent acute rejection after kidney transplantation. *Transplantation* 60: 248–252
19 Nashan B, Schlitt HJ, Schwinzer R, Ringe B, Kuse E, Tusch G, Wonigeit K, Pichlmayr R (1996) Immunoprophylaxis with a monoclonal anti-IL-2 receptor antibody in liver transplant patients. *Transplantation* 61: 546–554
20 Langren JM, Nussler NC, Neumann U, Guckelberger O, Lohmann R, Radtke A, Jonas S, Klupp J, Steinmuller T, Lobeck H et al (1997) A prospective randomized trial comparing interleukin-2 receptor antibody *versus* antithymocyte globulin as part of a quadruple immunosuppressive induction therapy following orthopic liver transplantation. *Transplantation* 63: 1772–1781
21 Amlot PL, Rawslings E, Fernando ON, Griffin PH, Heinrich G, Schreier MH, Castaigne JP, Moore R, Sceny P (1995) Prolonged action of a chimeric interleukin-2 receptor [CD25] monoclonal antibody used in cadaveric renal transplantation. *Transplantation* 60: 748–756
22 Queen C, Schneider WP, Selick HE, Payne PW, Landolfi NF, Duncan JF, Avdalovic NM, Levitt M, Junghans RP, Waldmann TA (1989) A humanized antibody that binds to the interleukin 2 receptor. *Proc Natl Acad Sci USA* 86: 10 029–10 033
23 Kahan BD, Rajagopalan PR, Hall M (1999) Reduction of the occurrence of acute cellular rejection among renal allograft recipients treated with basiliximab, a chimeric anti-interleukin-2-receptor monoclonal antibody. United States Simulect Renal Study Group. *Transplantation* 72: 276–284
24 Nashan B, Moore R, Amlot P, Schmidt A-G, Abaywickrama K, Soulillou J-P for the CHIB 201 International Study Group (1997) Randomised trial of basiliximab *versus* placebo for control of acute cellular rejection in renal allograft recipients. *Lancet* 350: 1193–1198
25 Vincenti F, Kirkman R, Light S, Bumgardner G, Pescovitz M, Halloran P, Neylan J, Wilkinson A, Ekberg H, Gaston R et al (1998) Interleukin-2 receptor blockade with daclizumab to prevent acute rejection in renal transplantation. *N Engl J Med* 338: 161–165
26 Choe S, Bennett MJ, Fujii G, Curmi PM, Kantardjieff KA, Collier RJ, Eisenberg D (1992) The crystal structure of diphtheria toxin. *Nature* 357: 216–222

27 Pastan I, Willingham MC, FitzGerald DJ (1986) Immunotoxins. *Cell* 47: 641–648
28 Olsnes S, Sandrig K, Petersen OW, VanDeurs B (1989) Immunotoxins – entry into cells and mechanisms of action. *Immunol Today* 10: 291–295
29 Williams DP, Regier D, Akiyoshi D, Genbauffe F, Murphy JR (1988) Design, synthesis and expression of a human interleukin-2 gene-incorporating the codon usage bias found in highly expressed *Escherichia coli* genes. *Nucl Acid Res* 16: 10 453–10 467
30 Siegall CB, Chaudhary VK, FitzGerald DJ, Pastan I (1988) Cytotoxic activity of an interleukin-6 *Pseudomonas* exotoxin fusion protein on human myeloma cells. *Proc Natl Acad Sci USA* 85: 9738–9742
31 Williams DP, Parker K, Bacha P, Bishai W, Borowski M, Genbauffe F, Strom TB, Murphy JR (1987) Diphtheria toxin receptor binding domain substitution with interleukin-2: genetic construction and properties of a diphtheria toxin-related interleukin-2 fusion protein. *Protein Eng* 1: 493–498
32 Williams DPSnider CE, Strom TB, Murphy JR (1990) Structure/function analysis of interleukin-2-toxin (DAB$_{486}$-IL-2). Fragment B sequences required for the delivery of fragment A to the cytosol of target cells. *J Biol Chem* 265: 11 885–11 889
33 Lorberboum-Gaiski H, FitzGerald D, Chaudhary V, Adhya S Pastan I (1988) Cytotoxic activity of an interleukin-2 *Pseudomonas* exotoxin chimeric protein produced in *Escherichia coli*. *Proc Natl Acad Sci USA* 85: 1922–1926
34 Murphy JR, Bishai W, Borowski A, Miyanohara A, Boyd J, Nagle S (1986) Genetic construction, expression, and melanoma-selective cytotoxicity of a diphtheria toxin-related alpha-melanocyte-stimulating hormone fusion protein. *Proc Natl Acad Sci USA* 83: 8258–8262
35 Chaudhary VK, FitzGerald DJ, Adhya S, Pastan I. Activity of a recombinant fusion protein between transforming growth factor type alpha and *Pseudomonas* toxin. *Proc Natl Acad Sci USA* 84: 4538–4542
36 Chaudhary VK, Mizukami T, Fuerst TR, FitzGerald DJ, Moss B, Pastan I, Berger EA (1988) Selective killing of HIV-infected cells by recombinant human CD4-*Pseudomonas* exotoxin hybrid protein. *Nature* 335: 369–372
37 Bacha P, Williams DP, Waters C, Williams JM, Murphy JR, Strom TB (1988) Interleukin-2 receptor targeted cytotoxicity: interleukin-2 receptor mediated action of a diphtheria toxin-related interleukin-2 fusion protein. *J Exp Med* 67: 612–622
38 LeMaistre CF, Saleh MN, Kuzel TM, Foss F, Platanias LC, Schwartz G, Ratain M, Rook A, Freytes CO, Craig F et al (1988) Phase I trial of a ligand fusion-protein (DAB$_{389}$IL-2) in lymphomas expressing the receptor for interleukin-2. *Blood* 91: 399–405
39 Gottlieb SL, Gilicaudeau P, Johnson R, Eftis A, Woodworth TG, Gottlieb AB, Kreuger JG (1995) The response of psoriasis to a lymphocyte selective toxin DAB389 IL-2 suggests a primary immune but not keratinocyte, pathogenic basis. *Nat Med* 1: 442–447

New avenues in immunosuppression

Modern Immunosuppressives
ed. by H.-J Schuurman, G. Feutren and J.-F. Bach
© 2001 Birkhäuser Verlag/Switzerland

Emerging therapeutic strategies for the prevention and treatment of chronic allograft rejection

Pekka Häyry, Hanna Savolainen, Serdar Yilmaz and Einari Aavik

Transplantation Laboratory m and Rational Drug Design Program, Biomedicum, University of Helsinki and Helsinki University Central Hospital, P.O. Box 21 (Haartmaninkatu 3), FIN-00014 Helsinki, Finland

Introduction

Concomitantly with the introduction of calcineurin inhibitors the short-term survival of organ allografts has dramatically increased. However, this is less reflected in the half-life of the transplant after the first year, and late graft failure has emerged as the major reason for graft loss. In renal transplantation, approximately half of late failures are due to death of the patient with functioning transplant – mostly because of cardiovascular reasons. Of the other half, most transplants are lost due to chronic allograft rejection. This is particularly the case for kidney and heart transplants, where protocol biopsies and/or coronary angiography/ultrasound studies have demonstrated an approximately 30–50% frequency of chronic alterations between 3 and 5 years post transplantation. Instead, the liver seems to be virtually "immune" to chronic rejection [1].

Several studies have demonstrated that the frequency and/or timing of acute episodes of rejection correlate with subsequent long-term graft outcome [2–5]. These observations, confirmed later in experimental studies [6, 7] are based on registry data or are retrospective in nature. Thus, the studies do not take into account the type of acute rejection, nor do they answer the question whether all acute rejections – or only a fraction of them – provide the risk for subsequent graft outcome.

Acute rejection is not a single entity. It may display itself with different intensities, length and histological pattern and at different time points after transplantation. Late acute rejections are considered more harmful than early acute rejections [4]. Of paramount importance is the histological pattern. Van Saase et al. [8] and Olsen, Hansen and Madsen (personal communication) have investigated the impact of the histological pattern of rejection to long-term graft survival. Both groups demonstrate that particularly a vascular pattern of acute rejection, but less a tubulointerstitial pattern, predicts inferior long-term graft survival. In other words, late graft function is highly dependent on the intensity of vasculitis in the acute biopsy histology.

There are still high hopes, particularly among pharmaceutical industry, that further improvement of immunosuppressive therapy will also improve the long-term graft outcome. This may be the case, especially if a new drug has additional vasculoprotective properties, as has been suggested to be the case, e.g., for mycophenolate mofetil [9], leflunomide [10] and rapamycin [11–14], or if a new drug has potentially less fibrogenic properties than the current calcineurin inhibitors [15]. At any rate, any such new drug candidate should reduce the vascular component in acute rejection. We consider it therefore imperative that in future trials aiming to improve immunosuppression the impact of experimental therapy on the histological pattern of acute rejection should be taken into account, if an impact on long-term graft function is to be predicted. Even then, one should not forget that half of the grafts are lost *via* death of the patient for cardiovascular reasons.

Pathophysiology

Before proceeding any further on potential future venues of therapy, it is obligatory to shortly consider the differences in acute and chronic rejection, and summarize some of the pertinent features of chronic rejection.

Risk factors and histological features of acute versus chronic rejection

Acute and chronic rejection are entirely different entities, as reflected by differences in their histological appearance and predisposing factors. The well-known risk factors for acute rejection are histoincompatibility and insufficient immunosuppression. Instead, retrospective clinical studies have demonstrated a variety of additional risk factors predisposing the graft to chronic rejection. These include alloantigen-related factors, such as histoincompatibility, insufficient immunosuppression, presence of anti-HLA-antibodies, lack of anti-idiotypic antibodies and acute rejection; alloantigen-unrelated factors, such as high and low donor age, preservation-reperfusion related injury, hyperlipidemia and donor/recipient size-incompatibility and infectious risk factors such as cytomegalovirus infection [16, 17]. Experimental studies suggest that some of the alloantigen unrelated and infectious risk factors may be confounding variables contributing *via* acute episodes of rejection [6].

The dominant histological feature of acute rejection is a lytic feature. The prominent features are lymphocytic and monocytic inflammation, invasion of inflammatory cells into the tissue and evidence of tissue destruction. Early and reversible patterns of rejection display high levels of lymphoid activation, whereas late and irreversible patterns of rejection (which under cyclosporine therapy are rarely seen) show high activation level of tissue macrophages and thrombocyte-endothelial aggregates in the transplant vessels [18, 19].

Table 1. Histopathology of chronic rejection in different organs

Heart	Kidney	Liver
Inflammation	Inflammation	Inflammation
Arteriosclerosis	Arteriosclerosis	Arteriosclerosis
Fibrosis	Basement membrane thickening	Hepatocellular ballooning
	Glomerular sclerosis	Vanishing bile ducts
	Tubular atrophy	Giant cell transformation
	Fibrosis	Fibrosis

Modified from Demetris [1]

The dominant histological feature of chronic rejection is a proliferative feature. Shared histopathology in all transplants undergoing chronic rejection, is persistent perivascular inflammation (sometimes subendothelial or transmural), fibrosis and concentric generalized arteriosclerosis affecting all intra-graft arteries to the level of arterioli (Tab. 1). These common histological changes are superimposed with organ-specific alterations, such as basement membrane thickening, glomerular sclerosis and tubular atrophy in the kidney, and hepatocellular ballooning, vanishing bile ducts and giant cell transformation in the liver [1]. In the perivascular/vascular inflammation, macrophages dominate over (activated) lymphoid cells and fragmentation of the internal elastic lamina and focal media necrosis is a rule. The cells migrating into the intima are virtually all α-actin-expressing smooth muscle cells (SMC) of the so-called "secretory" phenotype and atheroma formation or calcifications are not seen [20, 21] unless they have been present in graft vessels already at the time of grafting.

Immunological requirements of chronic rejection, gene expression and impact of experimental therapy

Studies in knock-out animals and usage of variations in experimental therapy have confirmed the alloantigen-related, alloantigen-unrelated and infectious etiologies of allograft vasculopathy. Mouse heart allografts transplanted to severe combined immune deficient (scid) mice generate no intimal response, but do so readily if the recipients are reconstituted with donor-directed cytotoxic antibody [22]. Depletion of T-cells, B-cells, CD4-cells and/or macrophages, all reduce allograft vasculopathy in knock-out mouse models [23].

In addition, reduction of allograft arteriosclerosis by immunosuppressive treatment with high-dose cyclosporine [24, 25], rapamycin [26], deoxyspergualin [27], mycophenolate mofetil [9] or CTLA4Ig [28] suggests an immunological origin of chronic rejection. On the other hand, triple anti-hypertensive drug treatment [29, 30], essential fatty-acid deficient diet [31], treatment with small-molecular weight heparins [32] and with anti-lipidemic 3-hydroxy-3-methyl-glutanyl-coenzyme A reductase inhibitors, results in inhibition of allograft vasculopathy. This is documented not only in rat models, but also in man [33], speaking for a non-immunological etiology of chronic rejection.

A number of genes are differentially expressed at the induction of and during allograft proliferative vasculopathy. Many of these genes are expected to be related to allograft response to trauma. There is increased expression of adhesion ligands and their receptors in the graft endothelium and in the inflammatory leukocytes, including members of the Ig-supergene family (ICAM, VCAM, class II), selectins, integrins and lectins [34]. Considering the chemotactic events of leukocytes through endothelium and SMCs towards the vessel lumen, it is not unexpected that a number of cytokine- and chemokine genes are also expressed [35]. Classical growth factor genes, known to be related SMC replication or migration and/or to endothelial repair after injury, and genes regulating their receptors, are prominently expressed in both human and rat allografts during chronic rejection [25]. Finally, and not unexpectedly, vasoactive hormones such as endothelin-1, matrix metalloproteinases, tissue inhibitors of matrix metalloproteinases and inducible nitric oxide synthetase are detected in high levels in these grafts [31, 36].

Differential display polymerase chain reaction studies by Paul and Russel have identified still additional differentially regulated genes (either up- or downregulated as a consequence of allograft vascular injury), including both known and previously unknown genes [37–39]. Using the more simple carotid denudation model in baboons and 9 500 clone human cDNA array chips, we found that approximately 5% of clones (genes) are significantly upregulated and 2.5% downregulated, but the differently-expressed genes were different early after injury and late after injury. In early specimens, genes related to cell migration and replication dominated, whereas late after injury the most differentially expressed genes were predomnatly genes related to connective tissue formation. Regardless of the fact that this search is only at its beginning, we may expect several hundred differentially expressed genes to be recorded when comparing chronically rejecting allografts to stabile allografts. The question remains, which of these genes are rate-limiting, i.e., potential targets of therapy.

Working hypothesis and "point of no return"

Having this information available, the following working hypothesis (Fig. 1) may be constructed. Several non-immunological factors such as ischemia, reperfusion injury, hypertension and infection, contribute to inflammation in the vascular wall, either directly or indirectly *via* upregulation of the pro-inflammatory molecules in the transplant and induction of acute episodes of rejection. The inflammatory leukocytes, particularly macrophages and throm-

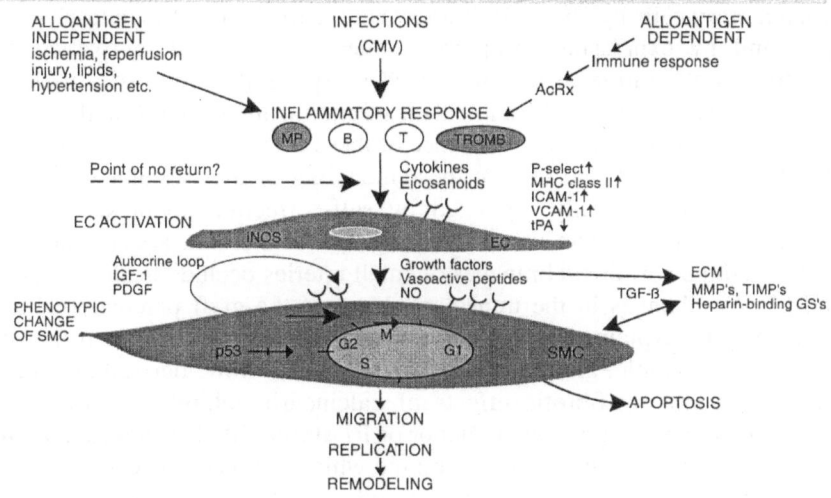

Figure 1. Summary of the major events of smooth muscle cell regulation in the generation of chronic rejection or allograft arteriosclerosis, and proven sites of intervention. The pathogenesis of chronic rejection is most likely multifactorial. Various mechanical, non-immune, immune and infectious factors generate inflammation in the transplant and induce a persistent low-grade damage to the vascular endothelium. The endothelium becomes activated, the endothelial cells express proinflammatory molecules on their surface and begin to secrete growth factors to repair the damage. This leads to paracrine and endocrine replication of vascular smooth muscle cells and their migration into the intima: this process culminates in the generation of a concentric intimal lesion (arteriosclerosis) throughout the entire length of allograft arteries (and to some extent also in the veins). Within the arterial wall, smooth muscle cells are embedded in and associated with a complex network of noncellular structural elements, called the extracellular matrix, which is in a steady-state of production and degradation. The degradation is mediated by a gene family of proteolytic enzymes including matrix metalloproteinases. These metalloproteinases are secreted as inactive zymogens, and are activated by proteolytic cleavage reactions. The activity of metalloproteinases is also regulated by a family of specific protein inhibitors, i.e., tissue inhibitors of metalloproteinases. The final events are remodeling and occlusion of the arteries and reduced blood flow leading to relative anoxia, damage of the graft structural components, fibrosis and loss of graft function. The identified sites of intervention are shown with arrows and boxes. Abbreviations: AcRx, acute rejection; CMV, cytomegalovirus; T, T-cells; B, B-cells; MP, macrophages; TROMB, thrombocytes; EC, endothelial cell; MHC, major histocompatibility complex; ICAM, intercellular adhesion molecule; VCAM, vascular cell adhesion molecule; tPA, tissue plasminogen activator; iNOS, inducible nitric oxide synthase; IGF-1, insulin-like growth factor-1; PDGF, platelet-derived growth factor; NO, nitrogen oxide; ECM, extracellular matrix; MMP, matrix metalloproteinase; TIMP, tissue inhibitor of metalloproteinases; HB-EGF, heparin binding epidermal growth factor; TGF transforming growth factor; SMC, smooth muscle cell.

bocytes, but also T- and B-cells, release cytokines and eicosanoids, leading to the activation of graft vascular endothelium. A vicious cycle is generated, whereby increased expression of pro-inflammatory molecules in the endothelium leads to increased leukocyte extravasation, increased inflammation and – again – increased expression of pro-inflammatory molecules. SMCs respond to growth factors and vasoactive peptides produced by the endothelial and

inflammatory cells by changing from a "contractile" into a "secretory" phenotype, and by expressing receptors to these ligands and by paracrine or
autocrine proliferation. In addition, SMCs express the genes of a variety of
proteolytic enzymes, which enable their migration and penetration through the
extracellular matrix. As a consequence of these events, the SMCs migrate into
the intima, replicate and initiate the remodeling of the vascular wall. These
events are only partially regulated by self-correcting apoptosis, affecting
inflammatory rather than vascular wall cells. As a result, arterial narrowing
occurs and the peripheral branches of small arteries occlude leading to anoxic
and fibrotic changes in the transplant. Most of the graft parenchymal alterations may be explained on the basis of anoxia and/or *via* shared responsiveness of, for example, glomerular mesangial cells to SMC-derived growth factors and/or *via* pro-fibrotic effects of calcineurin inhibitors. Furthermore,
retransplantation experiments to donor or F1-strain [40–42] suggest that there
is a "point of no return", once the trauma which initiated this cycle has exist-
ed sufficiently long and/or reached a given level. After this "point of no return"
the cycle becomes self-sustaining and independent of the original stimulus. In
kidney transplants, after sufficiently low levels of functioning nephrons have
been reached, self-sustaining intra-glomerular hypertension occurs leading to
an additional vicious cycle and further loss of functioning nephrons [16].
Finally, the paradigm that cells in the intima of the affected vessels derive from
the vascular media may be wrong: in bone marrow transplantation experiments
in recipients with denuded carotid arteries, we found suggestions that at least
some of these cells derive from the bone marrow, possibly from pluripotent
stem cells.

Prevention

At the moment, in the absence of specific therapy, only prophylactic measures
exist to avoid chronic rejection. Such measures may be considered under the
three etiologies of chronic rejection: alloantigen-related, alloantigen-unrelated
and infectious.

Avoiding known risk factors

Considering donor-related parameters, compromises are a rule and "best selection" is virtually never achieved both with regard to the alloantigen-related and
unrelated factors. Brain death [43–46] leads to significant endothelial trauma
which in turn leads to increased preservation-reperfusion injury. Elderly
donors are frequently used, perfect histocompatibility matches are seldom
obtained, and inadequate levels of immunosuppression can occur in noncom-
pliant recipients. Acute rejections still occur in about 50% of graft recipients

(depending somewhat on the racial composition of the region), though grafts are seldom lost any longer to acute rejections.

As all major classes of immunosuppressives have already been discussed in this book, they will not be considered here. Instead, we will shortly consider prophylaxis of infection.

CMV infection and prophylaxis with ganciclovir

Cytomegalovirus (CMV) [47–50], *Herpes simplex* virus (HSV) [51, 52] and other micro-organisms such as *Chlamydia pneumoniae* [53–55] have been associated with regular atherosclerosis in man [56–59]. CMV is one of the eight human herpes viruses. A link between herpesviruses and atherosclerosis is substantiated by the observations that Marek's disease herpesvirus, an avian herpesvirus, causes atherosclerotic lesions in chicken [60]. HSV mRNA has been recovered in the media and intimal cells of aortic specimens taken from patients with significant atherosclerosis [51]. In an electron microscopy study, virions of herpesviruses have been detected in the endothelial and SMC of the proximal aorta of arteriosclerotic patients [52].

Some years ago several groups reported that CMV infection is also related to enhanced cardiac allograft vasculopathy [24, 61–63]. We confirmed some of these findings in the prospective Helsinki Protocol Biopsy Study [64, 65], and demonstrated using protocol endomyocardial biopsies that CMV infection leads to early morphological endothelial activation preceding intimal proliferation and thickening.

In our first rat CMV (RCMV) infection model using DA rat aortic allografts transplanted into rats of the WF strain without immunosuppression afterwards, infection at the time of transplantation enhanced allograft arteriosclerosis, whereas late RCMV infection of allograft recipients or early RCMV infection of syngeneic graft recipients had no impact on aorta histology. RCMV infection induced an early prominent inflammatory episode in the allograft adventitia and doubled SMC proliferation and intimal arteriosclerotic alterations in the vascular wall [66]. The early intimal changes in RCMV-infected allografts were frequently associated with subendothelial infiltration (endothelialitis) of mononuclear cells [67]. In another experiment, we used heterotopic rat cardiac allografts in the same strain combination [68]. Again, RCMV infection accelerated the generation of cardiac allograft vasculopathy in triple-drug immunosuppressed rat heart transplants, particularly the occlusion of small intramyocardial arterioles. The vascular changes in both models were linked with increased perivascular and intramural inflammation and endovasculitis [68].

There are two likely mechanisms whereby CMV infection may stimulate vascular SMCs to form dysplastic lesions: either *via* a direct pro-proliferative effect on SMC or *via* an indirect pro-proliferative effect *via* induction of inflammation and cytokine and growth factor release by inflammatory and activated endothelial cells. These two mutually non-exclusive alternatives have been recently discussed [59].

In our first study on rat aortic allografts without immunosuppression of the recipient, we demonstrated that ganciclovir prophylaxis prevented RCMV infection and completely abolished the enhancing effect of CMV infection on aortic allograft arteriosclerosis. If ganciclovir treatment was initiated during ongoing infection, it only partially inhibited the development of intimal lesions [69]. We also tested the efficacy of ganciclovir prophylaxis on the prevention of RCMV infection-enhanced cardiac allograft vasculopathy during cyclosporine (CsA) immunosuppression. Ganciclovir prophylaxis reduced the intensity and magnitude of cardiac allograft vasculopathy in RCMV-infected animals by 50% of the level of noninfected CsA-immunosuppressed controls [69].

Most recently, these results have been confirmed in a clinical trial in man (Hannah Valantine, personal communication). In a study at Stanford University, 149 cardiac transplant recipients were randomized to receive either intravenous ganciclovir or placebo during the initial 28 days post-transplantation and were followed for 5 years. Even this relatively short course of ganciclovir therapy preceding the peak period of clinical CMV infection [70, 71], reduced the incidence of angiographically-detectable transplant coronary disease at 5 years by one-third, from 60 to 40%.

Heart, liver and lung allograft patients are more heavily immunosuppressed than renal allograft patients. Consequently, CMV infection is more common in the recipients of these transplants than in those of a kidney. On the other hand, acute rejections are more common in kidney than in heart transplants. This may be a likely reason why CMV has emerged as a major risk factor in cardiac transplantation, whereas in renal transplants it has been more difficult to verify the involvement of CMV, except for studies in experimental animal models [72]. At any rate, confirmation of the Stanford finding in a multicenter study possibly using the orally available valine-substituted ganciclovir seems clearly indicated.

Rate-limiting steps – potential targets for therapy?

Considering that several types of insult: alloantigen-dependent, alloantigen-independent and infectious, may lead to a common pattern of vascular response, we and others have investigated whether rate-limiting steps as potential sites for intervention may be defined downstream of the "point of no return", i.e., after the preventive measures to eliminate risk factors and the effect of acute rejection have failed. Needless to say, we also assume that the distal events in the cascade, leading to endothelial dysfunction and activation and formation of dysplastic lesions by the vascular SMCs, are common features and shared with other forms of proliferative vasculopathies. If this is the case, the therapies developed may be applicable not only to chronic allograft vasculopathy, but also be of potential use in other forms of vasculopathies including the major causes for late graft loss, death for cardiovascular reasons, but with a functioning graft.

Rate-limiting steps after the "point of no return"

In order to define rate-limiting steps in the allograft vascular response, investigators have focused on the differentially-expressed genes and gene products in the allograft parenchyma and in the vascular wall. In classical organ models, such as kidney or heart transplants, it is technically difficult to investigate gene expression in individual hollow structures, such as graft arteries or bronchioli, as this would require extensive dissection to produce sufficient amounts of RNA from them. Therefore, simple "tube models" have been developed, where only the hollow structures to be investigated are transplanted. This can be accomplished by aorta allografts [73] or tracheal allografts [74, 75]. Even more simple methods are endothelial trauma models to induce the intimal dysplastic response like denudation of carotid artery or aorta [76–78]. The "tube models" can be complemented with *in vitro* models of SMC migration and replication [79, 80]. The most common experimental animal species are mice (knock-out models), rats and rabbits. Finally, the results with tube models must be confirmed with regular organ models, first in rodents and then in large animals.

The past methods for differential gene expression, based on the analysis of subtraction cDNA libraries or differential-display RT-PCR, are being replaced with high-throughput cDNA array (microchip) technologies [81, 82]. These technologies allow the analysis of the expression of several thousand genes concomitantly. In addition to known genes, particularly interesting are the expressed sequence tags (EST), representing (possibly) unknown genes.

The sole over- or under-expression of a given gene, does not indicate that the gene is rate-limiting, i.e., a potential target for therapy. This must be verified by blocking or overexpressing the gene and by demonstrating the altered pattern of the vascular response. In the case that we limit ourselves to vascular wall physiology only, initial experiments may be conveniently done by using the *in vitro* models of SMC migration and replication, endothelial activation and antisense oligonucleotide technology or gene transfection *in vitro*. These various steps are summarized in Figure 2; in the following some of the results are summarized.

Regulation of smooth muscle cell response to mitogens

A variety of molecules (vasoactive peptides, cytokines, chemokines and growth factors) derived from endothelial cells, inflammatory cells and SMCs provide pro-mitogenic and pro-migratory signals to SMCs. These ligands and many of their receptors are prominently expressed in the vessels of chronical-

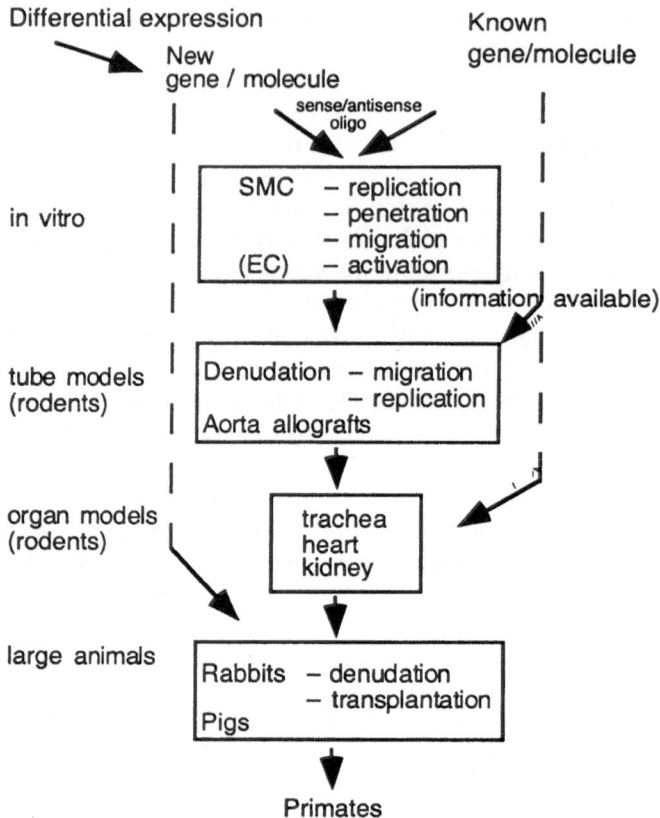

Figure 2. Identification of rate-limiting steps in proliferative vasculopathy. For details, see the text.

ly rejecting allografts. As these have recently been reviewed in depth by Raines and Ross [83], the information is not repeated here.

In our previous studies with chronically-rejecting rat cardiac allografts [68] we demonstrated that the expression of platelet-derived growth factor (PDGF)-A in the media and intima and of PDGF receptor-α and -β in the intima and endothelium significantly correlated to intimal thickening. It was, therefore, of interest to investigate whether altered responses to PDGF would inhibit the pathological changes in chronically rejecting organ allografts. PDGF is the major polypeptide mitogen in serum for cells of mesenchymal origin. PDGF is the critical mediator of vascular SMC proliferation and migration [84]. On the other hand, PDGF may set mechanisms in motion that limit the magnitude of the mitogenic response. Efficient inhibition of intimal thickening in tube models has been achieved by using anti-PDGF antibodies in rodents [85, 86] and baboon [87], as well as using PDGF-antisense oligonucleotides [88, 89].

Considering that ligands would be amply available, we reasoned that the receptor rather than the ligand would be the likely rate-limiting target in receptor-ligand interaction. Furthermore, we wanted to use small-molecular weight compounds which would be reasonably specific to the PDGF receptor, in order to exlude the use of antibodies. It is obvious that the more proximal in the signaling cascade one operates, the more selective is the effect to a given cell type and the higher is the likelihood for specific intervention. Highly specific protein tyrosine kinase (PTK) inhibitors have been generated by a number of pharmaceutical companies and in different laboratories [90] providing reasonably specific tools to test the hypothesis. In these experiments, a highly specific PTK inhibitor to PDGF receptor developed by Ciba-Geigy (CGP 53716, [91]) was used. The molecule was first tested *in vitro*, and thereafter in the rat carotid denudation model. CGP 53716 inhibited PDGF-A and -B -induced rat vascular SMC replication and migration *in vitro*, and smooth muscle cell replication and migration *in vivo*. At a dose of 50 mg/kg/d the compound also inhibited intimal thickening after carotid artery endothelial injury in the rat [92]. This result has since then been confirmed with another PDGF-receptor PTK inihibitor in the porcine carotid artery endothelial injury model [93].

Thereafter, we have repeated the experiment in the chronic rat heart allograft rejection model. Hearts from DA rats were transplanted to WF rat recipients which were suboptimally immunosuppressed with CsA, leading to characteristic histological obliteration of the allograft arteries. The recipients received 50 mg/kg/d of CGP 53716. Both the number of affected vessels and the mean index of intimal obliteration in rat cardiac allografts were reduced by approximately 50% at 60 days post-transplantation [94, 95]. These observations now need to be confirmed in large animal models.

Inhibition of proteolytic activity

Matrix metalloproteinases (MMP) are necessary for SMC locomotion and penetration through the extracellular matrix and the internal elastic lamina. Inhibition of MMP inhibits SMC migration into the neointima in trauma models [96] and after heart transplantation in rats and rabbits [97]. In all models this does not necessarily end up with intimal size reduction [98] of the injured vessels, as MMP-2 has been shown to cleave the ectodomain of the fibroblast growth factor (FGF)-receptor [99] and this might explain the increased replication rate in neointima [98]. Divergent effects have been seen in the case of overexpression of tissue inhibitors of metalloproteinases [100]. Overproduction of TIMP-1 in rat carotid arteries increases local elastin accumulation [101] and may, therefore, enhance fibrosis.

Exploitation of tissue-specific receptors of natural hormones

As described by Raines and Ross [83], a whole variety of pro-proliferative and pro-migratory signals, including cytokines, chemokines, vasoactive peptides and growth factors, are provided to SMCs as a consequence of endothelial activation after injury. Many of these signals can be inihibited, and the inhibition nearly invariably results in at least some level of inhibition of SMC functions *in vitro* and of intimal dysplasia *in vivo*. However, in most approaches, the inhibition of the intimal response achieved *in vivo* has been relatively modest, of the order of 30–50%, only.

On the other hand, evidence exists that there are vasculoprotective natural molecules, hormones which modulate several of these events concomitantly. Such hormones include somatostatin and estrogen. Both hormones have, however, pleiotropic actions on multiple tissues. The unwanted effects have excluded the use of estrogen for vasculoprotection (except in post-menopausal women – see later).

We generated a paradigm that the multiple effects of these natural hormones in multiple tissues, may be regulated by multiple receptors and that each tissue in resting and activated state expresses only a limited receptor repertoire. If this would be the case, targeting to the receptor subset(s) expressed (predominantly or exclusively) in vascular tissue but not, for example, in the alimentary tract or sex organs, would make it possible to generate drugs with a specific vasculoprotective effect and minimal side-effects.

Somatostatin receptors

Somatostatin (SST) is a neurohormone that is produced widely in the body. It acts both systemically *via* the circulation, as well as locally to inhibit cell proliferation as well as the secretion of various hormones, growth factors, and neurotransmitter substances [102, 103]. SST and its metabolically stable synthetic analogs like octapeptides (SMS201-995, octreotide, sandostatin; and BIM23014, lanreotide, angiopeptin) exert several vascular effects such as vasoconstriction in the gut and inhibition of angiogenesis [104, 105].

The actions of SST are mediated by a family of five G-protein-coupled receptors with seven helical transmembrane segments called SSTR1-5 [103]. All five SSTRs are functionally coupled to inhibition of adenylyl cyclase [103]. Some of the receptor isotypes also modulate other effectors, for example phosphotyrosine phosphatase, K^+ and voltage-dependent Ca^{2+} ion channels, a Na^+/H^+ exchanger, phospholipase C, phospholipase A2, and MAP kinase (MAPK) [103]. Based on structural similarity and its ability to react with octapeptide and hexapeptide SST analogs, the receptor family can be subdivided into two subclasses: the SSTR2,5 subclass which reacts strongly with these analogs and the SSTR1,(3),4 subclass which reacts poorly with these compounds [103].

In animal experiments using arterial, venous and vascular transplantation models, administration of octreotide and lanreotide usually prevents the formation of dysplastic lesions [106–111]. These results, however, have been inconsistent in other experimental models. In randomized placebo-controlled clinical trials, lanreotide in some studies prevented restenosis after subcutaneous transluminal angioplasty, as quantitated by angiography or as clinical events [112, 113], whereas the same success has not been achieved with octreotide [114].

To target the analogs for better vasculoprotection, we investigated [115] the pattern of expression of all five SSTR subtypes in rat thoracic aorta in resting state and at 15 min and 3, 7, and 14 days after balloon endothelial denudation injury. The SSTR1-5 expression level was determined as mRNA by RT-PCR and the protein was localized in the tissue by immunohistochemistry. All five SSTRs were expressed in rat aorta both as mRNA and as protein; SSTR1, 3 and 4 prominently and SSTR2 and 5 only in minute quantities. SSTR1, 3 and 4 displayed time-dependent, subtype-selective responses to endothelial denudation. SSTR1 mRNA increased significantly on days 3 and 7, coinciding with the proliferative response of SMC, and declined to basal levels by day 14. SSTR3 and 4 mRNA showed a different pattern coinciding with the migratory response following proliferation, with a more gradual increase beginning on day 3–7 and remaining elevated thereafter. SSTR2 and 5 mRNA was constitutively expressed at a very low level and showed almost no change post-injury (Fig. 3). By immunohistochemistry, SSTR1-5 antigens were localized pre-

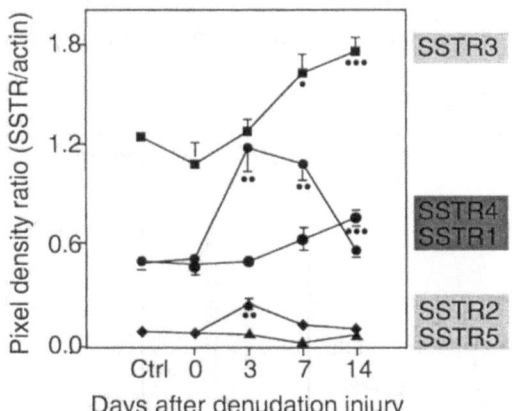

Figure 3. Time-course of somatostatin receptors SSTR1-5 mRNA expression in the vascular wall after trauma. SSTR1-5 mRNA was quantitated from Southern hybridization signals of RT-PCR products by densitometry using a Java Video Analysis. The arbitrary pixel density values were collected for background and expressed as a ratio of actin mRNA. Legend: ● SSTR1; ◆ SSTR2; ■ SSTR3; ● SSTR4; ▲ SSTR5. Statistical significance of difference from control nondenuded samples (Ctrl): • $p < 0.05$; •• $p < 0.01$; ••• $p < 0.001$. Time O represents samples collected 15 min after denudation. Data presented are mean values ± SE of at least six measurements of pixel densities of hybridization signals from three separate experiments. (From [115], courtesy of FASEB J).

dominantly in SMC that were present in the media, or which hád migrated into the intima, and the antigen expression correlated with receptor mRNA expression. Notably, only SSTR1, 3 and 4 were expressed in the intima, SSTR1 and 4 during the proliferative burst and SSTR3 and 4 after the proliferation when SMC continue to migrate into the intima. These results demonstrate subtype-specific tissue localization and dynamic changes in SSTR1-5 expression after vascular trauma and localize the receptors to areas of vascular SMC migration and replication. In view of their early prominent induction, SSTR subtype 1 may be the optimal subtype to target for inhibition of myointimal proliferation rather than the current ligands targeting to SSTR2; SSTR subtypes 3 and 4 may be exploited as potential target in migration and remodeling.

Estrogen receptors

The vasculoprotective effect of estrogen was first demonstrated in population studies in humans, where estrogen replacement therapy demonstrated a protective effect of atherosclerotic vascular disease in post-menopausal women [116, 117]. This was later confirmed in monkeys [118]. Later the vasculoprotective effect has been documented more in detail in animal models and *in vitro*. Estrogen inhibits intimal thickening after carotid balloon injury in rabbits [119], rats [120] and in mice [121], as well as the immunologically-induced vascular fibroproliferative dysplasia in rabbit aorta [122] and heart [123] allografts. *In vitro* estrogen inhibits migration and replication of vSMC [124–127]. These observations are consistant with the findings in reporter gene assays that functional estrogen receptors are expressed in vSMC of

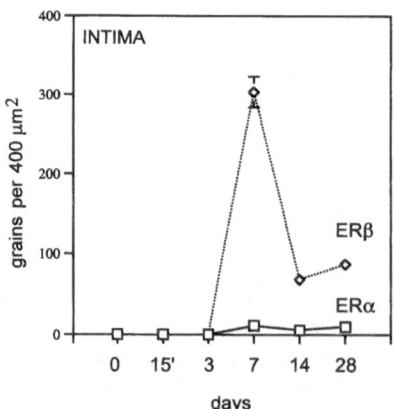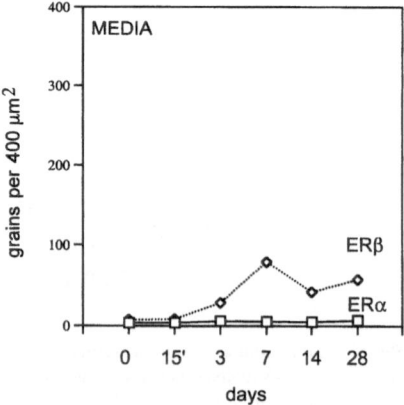

Figure 4. Expression of estrogen receptors ERα and ERβ mRNA in denuded male rat carotid at different time points after injury. Values represent number of grains per 400 μm² and are expressed as means from three rats per time point and three countings of each specimen ± SEM. (From [139], courtesy of Academy of Sciences, USA).

bovine [128], rat [129, 130], guinea pig [131], and human [132] origin.

In addition to the anti-proliferative and anti-migratory effect towards SMCs, estrogen may also display vasculoprotective effects *via* the vascular wall endothelium. Functional estrogen receptors have been demonstrated in endothelial cells [133], estrogen downregulates cytokine-induced adhesion molecule expression in human endothelium *in vitro* [134], it is anti-apoptotic to endothelial cells [135] and it enhances functional endothelial recovery after denudation *in vivo* [136]. There are also indirect pathways whereby estrogen may mediate vasculoprotective effects. Additional estrogen effects may be mediated indirectly *via* lipoprotein metabolism and systemically *via* promoting vasodilatation by stimulating prostacyclin and nitric oxide synthesis [137].

The development of vasculoprotective drug therapies based on the protective effect of estrogen has been difficult, as it has not been possible to differentiate the desired vasculoprotective effect of estrogen from its effects on the reproductive system. The discovery of a second estrogen receptor (ER) ERβ and the recent finding that disruption of the "classical" ERα gene in mice preserves the vasculoprotective effect of estrogen [138] offer better targeting of estrogen in vasculoprotective drug therapies.

Analogous with our paradigm already applied to the SSTR subsets, we investigated which of the known ER subsets are expressed in the vascular wall and how their expression level is regulated after cartorid artery injury. In a recent paper [139], we demonstrate that after endothelial denudation injury of rat carotid artery, the ERβ mRNA (and protein) are constitutively expressed at a low level in the vascular wall, whereas the expression of ERβ mRNA increases >30-fold after injury (Fig. 4). In *in situ* hybridization, the ERβ mRNA co-localizes with the replicating and migrating SMCs in the media and in the neointima. The results clearly suggest that ERβ rather than ERα would be a better candidate for vasculoprotective estrogen receptor.

In order to differentiate between the sex steroid (uterotrophic) and vasculoprotective effects, ligands with different binding affinities to ERα and ERβ were employed. Treatment of ovariectomized female rats on a soybean-deficient diet with the isoflavonic phytoestrogen genistein (which shows approximately 20 times higher binding affinity to ERβ than to ERα) and with 17β-estradiol (which does not differentiate between the two receptor subtypes) at a dose range between 0.0025 and 2.5 mg/kg/d, provided on both occasions a dose-dependent vasculoprotective effect (Fig. 5). However, only treatment with 17β-estradiol, but not with genistein, was accompanied with a dose-dependent uterotrophic effect. Thus, the vasculoprotective effect of estrogen can be differentiated from the uterotrophic effect using ligands with different binding affinity to ERβ and ERα. As genistein at this dose range is likely to function *via* ERβ and is devoid of the inhibitory effect on protein tyrosine kinases, we suggest that the vasculoprotective effect of genistein is mediated by ERβ. This observation will enable us, for the first time, to generate vasculoprotective estrogen mimetics without classical uterotrophic side-effects. A recent observation by the group of Mendelsohn [140], that the vasculoprotec-

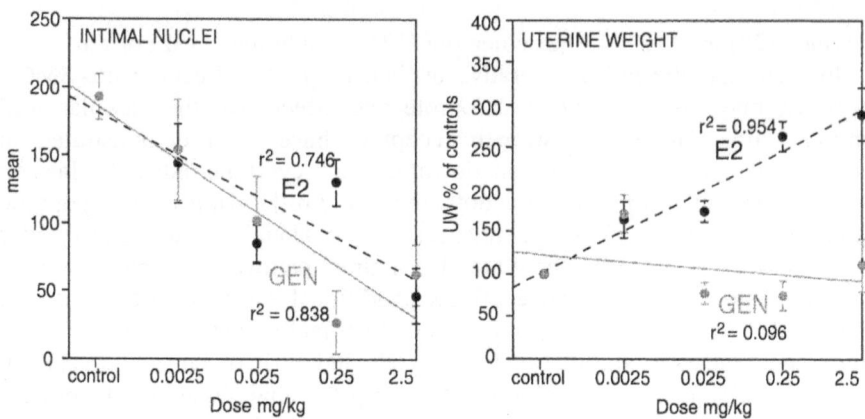

Figure 5. Left figure: dose-responses of 0.0025–2.5 mg/kg/d of 17β-estradiol (○) and genistein (●) on the nuclear number in the vascular intima 7 days after denudation injury of carotid arteries in ovariectomized female rats. The figures indicate the number of nuclei per vessel circumference. Data presented are mean values of 3 to 5 determinations per point ± SEM. In statistical analysis, the difference between regression coefficients (slopes) was not significant ($p = 0.5$). Right figure: dose-responses of 0.0025–2.5 mg/kg/d of 17β-estradiol (○) and genistein (●) on the uterine weight 7 days after denudation injury of carotid arteries in ovariectomized female rats. Data presented are mean values of three to five determinations per point ± SEM. In statistical analysis, the difference between regression coefficients (slopes) was significant ($p = 0.0003$).

tive effect of estrogen is preserved in ERβ knockout mice, invalidates our original paradigm that the vasculoprotective effect is mediated *via* ERβ, and suggests that both receptors can mediate the effect (unless a third receptor is involved). Double knock-out mice may resolve this question; for now it may be expected that Erβ-specific agonists are good drug candidates for vasculoprotective estrogens without uterotrophic effects.

Rational drug design

For targeted drug design, aiming to agonize or antagonize a given receptor, ligand or enzyme, the following four modalities exist. Gene therapy is highly specific, but the delivery of genes to the target organ and site has been difficult regardless whether live attenuated virus or conventional plasmid vectors are employed. The extreme selectivity and specificity of the immune system has been exploited to develop monoclonal antibodies, chimeric or humanized, to target (usually cell surface) proteins. Regardless of these modifications and their high specificity, monoclonal antibodies are not particularly good drugs; they require parenteral administration and they are prone to generate anti-antibodies blocking their action in long-term use. This may be partially overcome by using non-degradable peptides based on D- rather than L-amino acids [141]. Although these drugs have also to be administered parenterally, they do not usually evoke immune responses.

Peptidomimetics, which are organic compounds lacking the peptide bond, would be even better, but their development is particularly demanding and requires extensive modeling and combinatorial chemistry facilities. Only the last approach will generate credible orally-available drug candidates. However, this approach will need reliable modeling of the target receptor, combinatorial chemistry and high throughput screens using cell lines permanently overexpressing the desired genes.

In regard to 7-transmembrane G-protein coupled receptors, the modeling of SSTR subtypes will be a particularly demanding task, as the receptor cannot be crystallized. With regard to ER subtypes, the ligand-binding domain has already been crystallized. There is a high demand for new specific drugs for vasculoprotection. Indications for these drugs would not be limited to transplantation, but will also include other forms of fibroproliferative vasculopaties, such as complications of bypass surgery, percutaneous transluminal coronary angioplasty procedures, autoimmune and diabetic vasculopathies and possibly variations of the common form of atherosclerosis.

Acknowledgement
This chapter is based on Plenary Presentations at the Winter Symposium of American Society of Transplant Phycisians in Puerto Rico in 1997 [142], the recently published results presented at the World Congress of The Transplantation Society in Montreal in 1998 [115, 139], and on the Doctoral Thesis of Serdar Yilmaz at the University of Helsinki (1999).

References

1 Demetris AJ, Zerbe T, Banner B (1989) Morphology of solid organ allograft arteriopathy: identification of proliferating intimal cell populations. *Transplant Proc* 21: 3667–3669
2 Abele R, Novick AC, Braun WE, Steinmuller D, Buszta C, Greenstreet R, Hinton J (1982) Long-term results of renal transplantation in recipients with a functioning graft for 2 years. *Transplantation* 34: 264–267
3 Cecka MJ, Terasaki PI (1989) Early rejection episodes. *In*: PI Terasaki (ed.): *Clinical transplants*. UCLA Tissue typing laboratory, Los Angeles, 425–434
4 Basadonna GP, Matas AJ, Gillingham KJ, Payne WD, Dunn DL, Sutherland DE, Gores PF, Gruessner RW, Najarian JS (1993) Early *versus* late acute renal allograft rejection: impact on chronic rejection. *Transplantation* 55: 993–995
5 Lindholm A, Ohlman S, Albrechtsen D, Tufveson G, Persson H, Persson NH (1993) The impact of acute rejection episodes on long-term graft function and outcome in 1347 primary renal transplants treated by 3 cyclosporine regimens. *Transplantation* 56: 307–315
6 Yilmaz S, Häyry P (1993) The impact of acute episodes of rejection on the generation of chronic rejection in rat renal allografts. *Transplantation* 56: 1153–1156
7 Yilmaz A, Yilmaz S, Kallio E, Rapola J, Häyry P (1995) Evolution of glomerular basement membrane changes in chronic rejection. *Transplantation* 60: 1314–1322
8 Van Saase JL, Van der Woude FJ, Thorogood J, Hollander AA, Van Es LA, Weening JJ, Van Bockel J, Bruijn JA (1995) The relation between acute vascular and interstitial renal allograft rejection and subsequent chronic rejection. *Transplantation* 59: 1280–1285
9 Räisänen-Sokolowski A, Vuoristo P, Myllärniemi M, Yilmaz S, Kallio E, Häyry P (1995) Mycophenolate mofetil (MMF, RS-61443) inhibits inflammation and smooth muscle cell proliferation in rat aortic allografts. *Transpl Immunol* 3: 342–351
10 Nair RV, Cao W, Morris RE (1996) The antiproliferative effect of leflunomide on vascular smooth muscle cells *in vitro* is mediated by selective inhibition of pyrimidine biosynthesis. *Transplant Proc* 28: 3081

11 Cao W, Mohacsi P, Shorthouse R, Pratt R, Morris RE (1995) Effects of rapamycin on growth factor-stimulated vascular smooth muscle cell DNA synthesis. Inhibition of basic fibroblast growth factor and platelet-derived growth factor action and antagonism of rapamycin by FK506. *Transplantation* 59: 390–395

12 Sehgal SN (1998) Rapamune (RAPA, rapamycin, sirolimus): mechanism of action immunosuppressive effect results from blockade of signal transduction and inhibition of cell cycle progression. *Clin Biochem* 31: 335–340

13 Morris RE (1996) Mechanisms of action of new immunosuppressive drugs. *Kidney Int* Suppl 53: S26-S38

14 Brazelton TR, Morris RE (1996) Molecular mechanisms of action of new xenobiotic immunosuppressive drugs: tacrolimus (FK506), sirolimus (rapamycin), mycophenolate mofetil and leflunomide. *Curr Opin Immunol* 8: 710–720

15 Luo Z, Shyu K, Gualberto A, Walsh K (1998) Calcineurin inhibitors and cardiac hypertrophy. *Nat Med* 4: 1092–1093

16 Mackenzie HS, Tullius SG, Heemann UW, Azuma H, Rennke HG, Brenner BM, Tilney NL (1994) Nephron supply is a major determinant of long-term renal allograft outcome in rats. *J Clin Invest* 94: 2148–2152

17 Matas AJ (1994) Chronic rejection – definition and correlates. *Clin Transplant* 162–167

18 Von Willebrand E, Zola H, Häyry P (1985) Thrombocyte aggregates in renal allografts. Analysis with fine-needle aspiration biopsy and monoclonal antithrombocyte antibodies. *Transplantation* 39: 258–262

19 Häyry P, Von Willebrand E, Parthenais E, Nemlander A, Soots A, Lautenschlager I, Alfoldy P, Renkonen R (1984) The inflammatory mechanisms of allograft rejection. *Immunol Rev* 77: 85–142

20 Lemström K, Koskinen P, Häyry P (1995) Molecular mechanisms of chronic renal allograft rejection. *Kidney Int* Suppl 52: S2-S10

21 Räisänen-Sokolowski A, Häyry P (1996) Chronic allograft arteriosclerosis: contributing factors and molecular mechanisms in the light of experimental studies. *Transpl Immunol* 4: 91–98

22 Russell PS, Chase CM, Winn HJ, Colvin RB (1994) Coronary atherosclerosis in transplanted mouse hearts. II. Importance of humoral immunity. *J Immunol* 152: 5135–5141

23 Shi C, Lee WS, He Q, Zhang D, Fletcher DJ, Newell JB, Haber E (1996) Immunologic basis of transplant-associated arteriosclerosis. *Proc Natl Acad Sci USA* 93: 4051–4056

24 MacDonald AS, Sabr K, MacAuley MA, McAlister VC, Bitter SH, Lee T (1994) Effects of leflunomide and cyclosporine on aortic allograft chronic rejection in the rat. *Transplant Proc* 26: 3244–3245

25 Koskinen PK, Lemström KB, Häyry PJ (1995) How cyclosporine modifies histological and molecular events in the vascular wall during chronic rejection of rat cardiac allografts. *Amer J Pathol* 146: 972–980

26 Gregory CR, Huang X, Pratt RE, Dzau VJ, Shorthouse R, Billingham ME, Morris RE (1995) Treatment with rapamycin and mycophenolic acid reduces arterial intimal thickening produced by mechanical injury and allows endothelial replacement. *Transplantation* 59: 655–661

27 Räisänen-Sokolowski A, Yilmaz S, Tufveson G, Häyry P (1994) Partial inhibition of allograft arteriosclerosis (chronic rejection) by 15-deoxyspergualin. *Transplantation* 57: 1772–1777

28 Russell ME, Hancock WW, Akalin E, Wallace AF, Glysing JT, Willett TA, Sayegh MH (1996) Chronic cardiac rejection in the LEW to F344 rat model. Blockade of CD28-B7 costimulation by CTLA4Ig modulates T cell and macrophage activation and attenuates arteriosclerosis. *J Clin Invest* 97: 833–838

29 Kingma I, Chea R, Davidoff A, Benediktsson H, Paul LC (1993) Glomerular capillary pressures in long-surviving rat renal allografts. *Transplantation* 56: 53–60

30 Benediktsson H, Chea R, Davidoff A, Paul LC (1996) Antihypertensive drug treatment in chronic renal allograft rejection in the rat. Effect on structure and function. *Transplantation* 62: 1634–1642

31 Russell ME, Wallace AF, Wyner LR, Newell JB, Karnovsky MJ (1995) Upregulation and modulation of inducible nitric oxide synthase in rat cardiac allografts with chronic rejection and transplant arteriosclerosis. *Circulation* 92: 457–464

32 Akyurek LM, Funa K, Wanders A, Larsson E, Fellström BC (1995) Inhibition of transplant arteriosclerosis in rat aortic grafts by low molecular weight heparin derivatives. *Transplantation* 59: 1517–1524

33 Kobashigawa JA, Katznelson S, Laks H, Johnson JA, Yeatman L, Wang XM, Chia D, Terasaki PI, Sabad A, Cogert GA et al (1995) Effect of pravastatin on outcomes after cardiac transplantation. *N Engl J Med* 333: 621–627

34 Koskinen PK, Lemstrom KB (1997) Adhesion molecule P-selectin and vascular cell adhesion molecule-1 in enhanced heart allograft arteriosclerosis in the rat. *Circulation* 95: 191–196

35 Russell ME, Wallace AF, Hancock WW, Sayegh MH, Adams DH, Sibinga NE, Wyner LR, Karnovsky MJ (1995) Upregulation of cytokines associated with macrophage activation in the Lewis-to-F344 rat transplantation model of chronic cardiac rejection. *Transplantation* 59: 572–578

36 Watschinger B, Sayegh MH, Hancock WW, Russell ME (1995) Up-regulation of endothelin-1 mRNA and peptide expression in rat cardiac allografts with rejection and arteriosclerosis. *Amer J Pathol* 146: 1065–1072

37 Utans U, Liang P, Wyner LR, Karnovsky MJ, Russell ME (1994) Chronic cardiac rejection: identification of five upregulated genes in transplanted hearts by differential mRNA display. *Proc Natl Acad Sci USA* 91: 6463–6467

38 Chen J, Myllarniemi M, Akyurek LM, Hayry P, Marsden PA, Paul LC (1996) Identification of differentially expressed genes in rat aortic allograft vasculopathy. *Amer J Pathol* 149: 597–611

39 Chen J, Akyurek LM, Fellstrom B, Hayry P, Paul LC (1998) Eotaxin and capping protein in experimental vasculopathy. *Amer J Pathol* 153: 81–90

40 Brazelton TR, Adams BA, Cheung AC, Morris RE (1997) Progression of obliterative airway disease occurs despite the removal of immune reactivity by retransplantation. *Transplant Proc* 29: 2613

41 Mennander A, Häyry P (1996) Reversibility of allograft arteriosclerosis after retransplantation to donor strain. *Transplantation* 62: 526–529

42 Tullius SG, Hancock WW, Heemann U, Azuma H, Tilney NL (1994) Reversibility of chronic renal allograft rejection. Critical effect of time after transplantation suggests both host immune dependent and independent phases of progressive injury. *Transplantation* 58: 93–99

43 Novitzky D (1997) Donor management: state of the art. *Transplant Proc* 29: 3773–3775

44 Novitzky D (1996) Selection and management of cardiac allograft donors. *Curr Opin Cardiol* 11: 174–182

45 Takada M, Nadeau KC, Hancock WW, Mackenzie HS, Shaw GD, Waaga AM, Chandraker A, Sayegh MH, Tilney NL (1998) Effects of explosive brain death on cytokine activation of peripheral organs in the rat. *Transplantation* 65: 1533–1542

46 Pratschke J, Wilhelm MJ, Kusaka M, Basker M, Cooper DK, Hancock WW, Tilney NL (1999) Brain death and its influence on donor organ quality and outcome after transplantation. *Transplantation* 67: 343–348

47 Melnick JL, Petrie BL, Dreesman GR, Burek J, McCollum CH, DeBakey ME (1983) Cytomegalovirus antigen within human arterial smooth muscle cells. *Lancet* 2: 644–647

48 Hendrix MG, Dormans PH, Kitslaar P, Bosman F, Bruggeman CA (1989) The presence of cytomegalovirus nucleic acids in arterial walls of atherosclerotic and nonatherosclerotic patients. *Amer J Pathol* 134: 1151–1157

49 Hendrix MG, Salimans MM, Van Boven CP, Bruggeman CA (1990) High prevalence of latently present cytomegalovirus in arterial walls of patients suffering from grade III atherosclerosis. *Amer J Pathol* 136: 23–28

50 Melnick JL, Adam E, DeBakey ME (1990) Possible role of cytomegalovirus in atherogenesis. *JAMA* 263: 2204–2207

51 Benditt EP, Barrett T, McDougall JK (1983) Viruses in the etiology of atherosclerosis. *Proc Natl Acad Sci USA* 80: 6386–6389

52 Gyorkey F, Melnick JL, Guinn GA, Gyorkey P, DeBakey ME (1984) Herpesviridae in the endothelial and smooth muscle cells of the proximal aorta in arteriosclerotic patients. *Exp Mol Pathol* 40: 328–339

53 Saikku P, Leinonen M, Tenkanen L, Linnanmäki E, Ekman MR, Manninen V, Manttari M, Frick MH, Huttunen JK (1992) Chronic *Chlamydia pneumoniae* infection as a risk factor for coronary heart disease in the Helsinki Heart Study (see comments). *Ann Intern Med* 116: 273–278

54 Miettinen H, Lehto S, Saikku P, Haffner SM, Ronnemaa T, Pyörälä K, Laakso M (1996) Association of *Chlamydia pneumoniae* and acute coronary heart disease events in non-insulin dependent diabetic and non-diabetic subjects in Finland. *Eur Heart J* 17: 682–688

55 Muhlestein JB, Hammond EH, Carlquist JF, Radicke E, Thomson MJ, Karagounis LA, Woods

ML, Anderson JL (1996) Increased incidence of *Chlamydia* species within the coronary arteries of patients with symptomatic atherosclerotic *versus* other forms of cardiovascular disease. *J Amer Coll Cardiol* 27: 1555–1561

56 Rubin RH (1990) Impact of cytomegalovirus infection on organ transplant recipients. *Rev Infect Dis* 12: S754–766

57 Rubin RH (1993) Infectious disease complications of renal transplantation. *Kidney Int* 44: 221–236

58 Tolkoff-Rubin NE, Rubin H (1995) New strategies for the control of viral infection in organ transplantation. *Clin Transplant* 9: 255–259

59 Koskinen P, Kallio E, Tikkanen J, Sihvola R, Häyry P, Lemström K (1999) Cytomegalovirus infection and cardiac allograft vasculopathy – a review. *Transplant Inf Dis* 1: 115–126

60 Fabricant CG, Fabricant J, Litrenta MM, Minick CR (1978) Virus-induced atherosclerosis. *J Exp Med* 148: 335–340

61 Grattan MT, Moreno CC, Starnes VA, Oyer PE, Stinson EB, Shumway NE (1989) Cytomegalovirus infection is associated with cardiac allograft rejection and atherosclerosis. *JAMA* 261: 3561–3566

62 Loebe M, Schuler S, Zais O, Warnecke H, Fleck E, Hetzer R (1990) Role of cytomegalovirus infection in the development of coronary artery disease in the transplanted heart. *J Heart Transplant* 9: 707–711

63 Everett JP, Hershberger RE, Norman DJ, Chou S, Ratkovec RM, Cobanoglu A, Ott GY, Hosenpud JD (1992) Prolonged cytomegalovirus infection with viremia is associated with development of cardiac allograft vasculopathy. *J Heart Lung Transplant* 11: S133-S137

64 Koskinen PK, Nieminen MS, Krogerus LA, Lemstrom KB, Mattila SP, Hayry PJ, Lautenschlager IT (1993) Cytomegalovirus infection accelerates cardiac allograft vasculopathy: correlation between angiographic and endomyocardial biopsy findings in heart transplant patients. *Transplant Int* 6: 341–347

65 Koskinen PK, Nieminen MS, Krogerus LA, Lemström KB, Mattila SP, Häyry PJ, Lautenschlager IT (1993) Cytomegalovirus infection and accelerated cardiac allograft vasculopathy in human cardiac allografts. *J Heart Lung Transplant* 12: 724–729

66 Lemström KB, Bruning JH, Bruggeman CA, Lautenschlager IT, Häyry PJ (1993) Cytomegalovirus infection enhances smooth muscle cell proliferation and intimal thickening of rat aortic allografts. *J Clin Invest* 92: 549–558

67 Koskinen P, Lemström K, Bruggeman C, Lautenschlager I, Häyry P (1994) Acute cytomegalovirus infection induces a subendothelial inflammation (endothelialitis) in the allograft vascular wall. A possible linkage with enhanced allograft arteriosclerosis. *Amer J Pathol* 144: 41–50

68 Lemström KB, Koskinen PK (1997) Expression and localization of Platelet-Derived Growth Factor ligand and receptor protein during acute and chronic rejection of rat cardiac allografts. *Circulation* 96: 1240–1249

69 Lemström KB, Bruning JH, Bruggeman CA, Koskinen PK, Aho PT, Yilmaz S, Lautenschlager IT, Häyry PJ (1994) Cytomegalovirus infection-enhanced allograft arteriosclerosis is prevented by DHPG prophylaxis in the rat. *Circulation* 90: 1969–1978

70 Fishman JA, Rubin RH (1998) Infection in organ-transplant recipients. *N Engl J Med* 338: 1741–1751

71 Thaler SJ, Rubin RH (1996) Opportunistic infections in the cardiac transplant patient. *Curr Opin Cardiol* 11: 191–203

72 Yilmaz S, Koskinen PK, Kallio E, Bruggeman CA, Häyry PJ, Lemström KB (1996) Cytomegalovirus infection-enhanced chronic kidney allograft rejection is linked with intercellular adhesion molecule-1 expression. *Kidney Int* 50: 526–537

73 Mennander A, Tiisala S, Halttunen J, Yilmaz S, Paavonen T, Häyry P (1991) Chronic rejection in rat aortic allografts. An experimental model for transplant arteriosclerosis. *Arterioscler Thromb* 11: 671–680

74 Beigel A, Muller-Ruchholtz W (1984) Tracheal transplantation. II. Influence of genetic difference and degree of sensitization on reactions to the tracheal transplant. *Arch Otorhinolaryngol* 240: 217–225

75 Davreux CJ, Chu NH, Waddell TK, Mayer E, Patterson GA (1993) Improved tracheal allograft viability in immunosuppressed rats. *Ann Thorac Surg* 55: 131–134

76 Reidy MA, Clowes AW, Schwartz SM (1983) Endothelial regeneration. V. Inhibition of endothelial regrowth in arteries of rat and rabbit. *Lab Invest* 49: 569–575

77 Clowes AW, Karnowsky MJ (1977) Suppression by heparin of smooth muscle cell proliferation in injured arteries. *Nature* 265: 625–626
78 Clowes AW, Reidy MA, Clowes MM (1983) Kinetics of cellular proliferation after arterial injury. I. Smooth muscle growth in the absence of endothelium. *Lab Invest* 49: 27–333
79 Grunwald J, Haudenschild CC (1984) Intimal injury *in vivo* activates vascular smooth muscle cell migration and explant outgrowth *in vitro. Arteriosclerosis* 4: 183–188
80 Majack RA, Grieshaber NA, Cook CL, Weiser MC, McFall RC, Grieshaber SS, Reidy MA, Reilly CF (1996) Smooth muscle cells isolated from the neointima after vascular injury exhibit altered responses to platelet-derived growth factor and other stimuli. *J Cell Physiol* 167: 106–112
81 Iyer VR, Eisen MB, Ross DT, Schuler G, Moore T, Lee JCF, Trent JM, Staudt LM, Hudson J Jr, Boguski MS et al (1999) The transcriptional program in the response of human fibroblasts to serum. *Science* 283: 83–87
82 Eisen MB, Spellman PT, Brown PO, Botstein D (1998) Cluster analysis and display of genome-wide expression patterns. *Proc Natl Acad Sci USA* 95: 14 863–14 868
83 Raines EW, Ross R (1996) Multiple growth factors are associated with lesions of atherosclerosis: specificity or redundancy? *Bioessays* 18: 271–282
84 Jawien A, Bowen-Pope DF, Lindner V, Schwartz SM, Clowes AW (1992) Platelet-derived growth factor promotes smooth muscle migration and intimal thickening in a rat model of balloon angioplasty. *J Clin Invest* 89: 507–511
85 Ferns G, Raines E, Sprugel K, Motani A, Reidy M, Ross R (1991) Inhibition of neointimal smooth muscle accumulation after angioplasty by an antibody to PDGF. *Science* 253: 1129–1132
86 Rutherford C, Martin W, Salame M, Carrier M, Anggard E, Ferns G (1997) Substantial inhibition of neo-intimal response to balloon injury in the rat carotid artery using a combination of antibodies to platelet- derived growth factor-BB and basic fibroblast growth factor. *Atherosclerosis* 130: 45–51
87 Hart CE, Kraiss LW, Vergel S, Gilbertson D, Kenagy R, Kirkman T, Crandall DL, Tickle S, Finney H, Yarranton G et al (1999) PDGFbeta receptor blockade inhibits intimal hyperplasia in the baboon. *Circulation* 99: 564–569
88 Fukuda N, Kubo A, Watanabe Y, Nakayama T, Soma M, Izumi Y, Kanmatsuse K (1997) Antisense oligodeoxynucleotide complementary to platelet-derived growth factor A-chain messenger RNA inhibits the arterial proliferation in spontaneously hypertensive rats without altering their blood pressures. *J Hypertension* 15: 1123–1136
89 Sirois MG, Simons M, Edelman ER (1997) Antisense oligonucleotide inhibition of PDGFR-beta receptor subunit expression directs suppression of intimal thickening. *Circulation* 95: 669–676
90 Levitzki A (1996) Targeting signal transduction for disease therapy. *Curr Opin Cell Biol* 8: 239–244
91 Buchdunger E, Zimmermann J, Mett H, Meyer T, Muller M, Regenass U, Lydon NB (1995) Selective inhibition of the platelet-derived growth factor signal transduction pathway by a protein-tyrosine kinase inhibitor of the 2- phenylaminopyrimidine class. *Proc Natl Acad Sci USA* 92: 2558–2562
92 Myllärniemi M, Calderon L, Lemstrom K, Buchdunger E, Häyry P (1997) Inhibition of platelet-derived growth factor receptor tyrosine kinase inhibits vascular smooth muscle cell migration and proliferation. *FASEB J* 11: 1119–1126
93 Banai S, Wolf Y, Golomb G, Pearle A, Waltenberger J, Fishbein I, Schneider A, Gazit A, Perez L, Huber R et al (1998) PDGF-receptor tyrosine kinase blocker AG1295 selectively attenuates smooth muscle cell growth *in vitro* and reduces neointimal formation after balloon angioplasty in swine. *Circulation* 97: 1960–1969
94 Koskinen P, Sihvola R, Myllärniemi M, Häyry P, Buchdunger E, Lemström K (1999) Prevention of cardiac allograft arteriosclerosis by protein-tyrosine kinase inhibitor selective for platelet-derived growth factor receptor. *Transplant Proc* 31: 102
95 Sihvola R, Koskinen P, Myllärniemi M, Loubtchenkov M, Häyry P, Buchdunger E, Lemström K (1999) Prevention of cardiac allograft arteriosclerosis by protein tyrosine kinase inhibitor selective for platelet-derived growth factor receptor. *Circulation* 99: 2295–2301
96 Zempo N, Kenagy RD, Au YP, Bendeck M, Clowes MM, Reidy MA, Clowes AW (1994) Matrix metalloproteinases of vascular wall cells are increased in balloon-injured rat carotid artery. *J Vasc Surg* 20: 209–217
97 Rabinovitch M (1995) Elastase and cell matrix interactions in the pathobiology of vascular disease. *Acta Paediat Jpn* 37: 657–666

98 Bendeck M, Irvin C, Reidy M (1996) Inhibition of matrix metalloproteinase activity inhibits smooth muscle cell migration but not neointimal thickening after arterial injury. *Circ Res* 78: 38–43

99 Levi E, Fridman R, Miao HQ, Ma YS, Yayon A, Vlodavsky I (1996) Matrix metalloproteinase 2 releases active soluble ectodomain of fibroblast growth factor receptor 1. *Proc Natl Acad Sci USA* 93: 7069–7074

100 Baker AH, Zaltsman AB, George SJ, Newby AC (1998) Divergent effects of tissue inhibitor of metalloproteinase-1, -2, or -3 overexpression on rat vascular smooth muscle cell invasion, proliferation, and death *in vitro*. TIMP-3 promotes apoptosis. *J Clin Invest* 101: 1478–1487

101 Forough R, Lea H, Starcher B, Allaire E, Clowes M, Hasenstab D, Clowes AW (1998) Metalloproteinase blockade by local overexpression of TIMP-1 increases elastin accumulation in rat carotid artery intima. *Arterioscler Thromb Vasc Biol* 18: 803–807

102 Reichlin S (1983) Somatostatin. *N Engl J Med* 309: 1495–1501

103 Patel YC, Greenwood M, Panetta R, Hukovic N, Grigorakis S, Robertson LA, Srikant CB (1996) Molecular biology of somatostatin receptor subtypes. *Metabolism* 45: 31–38

104 Wahren J (1976) Influence of somatostatin on carbohydrate disposal and absorption in diabetes mellitus. *Lancet* 2: 1213–1216

105 Woltering EA, Barrie R, O'Dorisio TM, Arce D, Ure T, Cramer A, Holmes D, Robertson J, Fassler J (1991) Somatostatin analogues inhibit angiogenesis in the chick chorioallantoic membrane. *J Surg Res* 50: 245–251

106 Hong MK, Bhatti T, Matthews BJ, Stark KS, Cathapermal SS, Foegh ML, Ramwell PW, Kent KM (1993) The effect of porous infusion balloon-delivered angiopeptin on myointimal hyperplasia after balloon injury in the rabbit. *Circulation* 88: 638–648

107 Lindner V, Reidy MA (1991) Proliferation of smooth muscle cells after vascular injury is inhibited by an antibody against basic fibroblast growth factor. *Proc Natl Acad Sci USA* 88: 3739–3743

108 Grant MB, Wargovich TJ, Ellis EA, Caballero S, Mansour M, Pepine CJ (1994) Localization of insulin-like growth factor I and inhibition of coronary smooth muscle cell growth by somatostatin analogues in human coronary smooth muscle cells. A potential treatment for restenosis? *Circulation* 89: 1511–1517

109 Leszczynski D, Josephs MD, Fournier RS, Foegh ML (1993) Angiopeptin, the octapeptide analogue of somatostatin, decreases rat heart endothelial cell adhesiveness for mononuclear cells. *Regul Peptides* 43: 131–140

110 Foegh ML, Asotra S, Conte JV, Howell M, Kagan E, Verma K, Ramwell PW (1994) Early inhibition of myointimal proliferation by angiopeptin after balloon catheter injury in the rabbit. *J Vasc Surg* 19: 1084–1091

111 Foegh ML, Lou H, Chen MF, Ramwell PW (1997) Angiopeptin induces beneficial vascular remodeling after balloon injury. *Transplant Proc* 29: 2605–2608

112 Emanuelsson H, Beatt KJ, Bagger JP, Balcon R, Heikkila J, Piessens J, Schaeffer M, Suryapranata H, Foegh M (1995) Long-term effects of angiopeptin treatment in coronary angioplasty. Reduction of clinical events but not angiographic restenosis. European Angiopeptin Study Group. *Circulation* 91: 1689–1696

113 Eriksen UH, Amtorp O, Bagger JP, Emanuelsson H, Foegh M, Henningsen P, Saunamaki K, Schaeffer M, Thayssen P, Orskov H et al (1995) Randomized double-blind Scandinavian trial of angiopeptin *versus* placebo for the prevention of clinical events and restenosis after coronary balloon angioplasty. *Amer Heart J* 130: 1–8

114 Von Essen R, Ostermaier R, Grube E, Maurer W, Tebbe U, Erbel R, Roth M, Oel W, Brom J, Weidinger G (1997) Effects of octreotide treatment on restenosis after coronary angioplasty: results of the VERAS study. Verringerung der Restenoserate nach Angioplastie durch ein Somatostatin-analogon. *Circulation* 96: 1482–1487

115 Khare S, Kumar U, Sasi R, Puebla L, Calderon L, Lemström K, Häyry P, Patel AY (1999) Differential regulation of somatostatin receptor types 1–5 in rat aorta after angioplasty. *FASEB J* 13: 387–394

116 Grady D, Rubin SM, Petitti DB, Fox CS, Black D, Ettinger B, Ernster VL, Cummings SR (1992) Hormone therapy to prevent disease and prolong life in postmenopausal women. *Ann Intern Med* 117: 1016–1037

117 Stampfer MJ, Colditz GA, Willett WC, Manson JE, Rosner B, Speizer FE, Hennekens CH (1991) Postmenopausal estrogen therapy and cardiovascular disease. Ten-year follow-up from the nurs-

es' health study. *N Engl J Med* 325: 756–762
118 Wagner JD, Cefalu WT, Anthony MS, Litwak KN, Zhang L, Clarkson TB (1997) Dietary soy protein and estrogen replacement therapy improve cardiovascular risk factors and decrease aortic cholesteryl ester content in ovariectomized cynomolgus monkeys. *Metabolism* 46: 698–705
119 Foegh ML, Asotra S, Howell MH, Ramwell PW (1994) Estradiol inhibition of arterial neointimal hyperplasia after balloon injury. *J Vasc Surg* 19: 722–726
120 Chen SJ, Li H, Durand J, Oparil S, Chen YF (1996) Estrogen reduces myointimal proliferation after balloon injury of rat carotid artery. *Circulation* 93: 577–584
121 Sullivan TJ, Karas RH, Aronovitz M, Faller GT, Ziar JP, Smith JJ, O'Donnell TJ, Mendelsohn ME (1995) Estrogen inhibits the response-to-injury in a mouse carotid artery model. *J Clin Invest* 96: 2482–2488
122 Cheng LP, Kuwahara M, Jacobsson J, Foegh ML (1991) Inhibition of myointimal hyperplasia and macrophage infiltration by estradiol in aorta allografts. *Transplantation* 52: 967–972
123 Foegh ML, Khirabadi BS, Nakanishi T, Vargas R, Ramwell PW (1987) Estradiol protects against experimental cardiac transplant atherosclerosis. *Transplant Proc* 19 (4 Suppl 5): 90–95
124 Akishita M, Ouchi Y, Miyoshi H, Kozaki K, Inoue S, Ishikawa M, Eto M, Toba K, Orimo H (1997) Estrogen inhibits cuff-induced intimal thickening of rat femoral artery: effects on migration and proliferation of vascular smooth muscle cells. *Atherosclerosis* 130: 1–10
125 Kolodgie FD, Jacob A, Wilson PS, Carlson GC, Farb A, Verma A, Virmani R (1996) Estradiol attenuates directed migration of vascular smooth muscle cells *in vitro*. *Amer J Pathol* 148: 969–976
126 Morey AK, Pedram A, Razandi M, Prins BA, Hu RM, Biesiada E, Levin ER (1997) Estrogen and progesterone inhibit vascular smooth muscle proliferation. *Endocrinology* 138: 3330–3339
127 Suzuki A, Mizuno K, Ino Y, Okada M, Kikkawa F, Mizutani S, Tomoda Y (1996) Effects of 17 beta-estradiol and progesterone on growth-factor-induced proliferation and migration in human female aortic smooth muscle cells *in vitro*. *Cardiovasc Res* 32: 516–523
128 Balica M, Bostrom K, Shin V, Tillisch K, Demer LL (1997) Calcifying subpopulation of bovine aortic smooth muscle cells is responsive to 17 beta-estradiol. *Circulation* 95: 1954–1960
129 Bayard F, Clamens S, Delsol G, Blaes N, Maret A, Faye JC (1995) Oestrogen synthesis, oestrogen metabolism and functional oestrogen receptors in bovine aortic endothelial cells. *Ciba Found Symp* 191: 122–132
130 Bei M, Lavigne MC, Foegh ML, Ramwell PW, Clarke R (1996) Specific binding of estradiol to rat coronary artery smooth muscle cells. *J Steroid Biochem Mol Biol* 58: 83–88
131 Bhalla RC, Toth KF, Bhatty RA, Thompson LP, Sharma RV (1997) Estrogen reduces proliferation and agonist-induced calcium increase in coronary artery smooth muscle cells. *Amer J Physiol* 272: H1996-H2003
132 Karas RH, Baur WE, van EM, Mendelsohn ME (1995) Human vascular smooth muscle cells express an estrogen receptor isoform. *FEBS Lett* 377: 103–108
133 Venkov CD, Rankin AB, Vaughan DE (1996) Identification of authentic estrogen receptor in cultured endothelial cells. A potential mechanism for steroid hormone regulation of endothelial function. *Circulation* 94: 727–733
134 Caulin GT, Watson CA, Pardi R, Bender JR (1996) Effects of 17beta-estradiol on cytokine-induced endothelial cell adhesion molecule expression. *J Clin Invest* 98: 36–42
135 Spyridopoulos I, Sullivan AB, Kearney M, Isner JM, Losordo DW (1997) Estrogen-receptor-mediated inhibition of human endothelial cell apoptosis. Estradiol as a survival factor. *Circulation* 95: 1505–1514
136 Krasinski K, Spyridopoulos I, Asahara T, van der Zee R, Isner JM, Losordo DW (1997) Estradiol accelerates functional endothelial recovery after arterial injury. *Circulation* 95: 1768–1772
137 Farhat MY, Lavigne MC, Ramwell PW (1996) The vascular protective effects of estrogen. *FASEB J* 10: 615–624
138 Iafrati MD, Karas RH, Aronovitz M, Kim S, Sullivan TJ, Lubahn DB, O'Donnell TJ, Korach KS, Mendelsohn ME (1997) Estrogen inhibits the vascular injury response in estrogen receptor alpha-deficient mice. *Nat Med* 3: 545–548
139 Mäkelä S, Savolainen H, Aavik E, Strauss L, Rylander T, Kuiper G, Warner M, Gustafsson J, Häyry P (1999) Selective vasculoprotective effect of estrogen is mediated *via* estrogen receptor beta. *Proc Natl Acad Sci USA* 96: 7077–708
140 Karas RH, Hodgin JB, Kwoun M, Krege JH, Aronovitz M, Mackey W, Gustafsson JA, Korach KS, Smithies O, Mendelsohn ME (1999) Estrogen inhibits the vascular injury response in estro-

gen receptor beta deficient female mice. *Proc Natl Acad Sci USA* 96: 15 133–15 136

141 Häyry P, Myllärniemi M, Aavik E, Alatalo S, Aho P, Yilmaz S, AR-S, Cozzone G, Jameson BA, Baserga R (1995) Stabile D-peptide analog of insulin-like growth factor-1 inhibits smooth muscle cell proliferation after carotid ballooning injury in the rat. *FASEB J* 9: 1336–1344

142 Häyry P, Aavik E, Loubtchenkov M, Myllärniemi M, Koskinen P, Lemström K (1998) Problem of chronic rejection. *Graft* 1: 154–160

Modern Immunosuppressives
ed. by H.-J Schuurman, G. Feutren and J.-F. Bach
© 2001 Birkhäuser Verlag/Switzerland

Tolerance induction

Stuart J. Knechtle and Majed M. Hamawy

Department of Surgery, University of Wisconsin Medical School, 600 Highland Avenue, Madison, WI 53792-7375, USA

Introduction

Transplantation tolerance can be defined as immune unresponsiveness of a recipient toward the donor in the absence of ongoing therapy, yet maintenance of normal immune responsiveness toward other non-self antigens. The first observation of an animal immunologically tolerant to cells of another individual was made by Owen [1] in studying blood group chimerism which he noted in dizygotic cattle twins (Fig. 1). He explained the stable presence of two blood groups in each twin based on the knowledge that they shared common placental circulation *in utero* (Fig. 2). In other words, the exposure of one twin to the other's different blood group during fetal life had led to persistence of these blood group progenitors into adult life and hence immunologic tolerance of the other's blood group antigens. This seminal observation formed the first building block in our understanding of transplantation tolerance.

Billingham, Brent, and Medawar [2] extended this observation by experimentally exposing neonatal mice to allogeneic lymphoid cells followed a month later by skin grafting from the donor strain mice. This resulted in acceptance of skin grafts for more than 100 days. Because humans and large animals are phylogenetically more advanced in their neonatal period than mice, this experiment could not be duplicated in either. Nevertheless, the studies by the Medawar group spawned an enormous interest in transplantation tolerance.

Explanation of how an individual's immune system avoids attacking itself remains poorly answered despite extensive work and publications in immunology. It is, therefore, not surprising that a reliable means of inducing transplantation tolerance is not yet available for clinical organ transplantation. However, considerable progress is being made in this area currently. Several examples of clinical transplantation tolerance have been achieved, although they tend to be isolated rare cases. Some of these are enumerated below. New strategies with success in non-human primates have been developed and will be summarized below. First, however, principles learned from basic immunology regarding tolerance induction will be summarized, and parallels in clinical transplant tolerance will be noted as correlates of these principles.

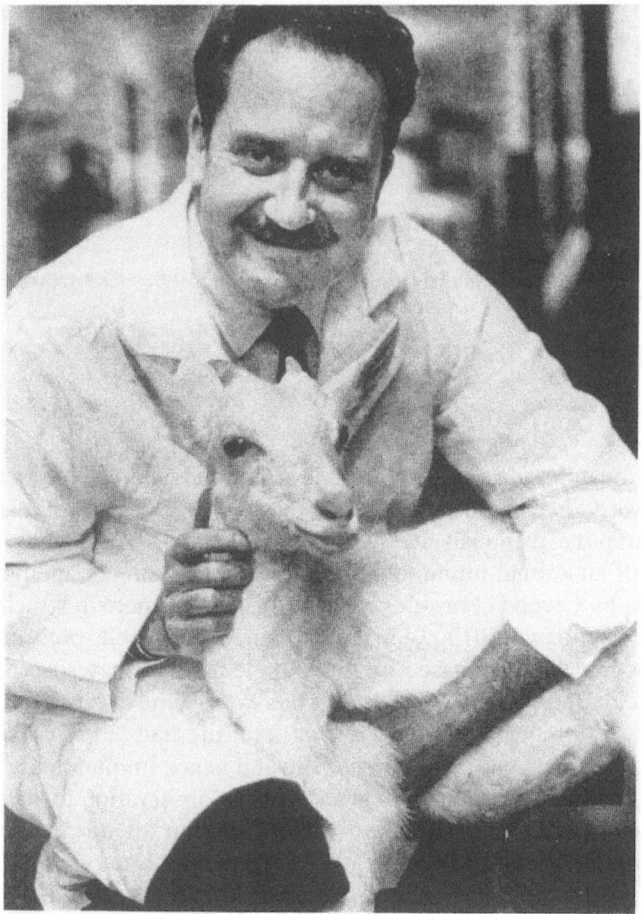

Figure 1. Ray Owen as an assistant professor of genetics at the University of Wisconsin, WI, USA.

Conditions favoring tolerance induction

State of lymphoid system

In experimental animal systems it is easier to induce tolerance with an immature lymphoid system (e.g., neonatal mice) or in a lymphoid system that has
been damaged by irradiation, antilymphocyte therapy, or immunologic senescence (advanced age). To induce tolerance in a fully mature immunorespon-
sive adult, either the animal's immune competence has to be impaired by treatment, or the antigen has to be administered in a nonimmunogenic form or by
a nonimmunizing route. Clinical correlates of this experimental observation
are that tolerance has been induced in a handful of patients treated with total

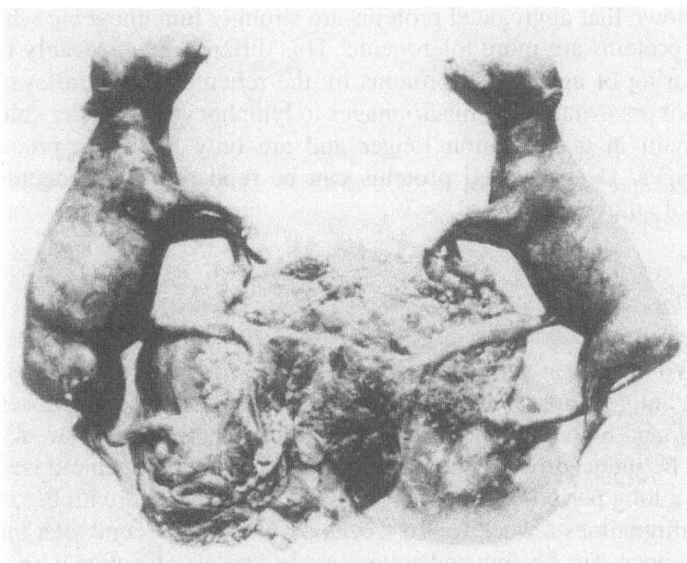

Figure 2. Dizygotic cattle twins fused at the placentae. Fusion of the placentae leads to exchange of blood cells in fetal life. Following separation, each animal permanently retains the cells of its twin. Although they are genetically different (dizygotic), each twin is permanently tolerant of the other's tissue type. (From Miller JFAP (1993) Immunological tolerance. In: IM Roitt, J Brostoff, DK Male (eds) *Immunology*, Third Edition. Mosby-Year Book Europe Limited, London, 10.1–10.10.)

lymphoid irradiation prior to renal transplantation. When antigen presentation (i.e., kidney transplantation) occurred during temporary impairment of the immune system, tolerance toward the graft developed despite later recovery of the immune system and regaining of immunocompetence [3]. Another clinical correlate is that allograft rejection is relatively less intense in frequency and severity in older patients compared to younger patients due to immunologic senescence impairing the vigor of the immune response [4].

Physicochemical properties of the antigen

The size of an antigen, whether it is monomeric or divalent, whether it is membrane-bound on a cell surface or soluble, are all factors that influence the immune response to an antigen. The type of organ transplanted influences the nature of the major histocompatibility complex (MHC) antigen associated with the graft. For instance, liver transplants are known to release a far larger amount of soluble MHC class I antigen than kidney or heart transplants [5]. This reflects a different route of MHC class I synthesis by hepatocytes [6]. Also, MHC antigens released by necrotic cells which have experienced preservation injury are different from MHC antigen recognized on viable donor cells.

It is known that aggregated proteins are strongly immunogenic while deaggregated proteins are more tolerogenic. This difference is probably related to rapid clearing of aggregated proteins by the reticuloendothelial system with subsequent presentation by macrophages to lymphocytes. Smaller soluble proteins remain in a circulation longer and are only gradually processed by macrophages. Deaggregated proteins can be rendered immunogenic by the addition of adjuvant [7].

Antigen dose

It is known that when antigen is injected over a wide range of concentrations, that low antigen doses often induce tolerance, intermediate doses induce immunity, and high antigen doses induce tolerance. So-called low-zone tolerance can be induced by frequent injection of nonimmunogenic doses of antigen over a long period of time. For instance, mice injected with bovine serum albumin three times a week for 16 weeks developed low-zone tolerance. Low-zone tolerance can be induced with a wide variety of antigens in newborn mice, whereas in adults only a few antigens work. Treatment of adults with irradiation or thymectomy renders adults more susceptible to low-zone tolerance. T-cells are apparently more susceptible to tolerization by low antigen doses than are B-cells [7].

A correlate of this principle in experimental transplantation is the observation that rat liver transplants are tolerated in strain combinations that would reject a liver or kidney transplant. When four simultaneous heart transplants are performed in the same strain combinations, they are tolerated presumably due to their larger load of donor antigen. This example of high-zone tolerance has a correlate in human transplantation in that liver transplants are less susceptible to rejection, and rejection is more easily reversed compared to pancreas, kidney, heart, or lung transplants. The mass of the liver is relatively great compared to these other organs. The principle of high-zone tolerance may, at least in part, account for these differences (Fig. 3) [8].

Route of antigen presentation

It is known from experimental transplantation that intradermal or subcutaneous injection of antigen is more immunogenic than intravenous injection of antigen. Still less immunogenic is portal vein injection of antigen. These differences are in part explained by the accessibility of antigen to macrophages. Macrophage-bound antigen is highly immunogenic. For instance, 1/1000th as much macrophage-bound bovine serum albumin as unbound antigen is required to immunize a mouse. Portal vein injection of donor blood cells, bone marrow cells, and islet cells has been used in experimental transplantation models to favor tolerance *versus* immunity. Similarly, donor blood transfu-

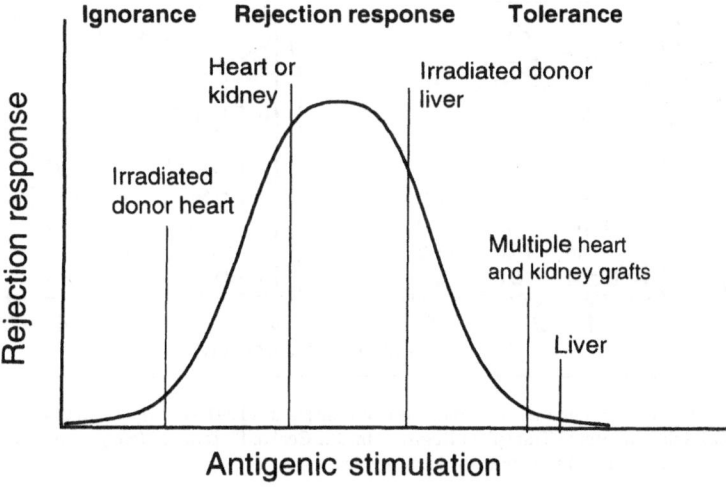

Figure 3. A proposed stimulus-response curve for transplanted organs showing high-dose tolerance. Increasing the antigenic stimulation increases the rejection response up to a point. Further increases in antigenic stimulation lead to overstimulation of the immune response, resulting in clonal exhaustion and a decreased rejection response. (From [8].)

sions by the intravenous route have been used to promote unresponsiveness. However, the relative advantage of donor-specific blood transfusions has been overshadowed by more potent strategies to induce tolerance [9].

Genetic constitution of the recipient

In experimental models, it has been observed that some MHC allotypes are strong stimulators of immunity while others are weak stimulators. Similarly, some MHC allotypes are strong responders while others are weak responders. While these differences have been clearly defined in inbred rodent strains, such differences have not been defined in outbred populations of large animals or humans. Clinical analogies to this experimental observation are that black recipients of organ transplants are relatively high responders, white recipients are intermediate, and Asian recipients are relatively low responders (Fig. 4) [4]. These differences hold true despite similar numbers of mismatched human leukocyte antigens (HLA) loci between donor and recipient. It has also been observed that donor-recipient pairs with only one HLA mismatch or even zero mismatch may undergo vigorous rejection responses. In fact, the relative advantages of better MHC matching in human renal allotransplantation have been difficult to observe, requiring very large cohorts of patients to even demonstrate a difference according to degree of matching. While this may be in part attributed to the multifactorial nature of the alloimmune response, it also speaks to the genetic heterogeneity of the alloimmune response in humans.

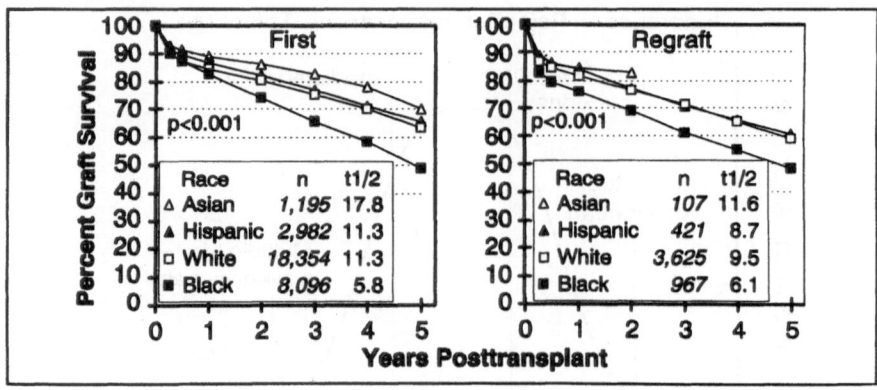

Figure 4. Effect of recipient race on cadaver donor transplants (1991–1995). (From Cecka JM (1997) The UNOS Scientific Renal Transplant Registry. In: JM Cecka, PI Terasaki (eds) *Clinical Transplants 1996*. UCLA Tissue Typing Laboratory, Los Angeles, 1-14.)

The nature of transplantation tolerance

Split tolerance

Tolerization of T-lymphocytes may require a different strategy than that of B-lymphocytes. For instance, mice inoculated with human gamma globulin develop B-cell tolerance following injection of a low dose of gamma globulin (1 to 10 mg), whereas T-cell tolerance in this model requires a higher dose (10 mg) of tolerogen [10]. An experimental analogy is that monkeys whose T-lymphocytes are rendered tolerant to renal allografts by immunotoxin (as demonstrated by subsequent acceptance of donor, but not third-party skin grafts; and suppression of donor, but not third-party mixed lymphocyte reaction (MLR) and cytotoxic T-lymphocyte (CTL) responses) may still produce alloantibody to the allograft. Such T-cell (but not B-cell) tolerance may permit long-term stable allograft function in some but not all cases (Tab. 1) [11]. The role of B-cell immunity in the absence of T-cell mediated rejection may be substantial in the etiology of chronic allograft rejection. Therefore, classical T-cell tolerance alone may not be sufficient to induce indefinite graft survival.

Robustness of tolerance

As mentioned above, animals tolerant of an allograft may produce antibody to the donor. When tolerance is measured simultaneously by several parameters, it may be present by one assay but not according to another. Split tolerance may occur with regard to T- *versus* B-cells, but also with regard to different immunoglobulin classes (i.e., suppression of some isotypes but not others). Tolerance may not be maintained indefinitely, but rather may be transient. The

Table 1. Alloreactive antibody and graft outcome in immunotoxin-treated monkeys

Animal	GST	Test[†]	ABX[‡]	ACC[§]	Outcome
AXF	51	51	1.3	ND	Creatinine < 2.0 mg/dl
1347	57	57	2.3	ND	IN
AXG	184	110	0.9	1	CR
WF6	287	98	6.3	243	CR
AKJ	133	133	1.2	1	CR
AXA	172	118	8.4	81	CR
XV3	307	120	1	1	CR
BED	630	125	2.5	>729	CR
2CP	435	120	1.6	1	CR
DFW	105	105	2.9	1	IN
EEF	>1441	112	0.8	1	Creatinine < 2.0 mg/dL

GST, graft survival time; ACC, antibody complement cytotoxicity; ABX, antibody crossmatch; IN, chronic interstitial nephritis; CR, chronic rejection; ND, not determined.
[†] Days after transplant from which sera were tested.
[‡] Ratio of the mean channel fluorescence of post-transplantation anti-human IgG reactive serum (1:100 dilution) binding to donor $CD3^+$ lymphocytes to the mean channel fluorescence of pretransplantation anti-human IgG reactive serum (1:100 dilution) binding to donor $CD3^+$ lymphocytes.
[§] Reciprocal end point titer of antibody complement cytotoxicity assay.
From [11].

continued presence of tolerogen may be an important requirement for the maintenance of tolerance. Exogenous factors may perturb the immune system such as infection, inflammation, or an experimentally added immunogen (immunization or vaccination). A powerful immunogen such as a skin graft may be able to break tolerance in a situation where it has already been demonstrated to be present [12]. Cross-reactive antigens may also break tolerance. For instance, when thyroglobulin of one species is injected to an animal of another species, the latter produces antibodies to epitopes shared by the two thyroglobulins and thus produces an autoimmune antibody response.

Mechanisms of tolerance

Hematopoietic chimerism

Animals undergoing successful bone marrow transplantation from allogeneic donors become hematopoietic chimeras. This implies persistence of detectable levels of donor bone marrow-derived elements in their peripheral blood. Stable hematopoietic chimeras such as this are examples of central or deletional tolerance. This experimental situation requires myeloablative regimens to deplete the host alloreactive lymphocytes. Following recovery and reconstitution of the host immune repertoire, donor-reactive clones are deleted in the thymus, permitting persistence of donor hematopoietic cells. This strategy has allowed successful allotransplantation of solid organs derived from the blood donor or genetically identical donor. Hematopoietic chimerism has been used effectively in rodents as well as large animal models to produce a robust form of tolerance to renal and cardiac allografts [13].

Immune deviation

All forms of tolerance other than that described above as central tolerance can be described as peripheral tolerance. Peripheral tolerance implies that the mechanism of tolerance occurs extrathymically by means other than depletion of donor-reactive clones from the host's immune repertoire. One of these forms of peripheral tolerance has been called immune deviation and refers to cytokine-mediated switching of the immune response to antigen from a T-helper-1-type (Th1) response to a T-helper-2-type (Th2) response. The Th1 response has been associated with interleukin-2 (IL-2) and interferon-γ elaboration by T helper cells, whereas the Th2 response is associated with IL-4 and IL-10 elaboration. In other words, the variables described above may combine in the same host to result in a Th2 rather than Th1 response. A Th2 response may favor unresponsiveness compared to a Th1 response which generally favors immunity. This is no doubt an oversimplification of the complex events surrounding T helper cell activation, although it has examples in experimental work. Until the complex cytokine pathways are better understood, this model will remain a useful standard [14].

Exhaustive immunization

Immune responsiveness induced by clonal exhaustion has been described for T-cell independent antigens. For instance, the antigen challenge may be so massive that all B-cells capable of recognizing the immunizing antigen differentiate to end-stage antibody-producing cells without generating memory cells. This results in no memory and no response to subsequent challenges with the same antigen.

Immune regulation

Immune regulation has replaced the term suppression to refer to the development of T-lymphocytes that actively down-regulate the immune response to antigen. The term suppressor T-cells has lost favor due to the lack of phenotypic correlation between such cells and lymphocyte surface markers. Nevertheless, in experimental models, populations of lymphocytes with specific down-regulatory function can be identified and may account for tolerance [15].

Anergy

Following engagement of the T-cell receptor by MHC antigen (first signal), a costimulatory or second signal is required for optimal T-cell activation. Furthermore, in the absence of this second signal, the T-cell enters an anergic state which may ultimately lead to apoptotic cell death. Pathways of costimulation include interaction between CD28 on a T-cell and B7-1 or B7-2 on the antigen-presenting cell. Conversely, interaction between CTLA4 on T-cells and B7 leads to inactivation. Another important costimulatory pathway is the interaction between CD40 ligand (CD154) on the T-cell and CD40 on the antigen-presenting cell. Blockade of these costimulatory pathways with either fusion protein CTLA4-Ig, anti-CD154 T antibody, or anti-B7 T antibody strategies has been shown to prolong allograft survival [16]. In addition, ongoing rejection may be reversed by such blockade (Fig. 5). These data suggest that costimulation is required for the induction and maintenance of a rejection response and that costimulation blockade may effectively promote unresponsiveness. Whether long-term tolerance can be induced by this strategy in large animals remains to be determined.

Strategies for tolerance induction in human organ transplantation

Total lymphoid irradiation

Total lymphoid irradiation (TLI) was originally used to treat Hodgkin's disease patients because of the potent cytotoxic effect of γ-irradiation on lymphocytes. Patients successfully treated for Hodgkin's disease following TLI were noted to have an inverted ratio of $CD4^+$ over $CD8^+$ lymphocytes (1:2 instead of the normal 2:1 ratio). The potential benefit of TLI as an immunosuppressive therapy in organ transplantation was then evaluated. Twenty-four patients were treated at Stanford University in the United States and in South Africa and were reported in 1989 [3]. Three of the 24 patients were successfully taken off immunosuppressive therapy for 10, 24, and 69 months, respectively, with stable graft function. All of the patients had HLA-mismatched grafts. At the time of the report, the grafts had survived for a total of 47, 55, and 94 months, respectively. While two of these patients ultimately lost their grafts due to technical reasons or to rejection, one patient remains off dialysis more than 10 years later (S. Strober, personal communication, 1998) demonstrating the principle that tolerance to an allogeneic renal allograft may occur in humans. Furthermore, it would appear that TLI in a small proportion of patients is able to effectively promote the development of tolerance.

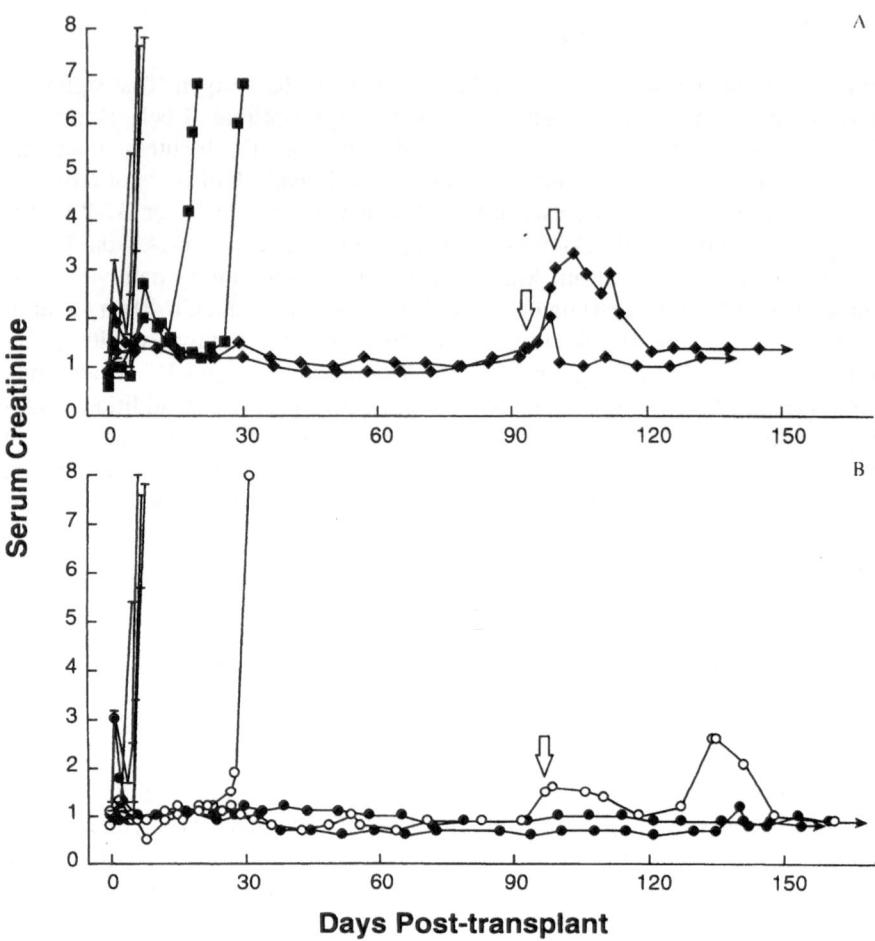

Figure 5. (A) Survival and renal function as determined by serum creatinine following unmodified allogeneic renal transplantation (–) or transplantation following induction with CTLA4-Ig alone (■) or anti-CD154 antibody 5C8 alone (◆). Open arrows indicate retreatment during biopsy-proven rejection. Solid arrows indicate continued survival. (B) Survival and renal function as determined by serum creatinine following unmodified allogeneic renal transplantation (–) or transplantation following induction with both CTLA4-Ig and 5C8. ○ indicate treatment on days 0, 2, 4, 6, 8, 10, and 12 posttransplant. ● indicate treatment on days 0, 2, 4, 6, 8, 12, 16, and 28 posttransplant. Open arrows indicate retreatment during biopsy-proven rejection for the animal depicted in ○. Solid arrows indicate continued survival free of rejection since transplantation. (From Kirk AD, Harlan DM, Armstrong NN et al. (1997) CTLA4-Ig and anti-CD40 ligand prevent renal allograft rejection in primates. *Proc Natl Acad Sci USA* 94: 8789–8794.)

Withdrawal of immunosuppression

An intriguing systematic study of withdrawal of immunosuppressive therapy from human liver transplant recipients was reported by Mazariegos et al. from the University of Pittsburgh [17]. Based on the observation that five liver transplant patients who had discontinued immunosuppression nevertheless avoided rejection, 95 liver transplant patients were prospectively withdrawn from immunosuppressive therapy. Criteria for study entry included compliance with immunosuppressive therapy, stable graft function for at least 2 years without rejection, at least 5 years post-transplantation, absence of acute or chronic rejection on a baseline liver biopsy, and exclusion of other diagnoses such as vascular or biliary tract complications or recurrence of original disease. The baseline immunosuppression in these patients comprised various combinations of azathioprine, prednisone, cyclosporine, and tacrolimus. Eighteen of the 95 patients in the prospective cohort were maintained off drugs for 8 months to 4.8 years. Another 18 patients developed rejection during weaning and had to return to immunosuppressive therapy. Twelve patients were withdrawn from the study due to noncompliance ($n = 8$), pregnancy ($n = 1$), renal failure requiring kidney transplantation ($n = 1$), and recurrence of primary biliary cirrhosis ($n = 2$). Patients originally on azathioprine, prednisone or on tacrolimus-based therapy were slightly more successful in coming off therapy than patients on cyclosporine-based therapy. The authors concluded that withdrawal of immunosuppression in such a trial should be done very slowly rather than abruptly as had been done at the beginning of the trial. The risk of recurrent autoimmune disease was also noted and caution advised in withdrawing such patients from immunosuppression. It should also be noted that although 18 patients were successfully withdrawn from immunosuppression in this study, they represent a small numerator in comparison to the large denominator of liver transplants performed at the University of Pittsburgh.

Microchimerism in a tolerant renal transplant patient

A single kidney transplant patient was studied in detail by Burlingham et al. [18] when it was noted that this patient had discontinued immunosuppressive therapy on his own by noncompliance, but maintained stable graft function. This patient had received a donor-specific blood transfusion from his mother under azathioprine coverage prior to receiving a haplo-identical living-related renal transplant. Initial postoperative immunosuppression consisted of cyclosporine, azathioprine and prednisone, but these were discontinued at 1 year post-transplantation. The patient continued to have excellent graft function while being off all immunosuppressive therapy for 8 years. Analysis of his peripheral blood post-transplantation demonstrated that it contained anergic $CD8^+$ cytotoxic lymphocytes and rare (approximately 1 in 10 000) inhibitory cells of donor origin. These donor cells were capable of suppressing recipient's CTL responses to donor lymphocytes even at this low frequency. Unfortunately, despite stable graft function for 8 years, this patient progressed to chronic rejection and returned to dialysis 8 years later. This example again raises the question of the durability of transplant tolerance and whether T-cell tolerance is adequate to prevent chronic rejection mediated by other pathways.

Non-inherited maternal HLA antigens

Burlingham et al. [19] retrospectively studied graft survival and rejection episodes in 205 patients undergoing living-related kidney transplantation from sibling donors bearing either maternal or paternal HLA antigens not inherited by the recipient. The donors mismatched for one HLA haplotype expressed either maternal (NIMA) or paternal (NIPA) HLA antigens not inherited by the recipient. Graft survival was higher 5 and 10 years after transplantation in recipients of kidneys from siblings expressing NIMA HLA antigens than in recipients of kidneys from siblings expressing NIPA HLA antigens. There was a higher incidence of early rejection in the recipients of kidneys from siblings expressing NIMA, suggesting that fetal and neonatal exposure to maternal antigens results in immunologic priming. Pretransplant donor-specific blood transfusions reduce the incidence of acute rejection and preserve the beneficial effect of tolerance to NIMA on graft survival. Although new immunosuppressive drugs have lessened the long-term survival advantage of grafts expressing NIMA, the long-term advantage remains just as great in the cyclosporine era. Interestingly, grafts from sibling donors expressing NIMA had equivalent survival to HLA-identical sibling donor grafts in this study of 205 patients (Fig. 6). These data are reminiscent of the findings of Owen which suggested that antigen exposure *in utero* was critical for tolerance induction. In this case, the beneficial effect of blood transfusions on kidney transplant survival was shown to be directly dependent on *in utero* exposure to noninherited antigen.

Anti-CD52

The potent antileukocyte antibody, CAMPATH-1H (humanized anti-CD52, H. Waldmann) has been used clinically as an induction strategy in human renal transplant recipients [20]. Two doses of the antibody were given, on day 0 and day 1. Low-dose cyclosporine and prednisone were given in a manner to maintain cyclosporine levels roughly half of the target concentration that is normally recommended. Only two patients had rejection episodes, on day 35 and day 60, with the former patient being switched to prednisone and azathioprine after the rejection episode. Despite profound depletion of circulating lymphocytes, all patients have recovered between 2 and 6 months postoperatively without any lymphoproliferative disorder or serious infections. These intriguing early results await further trials to evaluate the potential role of severe transient lymphocyte depletion in humans as a strategy to induce tolerance to solid

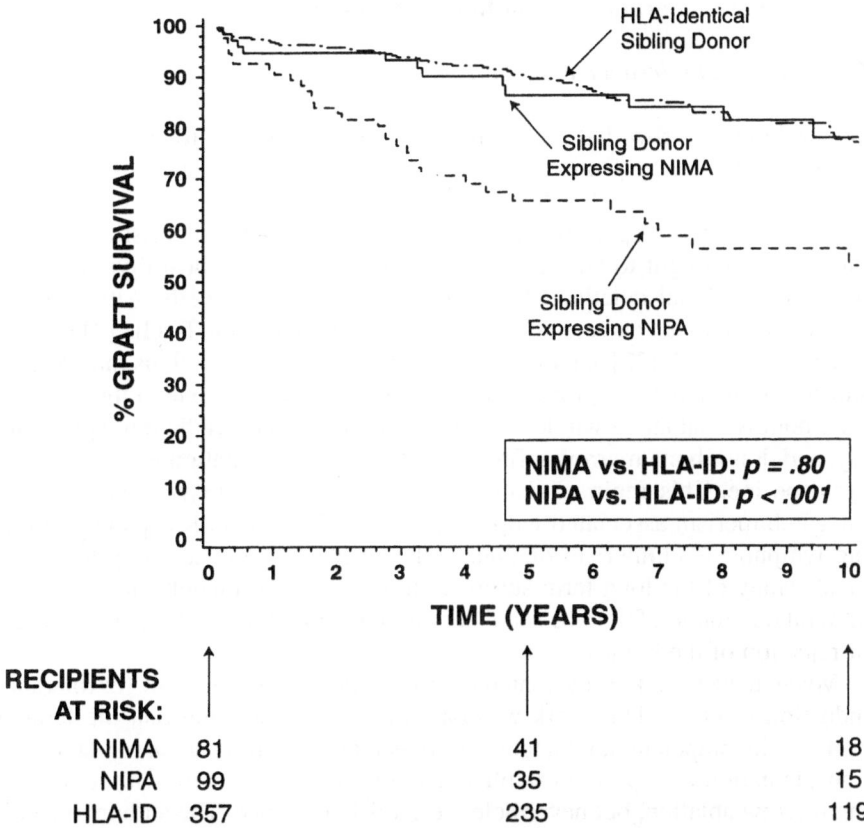

Figure 6: Graft survival in recipients of kidney transplants from HLA-identical sibling donors and sibling donors mismatched for one HLA haplotype. Transplants were performed at the five Pacific Northwest Centers, the University of Wisconsin Hospital, and the University of Leiden Hospital. The donors mismatched for one HLA haplotype expressed either maternal (NIMA) or paternal (NIPA) HLA antigens not inherited by the recipient. The results in a concurrent series of transplants from HLA-identical sibling donors at the same centers are shown for comparison. The numbers below the graph indicate the numbers of recipients at risk for graft loss at the time of transplantation (0) and 5 and 10 years thereafter. (From [19])

organ transplants. The anti-CD52 antibody differs from OKT3 (Ortho, Raritan, NJ) in that the latter is restricted to $CD3^+$ T-cells and depletes peripheral blood T-cells transiently. OKT3 has not been shown to induce tolerance in humans.

Experimental tolerance in non-human primates

Chimerism and tolerance induction

Donor bone marrow has been used by several groups to achieve mixed chimerism tolerance. Donor bone marrow-derived chimerism requires T-cell depletion of the recipient and partial or complete ablation of the recipient lympho-hematopoietic repertoire. The mechanism by which chimerism maintains tolerance is thought to be migration of donor cells to the host thymus where they induce clonal deletion of developing alloreactive T-cells. Alternatively, donor cells may act as veto cells by eliminating anti-donor T-cells [21].

Kimikawa et al. [22] achieved mixed chimerism in cynomolgus monkeys by subjecting the animals before transplantation to antithymocyte globulin injection, nonmyeloablative whole body irradiation, thymic irradiation, splenectomy, and donor bone marrow infusion, and after transplantation to therapy with cyclosporine. This regimen depleted most donor lymphocytes and induced mixed chimerism associated with long-term graft survival. Recipients achieving lymphocyte chimerism of greater than 1.5% experienced long-term survival. Many of the long-term survivors in this study ultimately succumbed to ureteral obstruction felt to be secondary to rejection of the ureter in the absence of rejection of the kidney.

Mychaliska et al. [23] evaluated the role of donor bone marrow for tolerance induction *in utero*. This work was based on the observation that the fetus is immuno-incompetent and unable to reject an allograft. *In utero* stem-cell transplantation may permit establishment of a hematochimera without requiring marrow ablation, but nevertheless establish tolerance. The authors injected T-cell-depleted paternal bone marrow *in utero* into the peritoneal cavity of female fetal rhesus monkeys at 61 days of gestation. Engraftment of less than 1% of donor cells was detectable by PCR assay for the rhesus Y chromosome, showing paternal bone marrow in the bone marrow of female recipients. Chimerism was detected in the newborn infants as early as 6 weeks of age and until 2 years of age. Two chimeric female monkeys, aged 2 and 3 years, underwent renal transplantation from paternal donors. Chimeric recipients had prolonged graft survival compared to controls, without evidence of rejection for 7 weeks post-transplantation. However, biopsies performed 1 to 4 weeks post-transplant showed evidence of moderate acute rejection. In parallel, *in vitro* MLR testing showed reduced MLR responses of recipient lymphocytes to donor cells compared to MLR responses to third-party cells [23].

Sablinski et al. [24] reported on the use of donor bone marrow in prolonging pig-to-primate kidney xenograft survival. Sublethal whole-body irradiation, antithymocyte globulin, and thymic irradiation were used as induction therapy prior to infusion of porcine bone marrow at the time of renal transplantation. Recipients were splenectomized and anti-pig natural antibodies removed using perfusion of the monkeys' blood through a pig liver or by using an anti-Gal-α(1,3)-Gal adsorption column. Post-transplantation the recipients received deoxyspergualin (DSG) and cyclosporine for 14 days. Seven of 11 monkeys survived more than 6 days in contrast to untreated animals that hyperacutely rejected the xenografts within hours. The role of mixed chimerism in maintaining graft survival was unclear as pig lymphocytes in peripheral blood of monkeys was demonstrable in only one monkey.

Costimulation blockade to prolong allograft survival

Engagement of the T-cell receptor by MHC antigen is a necessary and sufficient signal to activate T-cells. However, optimal proliferation and cytokine release occurs only after engagement of other costimulatory molecules on T-cells [25]. Engagement of the costimulatory molecules and their ligands initiates important intracellular signaling pathways in T-lymphocytes. Blockade of these costimulatory molecules has been viewed as a strategy to design therapeutic regimens to prevent allograft rejection [26]. The number of these costimulatory molecules described is increasing and their roles continue to be more accurately defined. Two of these molecules, CD28 and CD154 are discussed below.

CD28 is expressed mainly on T-cells [27] and binds B7.1 and B7.2 on antigen-presenting cells. CD154 (also known previously as CD40 ligand or gp39) is expressed on T-cells, B-cells, platelets, mast cells, and basophils [28, 29]. CD28 and CD154 functionally interact in that activation of one molecule augments the function of the other. For instance, T-cell activation increases expression of CD154 on T-cells. Enhanced CD154-CD40 interaction increases the expression of B7 molecules on antigen-presenting cells. This in turn enables increased engagement by antigen-presenting cells of CD28 on T-cells. This in turn augments TCR signaling with enhanced T-cell proliferation and cytokine elaboration. In rodent transplantation models involving skin, kidney and heart, blockade of the CD28-B7 and the CD154-CD40 interactions has been shown to substantially prolong allograft survival [30, 31].

The utility of blocking the CD28-B7 and the CD154-CD40 interactions in non-human primate renal allografts was examined by Kirk et al. [32]. Untreated control renal allografts in this model reject at 7 days. Monkeys receiving the B7 antagonistic fusion protein (CTLA4-Ig) alone had graft survival prolonged to 30 days. Animals treated with anti-CD154 monoclonal antibody (5C8, Biogen, Cambridge, MA) had rejection-free survival for 95 to 100 days. Kidney transplant biopsies at the time of rejection demonstrated acute cellular rejection. When two rejecting animals were retreated with 5C8, graft function returned to normal. This result suggests that the CD154-CD40 interaction is not only necessary for initiation of T-cell-mediated rejection, but also is necessary for maintaining a rejection response. The addition of CTLA4-Ig to 5C8 therapy did not provide a substantial benefit to treatment with 5C8 alone as had been reported in rodents, although this observation may be dependent on antibody dose levels. Interestingly, monkeys with stable renal allograft function following 5C8 and/or CTLA4-Ig treatment maintained a vigorous anti-donor MLR response, as well as MLR response to third-party cells. Presumably, this observation is related to differences between *in vivo* alloactivation and *in vitro* MLR responses. Because of the presence of CD154 on cells other than T-cells as noted above, blockade of the CD154-CD40 interaction may modulate the function of cells other than T-cells and, in this way, promote allograft survival. Continuing studies of anti-CD154 antibodies have suggested that addition of calcineurin inhibitors may decrease their efficacy in preventing rejection.

Anti-CD4 and toxin-conjugated anti-CD3 monoclonal antibodies

CD4 is expressed on the surface of T-lymphocytes and binds to MHC class II molecules on antigen-presenting cells. The cytoplasmic portion of CD4 associates with the protein tyrosine kinase $p56^{lck}$ [33]. The role of CD4 blockade on renal allograft survival was evaluated by Mourad et al. in cynomolgus monkeys [34]. Humanized anti-CD4 monoclonal antibodies were constructed based on a murine anti-human CD4, one as an IgG1 and the other as an IgG4. The IgG1 isotype caused marked depletion of $CD4^+$ lymphocytes from peripheral blood and lymph node. The IgG1 isotype was non-depleting, but both antibodies coated $CD4^+$ T-cells and both prolonged survival of cynomolgus monkey renal allografts. This is consistent with rodent data by Wood et al. [35] showing that depletion of $CD4^+$ T-cells is not necessary for the beneficial effect of CD4 blockade in prolonging graft survival. The efficacy of nondepleting anti-CD4 monoclonal antibodies may relate to their ability to block or modulate the CD4 molecule, hence interfering with effective TCR binding to the MHC-peptide complex or by influencing the role of $p56^{lck}$ in TCR signaling.

Krieger et al. [36] examined the combined use of anti-CD4 polyclonal antibodies affecting cardiac allograft survival in rhesus monkeys. Two monkeys had graft survival prolonged to 42 and 52 days. Again, untreated controls rejected in 7 days. A single dose of anti-CD4 antibody was unable to induce long-term survival, but prolonged administration of anti-CD4 maintained cardiac allograft survival until the antibody was cleared from peripheral blood. The CD4 antibody used resulted in complete depletion of $CD4^+$ cells 1 day after administration.

Neville et al. [37] developed a potent T-cell depleting agent by coupling a diphtheria toxin binding site mutant, CRM9, to a murine antibody recognizing rhesus monkey CD3. Our laboratory first evaluated this construct in a rhesus monkey renal allograft model using the immunotoxin (IT) to deplete T-cells pre-transplantation. MHC class I and class II mismatched donor-recipient pairs were selected, and untreated controls rejected in 7 days. When IT was administered at a total dose of 0.2 mg/kg in three divided daily doses beginning 1 week prior to transplantation, most monkeys had indefinite graft survival with no additional treatment. Most IT-treated monkeys accepted donor skin grafts for at least 100 days while rejecting third-party skin grafts in less than 2 weeks. There was no evidence of fever, rash, diarrhea, or respiratory difficulty in IT-treated animals. However, wasting was seen in three monkeys, characterized by progressive weight loss and appetite loss despite normal liver and renal function. IT-treated animals retained the ability to mount a T-cell dependent immune response despite the sharp decrease in $CD3^+$ cells. Within 1 to 3 months, most monkeys produced antibodies to tetanus, diphtheria, and the murine components of IT. Alloantibody also developed in most tested monkeys including complement-fixing antibody, but the presence of these antibodies did not correlate with allograft function.

In a subsequent series of experiments administering IT on day 0, long-term tolerance was not as reliably induced and most animals succumbed to either acute or chronic rejection, or to interstitial nephritis between 50 and 150 days post-transplantation. Chronic rejection was typified by hyalinization of glomeruli with reduplication of the glomerular capillary basement membrane, vasculopathy with neointimal hyperplasia, and interstitial fibrosis. The histologic picture was reminiscent of chronic rejection seen in human renal allografts. Interstitial nephritis occurred in some recipients in the absence of rejection that was typified by interstitial infiltrates scattered throughout the graft and the absence of tubular or glomerular injury. Presumably dysfunction was caused by interstitial edema resulting in compromised capillary blood flow to the kidney and ischemic injury [11].

Thomas et al. also evaluated the IT developed by Neville in a rhesus monkey model but using different protocols. Donor bone marrow depleted of mature antigen-presenting cells and T-cells was injected on day 0 with IT and prolonged graft survival for at least 120 days [38]. A lower dose (0.16 mg/kg total) was administered, and in this study IT alone did not induce long-term graft survival. Although chimerism was observed in all IT-treated animals, including those that did not receive donor bone marrow, the level of chimerism did not correlate with graft survival. Thomas et al. have subsequently shown that the combination of IT plus DSG without bone marrow infusion enhances graft survival when IT is administered on day 0. DSG is also associated with an alteration of the cytokine profile elaborated by IT-treated monkeys.

IT induces rapid and profound depletion of $CD3^+$ cells from the blood and lymph node, changes that persist for 3 to 6 months [38, 39]. Initially, there is a substantial nonspecific decline in the CTL precursor frequency against donor and third-party cells [39]. However, there has been no correlation measurable between the decline in CTL precursors and rejection, as some animals rejected their grafts despite low levels of CTL precursors. When measured 3 months post-transplantation, there has been no significant decrease in the MLR responsiveness to donor or third-party cells [38, 39]. Additionally, no association has been detected between levels of CTL precursors and MLR pre-transplantation and the outcome post-transplantation. While some animals produce anti-donor antibodies and some of these antibodies are complement-fixing, there has been no correlation between alloantibody levels and transplant outcome [38, 39].

The mechanisms by which anti-CD3 IT prolongs graft survival are not clear. As mentioned previously, an impaired immune response at the time of alloantigen presentation favors tolerance induction. This may relate to the impaired ability of the recipient immune system to develop an alloimmune response to the graft. In the absence of a vigorous immune response, donor-derived cells may migrate to the thymus or other sites where they interact with newly emerging T-cells. This interaction between graft cells and immature recipient immune cells may lead to alloreactive T-cell silencing and/or deletion.

The IT effect may be mediated by generation of long-lasting anergic cells. Hamawy has shown that IT activates T-cells *in vitro* leading to extensive protein tyrosine phosphorylation [40]. Because T-cell activation in the absence of costimulation may lead to T-cell anergy *in vitro* [41], it is similarly possible that T-cell receptor aggregation with IT may also lead to T-cell anergy. Alternatively, the pattern of T-cell receptor crosslinking by IT may be modified in a manner such that modified signaling induces hyporesponsiveness. Anergic, hyporesponsive cells may then compete with newly developed alloreactive T-cells for alloantigen. These mechanisms together with the ability of the conjugated toxin to inhibit protein synthesis could be contributing to the potency of the IT. Regardless of the mechanism involved, IT appears to be a safe and effective means of prolonging allograft survival. Further efforts are directed at overcoming the problems of weight loss, interstitial nephritis, and rejection when drug is administered on day 0.

Concluding remarks

Lessons learned from *in vitro* studies of T-cell tolerance, rodent models of allograft and xenograft tolerance, and more recently nonhuman primate studies, all suggest that while tolerance is a difficult goal to achieve, it is not impossible. Enforcing this view is the sporadic development of tolerance in human transplantation. Exciting new clinical studies will evaluate the potential of costimulation blockade in human renal and islet cell transplantation and it is anticipated that clinical trials with anti-CD52 (CAMPATH 1H), anti-CD3 immunotoxin, and combination regimens including donor bone marrow and antilymphocyte therapy will occur in the near future. The future of immunosuppressive therapy in tolerance trials is the subject of intensive study. Clinical application of xenograft methods will importantly depend on successful development of tolerance strategies. We predict that the coming decade will see the successful implementation of reliable and robust tolerance strategies in human organ transplant patients.

References

1 Owen RD (1945) Immunogenetic consequences of vascular anastomoses between bovine twins. *Science* 102: 400–401
2 Billingham RE, Brent L, Medawar PB (1953) Actively acquired tolerance of foreign cells. *Nature* 172: 603–606
3 Strober S, Dhillon M, Schubert M, Holm B, Engleman E, Benike C, Hoppe R, Sibley R, Myburgh JA, Collins G et al (1989) Acquired immune tolerance to cadaveric renal allografts. A study of three patients treated with total lymphoid irradiation. *N Engl J Med* 321: 28–33
4 Cecka JM (1997) The UNOS Scientific Renal Transplant Registry. *In*: JM Cecka, PI Terasaki (eds): *Clinical transplants 1996*. UCLA Tissue Typing Laboratory, Los Angeles, 1–14
5 DeVito-Haynes LD, Jankowska-Gan E, Sollinger HW, Knechtle SJ, Burlingham WJ (1994) Monitoring of kidney and simultaneous pancreas-kidney transplantation rejection by release of donor-specific, soluble HLA class I. *Hum Immunol* 40: 191–201
6 Zhai Y, Hong X, Wang J, Fechner JH, Goodman RE, Johnson MC, Knechtle SJ (1998) Modulation of alloimmunity to major histocompatibility complex class I by cotransfer of cytokine genes *in vivo*. *Transpl Immunol* 6: 169–175
7 Klein J (1990) *Immunology*. Blackwells Scientific Publications, Boston
8 Bishop GA, Sun J, Sheil AG, McCaughan GW (1997) High-dose/activation-associated tolerance: a mechanism for allograft tolerance. *Transplantation* 64: 1377–1382
9 Burlingham WJ (2001) The blood transfusion effect. *In*: S Thiru, H Waldmann (eds): *Immunology and pathology of transplantation*. Blackwell Scientific Publications, Oxford, England, 92–115
10 Chiller JM, Habicht GS, Weigle WO (1971) Kinetic differences in unresponsiveness of thymus and bone marrow cells. *Science* 171: 813–815
11 Knechtle SJ, Fechner JH Jr, Dong Y, Stavrou S, Neville DM Jr, Oberley T, Buckley P, Armstrong N, Rusterholz K, Hong X et al (1998) Primate renal transplants using immunotoxin. *Surgery* 124: 438–447
12 Knechtle SJ, Vargo D, Fechner J, Zhai Y, Wang J, Hanaway MJ, Scharff J, Hu H, Knapp L, Watkins D et al (1997) FN18-CRM9 immunotoxin promotes tolerance in primate renal allografts. *Transplantation* 63: 1–6
13 Wood K, Sachs DH (1996) Chimerism and transplantation tolerance: cause and effect. *Immunol Today* 17: 584–588
14 Nickerson P, Steiger J, Zheng XX, Steele AW, Steurer W, Roy-Chaudhury P, Strom TB (1997) Manipulation of cytokine networks in transplantation: false hope or realistic opportunity for tolerance? *Transplantation* 63: 489–494
15 Knechtle SJ, Wang J, Graeb C, Zhai Y, Hong X, Fechner JH Jr, Geissler EK (1997) Direct MHC class I complementary DNA transfer to thymus induces donor-specific unresponsiveness, which involves multiple immunologic mechanisms. *J Immunol* 159: 152–158
16 Harlan DM, Kirk AD (1998) Anti-CD154 therapy to prevent graft rejection. *Graft* 1: 63–70
17 Mazariegos GV, Reyes J, Marino IR, Demetris AJ, Flynn B, Irish W, McMichael J, Fung JJ, Starzl TE (1997) Weaning of immunosuppression in liver transplant recipients. *Transplantation* 63: 243–249
18 Burlingham WJ, Grailer AP, Fechner JH Jr, Kusaka S, Trucco M, Kocova M, Belzer FO, Sollinger HW (1995) Microchimerism linked to cytotoxic T lymphocyte functional unresponsiveness (clonal anergy) in a tolerant renal transplant recipient. *Transplantation* 59: 1147–1155
19 Burlingham WJ, Grailer AP, Heisey DM, Claas FHJ, Norman D, Mohanakumar T, Brennan DC, de Fijter H, van Gelder T, Pirsch JD et al (1998) The effect of tolerance to noninherited maternal HLA antigens on the survival of renal transplants from sibling donors. *N Engl J Med* 339: 1657–1664
20 Calne R, Friend P, Moffatt S, Bradley A, Hale G, Firth J, Bradley J, Smith K, Waldmann H (1998) Prope tolerance, perioperative campath 1H, and low-dose cyclosporin monotherapy in renal allograft recipients. *Lancet* 351: 1701–1702
21 Nikolic B, Sykes M (1997) Bone marrow chimerism and transplantation tolerance. *Curr Opin Immunol* 9: 634–640
22 Kimikawa M, Sachs DH, Colvin RB, Bartholomew A, Kawai T, Cosimi AB (1997) Modifications of the conditioning regimen for achieving mixed chimerism and donor-specific tolerance in cynomolgus monkeys. *Transplantation* 64: 709–716
23 Mychaliska GB, Rice HE, Tarantal AF, Stock PG, Capper J, Garovoy MR, Olson JL, Cowan MJ,

Harrison MR (1997) *In utero* hematopoietic stem cell transplants prolong survival of postnatal kidney transplantation in monkeys. *J Pediat Surg* 32: 976–981

24 Sablinski T, Gianello PR, Bailin M, Bergen KS, Emery DW, Fishman JA, Foley A, Hatch T, Hawley RJ, Kozlowski T et al (1997) Pig to monkey bone marrow and kidney xenotransplantation. *Surgery* 121: 381–391

25 Schwartz RH (1996) Models of T cell anergy: is there a common molecular mechanism? *J Exp Med* 184: 1–8

26 Hamawy MM, Knechtle SJ (1998) Strategies for tolerance induction in nonhuman primates. *Curr Opin Immunol* 10: 513–517

27 Lenschow DJ, Walunas TL, Bluestone JA (1996) CD28/B7 system of T cell costimulation. *Annu Rev Immunol* 14: 233–258

28 Lederman S, Yellin MJ, Krichevsky A, Belko J, Lee JJ, Chess L (1992) Identification of a novel surface protein on activated CD4+ T cells that induces contact-dependent B-cell differentiation (help). *J Exp Med* 175: 1091–1101

29 Henn V, Slupsky JR, Grafe M, Anagnostopoulos I, Forster R, Muller-Berghaus G, Kroczek RA (1998) CD40 ligand on activated platelets triggers an inflammatory reaction of endothelial cells. *Nature* 391: 591–594

30 Sayegh MH, Akalin E, Hancock WW, Russell ME, Carpenter CB, Linsley PS, Turka LA (1995) CD28-B7 blockade after alloantigenic challenge *in vivo* inhibits Th1 cytokines but spares Th2. *J Exp Med* 181: 1869–1874

31 Larsen CP, Elwood ET, Alexander DZ, Ritchie SC, Hendrix R, Tucker-Burden C, Cho HR, Aruffo A, Hollenbaugh D, Linsley PS et al (1996) Long-term acceptance of skin and cardiac allografts after blocking CD40 and CD28 pathways. *Nature* 381: 434–438

32 Kirk AD, Harlan DM, Armstrong NN, Davis TA, Dong Y, Gray GS, Hong X, Thomas D, Fechner JH Jr, Knechtle SJ (1997) CTLA4-Ig and anti-CD40 ligand prevent renal allograft rejection in primates. *Proc Natl Acad Sci USA* 94: 8789–8794

33 Veillette A, Bookman MA, Horak EM, Bolen JB (1988) The CD4 and CD8 T cell surface antigens are associated with the internal membrane tyrosine-protein kinase p56[lck]. *Cell* 55: 301–308

34 Mourad GJ, Preffer FI, Wee Sl Powelson JA, Kawai T, Delmonico FL, Knowles RW, Cosimi AB, Colvin RB (1998) Humanized IgG1 and IgG4 anti-CD4 monoclonal antibodies: effects on lymphocytes in the blood, lymph nodes, and renal allografts in cynomolgus monkeys. *Transplantation* 65: 632–641

35 Saitovitch D, Bushell A, Mabbs DW, Morris PJ, Wood KJ (1996) Kinetics of induction of transplantation tolerance with a nondepleting anti-CD4 monoclonal antibody and donor-specific transfusion before transplantation. A critical period of time is required for development of immunological unresponsiveness. *Transplantation* 61: 1642–1647

36 Krieger NR, Yuh D, McIntyre B, Flavin TF, Yin D, Robbins R, Fathman CG (1998) Prolongation of cardiac graft survival with anti-CD4Ig plus hCTLA4Ig in primates. *Surgery* 76: 174–178

37 Neville DM Jr, Scharff J, Srinivasachar K (1992) *In vivo* T-cell ablation by a holo-immunotoxin directed at human CD3. *Proc Natl Acad Sci USA* 89: 2585–2589

38 Thomas JM, Neville DM, Contreras JL, Eckhoff DE, Meng G, Lobashevsky AL, Wang PX, Huang ZQ, Verbanac KM, Haisch CE, Thomas FT (1997) Preclinical studies of allograft tolerance in rhesus monkeys: a novel anti-CD3-immunotoxin given peritransplant with donor bone marrow induces operational tolerance to kidney allografts. *Transplantation* 64: 124–135

39 Fechner JH Jr, Vargo DJ, Geissler EK, Graeb C, Wang J, Hanaway MJ, Watkins DI, Piekarczyk M, Neville DM Jr, Knechtle SJ (1997) Split tolerance induced by immunotoxin in a rhesus kidney allograft model. *Transplantation* 63: 1339–1345

40 Hamawy MM, Tsuchida M, Manthei ER, Dong Y, Fechner JH, Knechtle JS (1999) Activation of T lymphocytes for adhesion and cytokine expression by toxin-conjugated anti-CD3 monoclonal antibodies. *Transplantation* 68: 693–698

41 Gajewski TF, Qian D, Fields P, Fitch FW (1994) Anergic T-lymphocyte clones have altered inositol phosphate, calcium, and tyrosine kinase signaling pathways. *Proc Natl Acad Sci USA* 91: 38–42

Modern Immunosuppressives
ed. by H.-J Schuurman, G. Feutren and J.-F. Bach
© 2001 Birkhäuser Verlag/Switzerland

Gene therapy approaches to immunosuppression

Reto A. Gadient, Thomas Bühler, Marcel Luyten and N. Rao Movva

Novartis Pharma Ltd., Transplantation Research, WSJ-386/906, P.O. Box, CH-4002 Basel, Switzerland

Introduction

Gene therapy is defined as the delivery of genetic material in the form of DNA. Its purpose is to correct a missing or disturbed gene function associated with a pathophysiological situation in patients. It is attractive compared to the conventional pharmacological therapy, as it can be applied more locally and thus should have fewer side-effects. Somatic gene therapy, the delivery of genetic material in a non-hereditary fashion to mostly an adult target tissue has been persued by the research community for the past 10 years with only moderate success. The methodology of gene therapy must be improved before it becomes a clinical reality. This is in terms of improved efficiency of gene transfer to the target tissue, as well as in tighter control of gene expression. The primary focus of gene therapy will be in correcting genetic disorders followed by its application to so far unmet medical needs, e.g., cancer treatment. The present review summarises the progress which has been made in the past several years in the therapeutic area of transplantation and highlights the potential future applications of gene therapy in enhancing graft survival.

Transplantation and immunosuppression

The current pharmacological interventions, e.g treatment with Cyclosporine A (CsA), to prevent rejection of a transplanted organ, is far from being optimal and has several limitations. First, a significant part of the immune system remains suppressed throughout the patient's life, thus causing susceptibility to a variety of infections. Second, many of the immunosuppressants currently in use exert unwanted side-effects that are detrimental to the graft itself. Third, they efficiently suppress acute graft rejection, but have very limited effects on chronic rejection, which is currently untreatable and for which the only therapeutic option is retransplantation.

Currently, many more donor organs are needed than are available. Xenotransplantation, with its present focus on porcine organs as donors, might provide a way to ameliorate this situation. However, xenotransplantation still remains an experimental paradigm which needs further technological development to become a viable therapy. One of the most promising new approaches for allo- and xenotransplantation is gene therapy, which should provide a significant advantage as compared to classical immunosuppressive treatment.

Gene therapy in transplantation

Gene therapy presents itself as an attractive option to locally introduce novel genes *ex vivo* into the donor organs prior to transplantation, as schematically shown (Fig. 1). Genes can be selected for their beneficial effects in prolonging graft survival by controlling the events of early and late rejection. The local expression of gene products for the desired benefits can be envisioned to have minimal systemic side-effects in comparison to oral drugs for a similar indication. Suitable vector systems and methods that allow the regulation of gene expression provide an additional option to control the events occurring during early or late graft loss, as needed. Gene therapy can also help to elucidate the pathophysiological mechanisms involved in graft rejection and thus help in the development of classical drugs.

In xenotransplantation, gene therapy provides the opportunity to rapidly evaluate the beneficial effects of therapeutic genes in graft survival in the

Graft protection through gene therapy

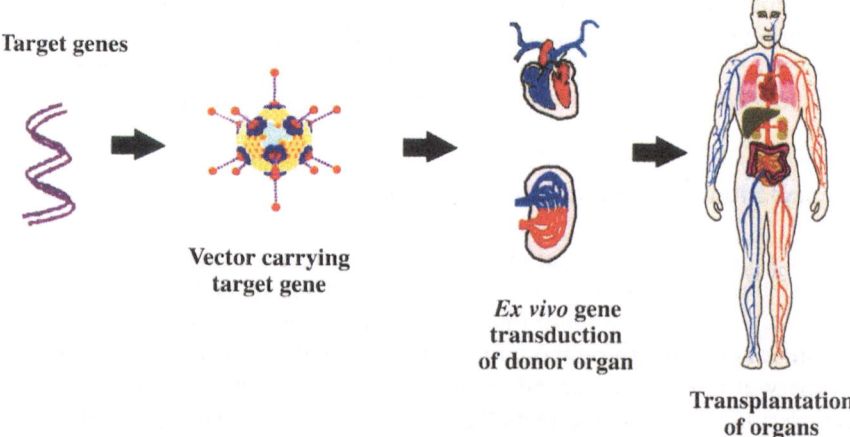

Figure 1. Schematic presentation of gene transfer into solid organs prior to transplantation. In this example the target genes are introduced using a recombinant adenovirus. Target genes are cloned into a shuttlevector and recombinant adenovirus carrying the transgene is produced. A solution containing this virus is then perfused through the organ prior to transplantation. After a short incubation period the viral solution is washed out and the organ transplanted. The target genes are expressed in the virally infected cells and thereby protect the transplanted organ.

absence of available novel agents. For these reasons, gene therapy in transplantation has become an important area of research. Several genes have been identified as therapeutically beneficial and have been evaluated in transplanted grafts in animal models. The rapid progress being made in this area is summarized (Tab. 1) in the following sections.

Table 1. Summary of target genes used in gene therapy in transplantation

Target gene	Location	References
TGF β1	Heart	[1–6]
	Liver	[10]
Viral IL-10	Heart	[1–6]
	Liver	[11]
	Pancreatic islets	[21]
Murine IL-10	Heart	[4]
	Lung	[16]
Human IL-10	Hepatocytes	[26]
FasL	Kidney	[8, 9]
	Pancreatic islets	[22–25]
CTLA4Ig	Liver	[12–14]
	Lung	[18]
	Pancreatic islets	[20]
Bcl-2	Liver	[15]
HSP-70	Lung	[19]
IL-12p40	Pancreatic islets	[21]

Solid organ transplantation

Heart transplantation
In several studies using murine cardiac allograft transplantation models Qin et al. [1–4] have reported beneficial effects of therapeutic gene transfer. Their studies focused on two immunosuppressive gene products, murine transforming growth factor TGF β1 and viral interleukin 10 (IL-10). In a first attempt, naked plasmid DNA engineered to express these proteins was injected into murine hearts, prior to syngeneic or allogeneic transplantation [1, 2]. A significant prolongation of graft survival (26.3 ± 2.5 days *versus* 12.6 ± 1.1 days) was demonstrated using murine TGF β1 under the control of the Simian virus 40 (SV40) promotor. Using the β-galactosidase reporter gene it was demonstrate that in this setting gene expression lasted for at least 2 weeks post-transplantation. Toxic side-effects of the injected plasmid DNA were not observed. Injection of the TGF β1 plasmid remote from the transplant did not increase graft survival.

In a second attempt, two different gene transfer methods in terms of trans-gene distribution and prolongation of graft survival were compared. Either naked plasmid DNA or different viral vectors, including retroviral, adenoviral and herpes simplex virus vectors were injected [3]. Using the β-galactosidase reporter gene it was shown that plasmid DNA is predominantly expressed in cardiac myocytes, whereas retroviral vectors directed expression excusively to the inflammatory infiltrate in the graft. Expressions of adenoviral and herpes simplex virus vectors were detected in both myocytes as well as in infiltrating inflammatory cells. As mentioned above, direct injection of plasmid DNA expressing murine TGF β1 significantly enhanced graft survival. A retroviral construct expressing viral IL-10 under the control of the Moloney leukemia virus (MoLV) promotor was even more potent in enhancing transplant survival (36.7 ± 1.3 days *versus* 13.5 ± 2.0 days). This effect was dose-dependent [4] and was reflected by a reduced number of graft-infiltrating T-lymphocytes. Repeated injection of the virus did only moderately enhance graft survival as compared to a single injection prior to transplantation.

In contrast, murine IL-10 which has additional T-cell costimulatory proper-ties compared to its viral counterpart does not prolong cardiac allograft sur-vival. In contrast to the retroviral gene transfer, a single injection of viral IL-10 protein prior to transplantation did not confer enhanced graft survival. Prolonged expression of viral IL-10 seemed to be required to protect the trans-planted organ. Measurements of the viral IL-10 transcripts showed that the gene was still expressed 7 days post transplantation.

Brauner et al. [5] compared the efficiency of adenoviral gene transfer in a rabbit model of heterotopic heart transplantation. A single intracoronary injec-tion was compared with slow infusion and not suprisingly it was found that slow infusion is roughly tenfold more efficient as a single bolus injection in establishing efficient gene transfer. Using the method of slow intracoronary infusion, TGF β1 and viral IL-10 were tested for prolongation of graft survival [6]. In this model, the effects of TGF β1 (11.1 ± 1.7 days *versus* 6.9 ± 0.9 days) and viral IL-10 (11.2 ± 3 days *versus* 6.9 ± 0.9 days) on graft survival were less pronounced. In addition, combination of viral transfer with systemic immunosuppression by CsA did not improve graft survival. On the contrary, CsA cotreatment reduced the survival of heart transplants after viral IL-10 gene transfer to control values, whereas TGF β1-treated grafts were unaffect-ed. Currently, it is unclear what is the mechanistic basis for the opposing actions of CsA and viral IL-10.

Kidney transplantation
Kidney loss after transplantation due to immunological injury still remains a major problem and gene therapy might provide the means to significantly improve this situation [7]. A potential therapeutic gene which fullfills these specifications is Fas ligand (FasL), a molecule shown to be important in T-cell development. Initially, Bellgrau et al. [8] showed that FasL-bearing Sertoli cell allografts, in contrast to Sertoli cells from FasL-deficient mice, survive indef-

initely, indicating that FasL is an important immunoprotective factor. FasL induces apoptosis in cells bearing the Fas receptor and its expression is shown to confer immune privilege to specific sites in the body. Transduction of rat renal allografts with an adenovirus carrying murine FasL immediately prior to transplantation significantly prolonged the survival of the transplant (27.8 days *versus* 11.6 days in controls) [9] in the absence of any systemic immunosuppression. Expression of FasL protein lasted for approximately 2 weeks after transplantation. Using PCR and Northern analysis, FasL transcripts were observed in the transduced but not in the control kidneys. In addition, FasL mRNA was detected in normal testis and spleen. There were only minimal inflammatory changes in graft vasculature observed in the FasL-transduced kidney, whereas the controls showed severe signs of arteritis. In contrast, interstitial inflammation was equally observed in both experimental conditions. The data suggest that FasL can be of therapeutic use to prolong graft survival.

Liver transplantation

TGF β1 [10] and viral IL-10 [11] were also studied in the context of rat liver transplantation. Cold preserved liver was perfused with a solution containing an adenoviral vector carrying the transgene and subsequently transplanted without immunosuppression. Intragraft levels of inflammatory cytokines, e.g., tumor necrosis factor (TNF)-α and interferon (IFN)-γ were measured and were found to be significantly reduced in livers transduced with TGF β1. Other candidate genes that have been investigated for their ability to prolong survival of liver grafts include soluble CTLA4Ig [12], which is a chimeric protein of the murine IgCγ2a fused with the murine CTLA4. Soluble CTLA4Ig molecules block costimulatory signals between T-cells and antigen-presenting cells. Treatment of rat livers with either a soluble CTLA4Ig protein or transduction with an adenovirus carrying the corresponding gene leads to sustained survival of the transplanted liver and the development of donor-specific unresponsiveness. In both cases, grafts treated with CTLAIg had a 5–10 fold longer survival as compared to controls which rejected around 11 days post transplantation. In addition, CTLA4Ig downregulates the immune response to adenoviral vectors in mouse liver and thereby prolongs the expression of the introduced genes (>5 months *versus* 2–7 weeks) [13, 14].

Recently, Bilbao et al. [15] reported for grafted liver that the anti-apoptotic gene Bcl-2 significantly improves organ damage due to preservation. The use of anti-apoptotic genes in transplantation addresses the problem of previous tissue damage, e.g., ischemia/reperfusion injury, which leads to extensive cell death in the grafted organ. Gene therapy with Bcl-2 significantly decreased the number of apoptotic cells in the graft, reduced the levels of biochemical markers of liver function like aspartate aminotransferase and lactate dehydrogenase after transplantation, and increased the protection of the cytoarchitecture after graft rewarming. Introduction of such genes will improve the overall function of a transplant and allow longer preservation times.

Lung transplantation

In lung transplantation a form of chronic allograft rejection, called bronchiolitis obliterans, is a serious limitation for prolonged graft survival. The disease is characterized by a progressive obliteration of the airways which usually leads to the death of the graft recipient. Murine IL-10 has been reported to significantly reduce the formation of bronchiolitis obliterans [16] in a rat heterotopic tracheal transplantation model. Recombinant mouse IL-10 was either given *via* a osmotic minipump, or by transduction with an adenoviral vector. Three weeks after transplantation, murine IL-10, given by either treatment, completely inhibited the obliteration of the airways. A single administration of the gene was sufficient to achieve this protective effect.

Although in this model a single administration was sufficient, it is often desirable to repetitively administer the adenoviral vector. The main problem in this respect is the formation of neutralizing anti-adenoviral antibodies, which reduce transduction efficiency and shortens the duration of gene expression. Treatment with recombinant IL-12 [17] or CTLA4Ig protein [18] significantly ameliorates stability of gene expression as well as increases the gene transfer efficiency in the absence of systemic immunesuppression. In addition, both treatments allow the repetitive administration of adenoviral vectors to the lung.

Recently, Hiratsuka et al. [19] have reported that transduction of lung allografts with an adenovirus carrying the heat-shock protein 70 (HSP70) gene decreased ischemia-reperfusion injury. Lungs which were transduced with HSP70 had significantly higher oxygenation levels as compared to controls. Lung presents itself as an attractive organ for gene therapy as repeat delivery to the graft following transplantation is readily possible with inhalation delivery systems. Moreover, the conventional immunosuppressive strategies are largely unsuccessful in preventing early graft loss in lung allograft transplantation due to the systemic toxicity associated with high levels of immunosuppression.

Tissue and cell therapy

Pancreatic islet transplantation

A major focus in transplantation is the potential of pancreatic islets grafts to treat diabetes and the design of novel immunosuppressives to make such a treatment possible. Chahine et al. [20] transplanted muscle cells which stably expressed CTLA4Ig together with pancreatic islets, into the renal subcapsular space of mice. They found a significant prolongation of islet survival (31.7 days *versus* 11.0 days) when cotransplanted myoblasts were syngeneic, but not when the myoblasts were of allogeneic origin. Moreover, additional blockage of LFA-1 by a neutralizing antibody was synergistic to CTLA4Ig in achieving prolongation of islet survival.

Yasuda et al. [21] showed that local production of the murine IL-12p40 subunit dramatically extended graft survival (87.0 days *versus* 9.6 days) in syngeneic islet grafts in diabetic NOD mice. In contrast, similarly delivered viral IL-10 did not show graft prolongation. The local production of IL-12p40 was associated with decreased IFN-γ and increased TGFβ production at the graft site. In addition, histology revealed a very small number of lymphocytes in the IL-12p40 transduced islets.

The effect of FasL in islet transplantation is controversial. Lau et al. [22] reported that cotransplantation of pancreatic islets together with genetically engineered myocytes expressing FasL prolongs islet survial. In contrast to this study, other research groups reported the opposite effect [23–25]. Transplantation of islets from transgenic mice expressing FasL in pancreatic β cells were rapidly rejected [23, 24] which was explained by a massive infiltration of inflammatory cells, mainly neutrophils and granulocytes. Similar findings were also made by Judge et al. [25] who transduced islets with a FasL-carrying adenovirus. These contradictory results are based on subtle differences in the various experimental models used, which remain to be resolved before an effective immunoprotective effect of Fas ligand can be firmly established.

Hepatocyte transplantation
Hepatocyte transplantation is considered as an alternative to liver transplantation. A major obstacle is the limited ability of hepatocytes to repopulate the liver after transplantation. Fabrega et al. [26] reported an enhanced survival of transplanted hepatocytes expressing human IL-10. The gene was introduced by cationic lipid-mediated transfer and was found to be expressed for only a short time after which the protective effect was lost.

A more efficient way to deliver genes into hepatocytes is by adenoviral vectors. Hammel et al. [27] have reported that hepatocytes transduced with complement receptor type 1 *via* an adenoviral vector are resistant to hyperacute rejection. As liver is an attractive secretory organ as well, hepatocyte gene transfection and transplantation will receive greater attention in future for systemic delivery of proteins. In this context immunosuppressive strategies will be further explored.

Neuronal cell transplantation
Gene therapy in the central nervous system (CNS) currently involves two different approaches. In one approach genes are directly applied into different areas of the CNS (for review see [28]), while in the other genetically altered cells are transplanted. The second approach is performed either by grafting of modified cells [29, 30], or by implantation of encapsulated cells [31, 32]. Polymer encapsulated cells were used to deliver soluble molecules such as neurotrophic factors or neurotransmitters like dopamine to the surrounding nervous tissue. The main limitation is the survival of the encapsulated cells and in case of insufficient nutrition, these cells can undergo necrotic cell death, thereby releasing toxic products into the local environment. The alternative is to directly transplant genetically-altered cells by stereotactic injection into the

brain. Due to the special characteristics of the CNS, transplanted cells should have a very limited or no growth potential.

Genetically-modified neuronal cells [33], astrocytes [34] and fibroblasts [35] have been grafted into the brains of mice, rats and primates, respectively. Although the CNS is thought to be an immunoprivileged site, immunosuppression increases the survival of grafted cells [36]. Okura et al. [37] studied the effect of T-cell depletion on the survival of cells isolated from the mouse ventral mesencephalon transplanted into the rat brain. It was found that treatment with anti-CD2 or anti T-cell receptor antibodies, or a combination of both, leads to graft survival for more than 100 days. Moreover, the combination of both antibodies induced tolerance to a second neural graft from the same donor strain, but not to a third-party donor strain. Cotransplanted Sertoli cells protected neural grafts in a rodent Parkinson model presumably due to the expression of the immuneprotective molecule FasL [38]. Thus many well established immunosuppressive molecules seem to confer similar benefits in the CNS, thus suggesting their therapeutic potential in neural transplants.

Delivery of genes

Methods of gene transfer

Currently, several different delivery systems, both of viral and non-viral nature, are being used to introduce genes into cells or solid organs (Tab. 2). The non-viral methods comprise classical transfection techniques, such as calcium precipitation, complex formation with different mixtures of cationic lipids or electroporation. Most of these techniques have been initially developed to introduce genes into cultured cells *in vitro*. In solid organs, successful gene therapy was also performed by local injection of naked plasmid DNA

Table 2: Comparison of gene transfer methods

	Adenovirus	Adeno associated virus (AAV)	Lentivirus	Nonviral (Plasmid)
Efficiency of gene transfer	high	high	high	poor
Level of gene expression	medium	medium	medium	low
Duration of gene expression	weeks	months	months	days
Safety	medium	medium	medium	high
Integration into the host genome	low frequency	high frequency	high frequency	low frequency
Immunogenicity	moderate	none	none	none

into the myocardium. The efficiency of gene transfer by these methods is usually quite low, however the expression of the protein can at times be sufficient to obtain a therapeutic effect.

Higher gene transfer efficiency is generally obtained using virus-based vectors. There are several types of gene therapy vectors based on retrovirus, adenovirus, adeno-associated virus (AAV), lentivirus, herpesvirus and baculovirus. Retrovirus and lentivirus are RNA viruses, which integrate into the host genome and thereby enable long-term expression of the transgene. Adenovirus is a non-integrating DNA virus, where as wildtype AAV, integrates to a specific site on human chromosome 19. AAV, adeno- and lentiviruses can transduce both resting as well as proliferating cells, whereas retroviruses can only transduce proliferating cells. All the different viral systems are genetically modified in such a way that they become replication-deficient. Specific vector sytems can be selected depending on the desired duration of expression, nature of the target tissue and the ease of vector production. Significant improvements need to be made in the rapid generation of vectors and their scale up prior to their consideration as therapeutic vectors. Enhanced gene transfer and specific targeting of the virus to different cells is the current major focus of vector development. A more detailed review on current gene therapy vectors has recently been presented [39].

Regulation of gene expression

Physiologically, gene expression is tightly controlled thereby avoiding unwanted side-effects. Similarly, it is important to consider ways of achieving therapeutically desired gene expression as well as its regulation. There are a variety of strategies to obtain high levels of gene expression. Currently, several constitutive promoters from viral systems such as simian virus 40 (SV40), the rous sarcoma (RSV) or the cytomegalovirus (CMV) promotors are routinely used. These viral promotors usually confer therapeutic protein expression at quite high levels and in a broad spectrum of cell types. Besides constitutively-expressed promotors tissue-specific promotors are worth mentioning. Examples for this group are promotors such as the immunoglobulin heavy chain enhancer which is expressed in B-lymphocytes, the Thy-1 promotor expressed by neurons, and the ICAM-2 promotor expressed by vascular endothelial cells. Expression of the gene is highly regulated and occurs only in a specific subpopulation of cells when placed under the control of these promotors [39, 40].

The last group of regulatory systems is the inducible promotors, natural as well as engineered promotor systems such as Tet-system, rapamycin-regulated system, metallothionine, ecdysone promotors which are based on small-molecule inducers like tetracycline, metals, steroids and dimerizing agents like FK-1012 or rapamycin. The presence or the absence of the inducer switches the gene on or off, thereby creating a tight control over the gene expression.

However, even in these systems a certain degree of leakiness of expression or non-responsiveness to the inducer can be seen depending on the cell type. These potential complications problems are currently a significant focus in this area of research [41, 42].

Concluding remarks

The area of gene therapy is rapidly evolving and has become a major focus of research in academic institutions as well as industry. In transplantation, the immediate goal of gene therapy will be to improve the treatment beyond the currently used immunosuppressive regimes in terms of preventing acute and chronic rejection of grafted organs and tissues. Moreover, gene therapy should provide us with a precise way to prolong graft survival by local delivery of pro-tective genes to the graft tissue itself prior to transplantation, thereby avoiding systemic side-effects.

The transplantation of xenografts, e.g., porcine organs, has gained signifi-cant attention recently as a means to provide unlimited and more easily acces-sible organs. Gene therapy should facilitate the therapeutic use of these organs by rapid evaluation and introduction of graft-protective concepts both at the experimental and therapeutic levels. The development of new and improved vector systems will be an essential prerequisite for the future success of gene therapy. Such systems should facilitate efficient gene transfer, enhance target-ing into desired cell populations, and should enable us to tightly regulate gene expression. In summary, much work has already been initiated to make gene therapy a clinical reality, and in the coming years we will witness exciting and novel gene therapeutic options in the realm of transplantation medicine.

References

1 Qin L, Chavin KD, Ding Y, Woodward JE, Favaro JP, Lin J, Bromberg JS (1994) Gene transfer for transplantation. Prolongation of allograft survival with transforming growth factor-beta 1. *Ann Surg* 220: 508–518
2 Qin L, Ding Y, Bromberg JS (1996) Gene transfer of transforming growth factor-beta 1 prolongs murine cardiac allograft survival by inhibiting cell-mediated immunity. *Hum Gene Ther* 7: 1981–1988
3 Qin L, Chavin KD, Ding Y, Favaro JP, Woodward JE, Lin J, Tahara H, Robbins P, Shaked A, Ho DY et al (1995) Multiple vectors effectively achieve gene transfer in a murine cardiac transplan-tation model. Immunosuppression with TGF-beta 1 or vIL-10. *Transplantation* 59: 809–816
4 Qin L, Chavin KD, Ding Y, Tahara H, Favaro JP, Woodward JE, Suzuki T, Robbins PD, Lotze MT, Bromberg JS (1996) Retrovirus-mediated transfer of viral IL-10 gene prolongs murine cardiac allograft survival. *J Immunol* 156: 2316–2323
5 Brauner R, Wu L, Laks H, Nonoyama M, Scholl F, Shvarts O, Berk A, Drinkwater-DCJ, Wang JL (1997) Intracoronary gene transfer of immunosuppressive cytokines to cardiac allografts: method and efficacy of adenovirus-mediated transduction. *J Thorac Cardiovasc Surg* 113: 1059–1066
6 Brauner R, Nonoyama M, Laks H, Drinkwater-DCJ, McCaffery S, Drake T, Berk AJ, Sen L, Wu L (1997) Intracoronary adenovirus-mediated transfer of immunosuppressive cytokine genes pro-

longs allograft survival. *J Thorac Cardiovasc Surg* 114: 923–933

7 Kelley VR, Sukhatme VP (1999) Gene transfer in the kidney. *Amer J Physiol* 276: F1-F9

8 Bellgrau D, Gold D, Selawry H, Moore J, Franzusoff A, Duke RC (1995) A role for CD95 ligand in preventing graft rejection. *Nature* 377: 630–632

9 Swenson KM, Ke B, Wang T, Markowitz JS, Maggard MA, Spear GS, Imagawa DK, Goss JA, Busuttil RW, Seu P (1998) Fas ligand gene transfer to renal allografts in rats: effects on allograft survival. *Transplantation* 65: 155–160

10 Drazan KE, Olthoff KM, Wu L, Shen XD, Gelman A, Shaked A (1996) Adenovirus-mediated gene transfer in the transplant setting: early events after orthotopic transplantation of liver allografts expressing TGF-beta1. *Transplantation* 62: 1080–1084

11 Drazan KE, Wu L, Olthoff KM, Jurim O, Busuttil RW, Shaked A (1995) Transduction of hepatic allografts achieves local levels of viral IL-10 which suppress alloreactivity *in vitro*. *J Surg Res* 59: 219–223

12 Olthoff KM, Judge TA, Gelman AE, da SX, Hancock WW, Turka LA, Shaked A (1998) Adenovirus-mediated gene transfer into cold-preserved liver allografts: survival pattern and unresponsiveness following transduction with CTLA4Ig. *Nat Med* 4: 194–200

13 Kay MA, Holterman AX, Meuse L, Gown A, Ochs HD, Linsley PS, Wilson CB (1995) Long-term hepatic adenovirus-mediated gene expression in mice following CTLA4Ig administration. *Nat Genet* 11: 191–197

14 Kay MA, Meuse L, Gown AM, Linsley P, Hollenbaugh D, Aruffo A, Ochs HD, Wilson CB (1997) Transient immunomodulation with anti-CD40 ligand antibody and CTLA4Ig enhances persistence and secondary adenovirus-mediated gene transfer into mouse liver. *Proc Natl Acad Sci USA* 94: 4686–4691

15 Bilbao G, Contreras JL, Gomez NJ, Eckhoff DE, Mikheeva G, Krasnykh V, Hynes T, Thomas FT, Thomas JM, Curiel DT (1999) Genetic modification of liver grafts with an adenoviral vector encoding the Bcl-2 gene improves organ preservation. *Transplantation* 67: 775–783

16 Boehler A, Chamberlain D, Xing Z, Slutsky AS, Jordana M, Gauldie J, Liu M, Keshavjee S (1998) Adenovirus-mediated interleukin-10 gene transfer inhibits post-transplant fibrous airway obliteration in an animal model of bronchiolitis obliterans. *Hum Gene Ther* 9: 541–551

17 Yang Y, Trinchieri G, Wilson JM (1995) Recombinant IL-12 prevents formation of blocking IgA antibodies to recombinant adenovirus and allows repeated gene therapy to mouse lung. *Nat Med* 1: 890–893

18 Jooss K, Turka LA, Wilson JM (1998) Blunting of immune responses to adenoviral vectors in mouse liver and lung with CTLA4Ig. *Gene Ther* 5: 309–319

19 Hiratsuka M, Mora BN, Yano M, Mohanakumar T, Patterson GA (1999) Gene transfer of heat shock protein 70 protects lung grafts from ischemia-reperfusion injury. *Ann Thorac Surg* 67: 1421–1427

20 Chahine AA, Yu M, McKernan MM, Stoeckert C, Lau HT (1995) Immunomodulation of pancreatic islet allografts in mice with CTLA4Ig secreting muscle cells. *Transplantation* 59: 1313–1318

21 Yasuda H, Nagata M, Arisawa K, Yoshida R, Fujihira K, Okamoto N, Moriyama H, Miki M, Saito I, Hamada H et al (1998) Local expression of immunoregulatory IL-12p40 gene prolonged syngeneic islet graft survival in diabetic NOD mice. *J Clin Invest* 102: 1807–1814

22 Lau HT, Yu M, Fontana A, Stoeckert-CJJ (1996) Prevention of islet allograft rejection with engineered myoblasts expressing FasL in mice. *Science* 273: 109–112

23 Allison J, Georgiou HM, Strasser A, Vaux DL (1997) Transgenic expression of CD95 ligand on islet beta cells induces a granulocytic infiltration but does not confer immune privilege upon islet allografts. *Proc Natl Acad Sci USA* 94: 3943–3947

24 Kang SM, Schneider DB, Lin Z, Hanahan D, Dichek DA, Stock PG, Baekkeskov S (1997) Fas ligand expression in islets of Langerhans does not confer immune privilege and instead targets them for rapid destruction. *Nat Med* 3: 738–743

25 Judge TA, Desai NM, Yang Z, Rostami S, Alonso L, Zhang H, Chen Y, Markman JF, DeMateo RP, Barker CF et al (1998) Utility of adenoviral-mediated Fas ligand gene transfer to modulate islet allograft survival. *Transplantation* 66: 426–434

26 Fabrega AJ, Fasbender AJ, Struble S, Zabner J (1996) Cationic lipid-mediated transfer of the hIL-10 gene prolongs survival of allogeneic hepatocytes in Nagase analbuminemic rats. *Transplantation* 62: 1866–1871

27 Hammel JM, Elfeki SK, Kobayashi N, Ito M, Cai J, Fearon DT, Graham FL, Fox IJ (1999) Transplanted hepatocytes infected with a complement receptor type 1 (CR1)-containing recombi-

nant adenovirus are resistant to hyperacute rejection. *Transplant Proc* 31: 939

28 Barkats M, Bilang BA, Buc CM, Castel BM, Corti O, Finiels F, Horellou P, Revah F, Sabate O, Mallet J (1998) Adenovirus in the bra*In*: recent advances of gene therapy for neurodegenerative diseases. *Prog Neurobiol* 55: 333–341

29 Flax JD, Aurora S, Yang C, Simonin C, Wills AM, Billinghurst LL, Jendoubi M, Sidman RL, Wolfe JH, Kim SU et al (1998) Engraftable human neural stem cells respond to developmental cues, replace neurons, and express foreign genes. *Nat Biotechnol* 16: 1033–1039

30 Martinez SA, Bjorklund A (1997) Immortalized neural progenitor cells for CNS gene transfer and repair. *Trends Neurosci* 20: 530–538

31 Aebischer P, Schluep M, Deglon N, Joseph JM, Hirt L, Heyd B, Goddard M, Hammang JP, Zurn AD, Kato AC et al (1996) Intrathecal delivery of CNTF using encapsulated genetically modified xenogeneic cells in amyotrophic lateral sclerosis patients. *Nat Med* 2: 696–699

32 Deglon N, Heyd B, Tan SA, Joseph JM, Zurn AD, Aebischer P (1996) Central nervous system delivery of recombinant ciliary neurotrophic factor by polymer encapsulated differentiated C2C12 myoblasts. *Hum Gene Ther* 7: 2135–2146

33 Andsberg G, Kokaia Z, Bjorklund A, Lindvall O, Martinez SA (1998) Amelioration of ischaemia-induced neuronal death in the rat striatum by NGF-secreting neural stem cells. *Eur J Neurosci* 10: 2026–2036

34 Ridet JL, Corti O, Pencalet P, Hanoun N, Hamon M, Philippon J, Mallet J (1999) Toward autologous *ex vivo* gene therapy for the central nervous system with human adult astrocytes. *Hum Gene Ther* 10: 271–280

35 Tuszynski MH, Roberts J, Senut MC, HS, Gage FH (1996) Gene therapy in the adult primate bra*In*: intraparenchymal grafts of cells genetically modified to produce nerve growth factor prevent cholinergic neuronal degeneration. *Gene Ther* 3: 305–314

36 Borlongan CV, Stahl CE, Cameron DF, Saporta S, Freeman TB, Cahill DW, Sanberg PR (1996) CNS immunological modulation of neural graft rejection and survival. *Neurol Res* 18: 297–304

37 Okura Y, Tanaka R, Ono K, Yoshida S, Tanuma N, Matsumoto Y (1997) Treatment of rat hemi-parkinson model with xenogeneic neural transplantation: tolerance induction by anti-T-cell antibodies. *J Neurosci* 48: 385–396

38 Sanberg PR, Borlongan CV, Saporta S, Cameron DF (1996) Testis-derived Sertoli cells survive and provide localized immunoprotection for xenografts in rat brain. *Nat Biotechnol* 14: 1692–1695

39 Robbins PD, Ghivizzani SC (1998) Viral vectors for gene therapy. *Pharmacol Ther* 80: 35–47

40 Walther W, Stein U (1996) Cell type specific and inducible promoters for vectors in gene therapy as an approach for cell targeting. *J Molec Med* 74: 379–392

41 Jane SM, Cunningham JM, Vanin EF (1998) Vector development: a major obstacle in human gene therapy. *Ann Med* 30: 413–415

42 Peng KW (1999) Strategies for targeting therapeutic gene delivery. *Mol Med Today* 5: 448–453

Perspectives

Modern Immunosuppressives
ed. by H.-J Schuurman, G. Feutren and J.-F. Bach
© 2001 Birkhäuser Verlag/Switzerland

A rigorous approach to the diagnosis of synergy among combination therapies of immunosuppressive agents

Ting-Chao Chou[1] and Barry D. Kahan[2]

[1] Molecular Pharmacology and Therapeutics Program, Memorial Sloan-Kettering Cancer Center, 1275 York Avenue, New York, NY 10021, USA
[2] Division of Immunology and Organ Transplantation, Department of Surgery, The University of Texas Medical School, 6431 Fannin, Suite 6.240, Houston, TX 77030, USA

Introduction

Historical considerations

The word "synergism" is derived from the Greek συνεργοσ (synergos), meaning "working together". The application of synergism to drug therapeutics as the law of compounds was espoused by the Persian physician Avicenna, who proposed that the addition of a second (or multiple) agent(s) to a drug regimen exponentially increased the efficacy of the treatment [1]. Averroes disputed this claim, recognizing the possibility that interactions between drugs might be only additive; indeed, the drug interactions might be antagonistic, or less than additive [2].

The modern era of analysis of drug interactions sought to establish optimally effective antibiotic combinations. For example, Thatcher [3] documented the benefit of adding sulfonamides to a regimen of another antibacterial agent. However, Lankford and Lacy [4] pointed out the caution that combinations of two antibiotics might be less effective than a single drug alone. Price documented another caution [5] after observing both a lack of correlation between *in vitro* and *in vivo* results, and the importance of selecting the proper concentrations (and ratios of two drugs) to document "synergism."

In 1950, Javetz et al found both *in vitro* [6] and *in vivo* [7] that the bacteriocidal effect of penicillin on enterococci was potentiated by streptomycin, which by itself was inactive. This effect contrasted with the antagonistic action of chloromycetin on penicillin antibiosis. They observed that different strains of a given organism showed variable degrees of susceptibility to a supra-additive interaction [8]. These findings suggested differences in interactions both between patients and among organisms that are targets of drug action. Furthermore, they recognized that in order to demonstrate a supra-additive effect at least one drug of a pair must show effects alone. They recognized that "drugs that were ineffective even in very high concentrations against a given organism will not allow the determination of synergism or antagonism, but instead be classified as potentiation (enhancement) or suppression (inhibition)" [9]. They suggested that antibiotics could be grouped into clusters based upon their mutual interactions and that "synergism" may be documented either when the drugs are present simultaneously or sequentially. They also recognized that direct application of the observations concerning *in vitro* bacterioci-dal actions of drug combinations may be obfuscated by the intervention of host resistance *in vivo*, which can exploit concomitant bacteriostatic effects (in the absence of bacteriocidal actions) to achieve cure from infection. In their analysis the authors found that "synergistic" drug combinations can achieve not only quantitatively greater but also qualitatively different effects from those obtained with each agent alone.

Jawetz [10] expanded his classification of antibiotic clusters, suggesting that the choice of therapeutic drugs should be based on *in vitro* testing against the infectious agent. The authors noted that it is important for a synergy analysis to determine the dose-response relation of each agent alone, since this relation is frequently non-linear and since in combinations drugs are used at concentrations in the low range of effective doses. In this range, the dose-effect curve may be hyperbolic, linear or sigmoidal in shape. Although the authors distinguished "indifference" (additivity) – namely, no effect of a combination of agents on an organism despite the presence (or absence) of an effect of each drug alone – from "antagonism", they failed to unequivocally distinguish it from synergism. Indeed they recognized that "there are no universally accepted definitions to separate additive from synergistic actions." Indeed, there has been a lot of confusion in this field of study.

The problem of defining "synergy" for antibiotic combinations was addressed by Garrett [11], who used dose-response curves to classify interactions. He showed that simple algebraic summation of response equivalents could not discern drug interactions unless the dose-response curves for each agent were linear, which is an exceedingly rare situation. Furthermore, he questioned the definition of antibiotic responses: was it the proportion of organisms killed, or the rate of the kill? Did a growth inhibition effect lead to the emergence of aged organisms that display a propensity toward death? Because the rate effects are linear, he suggested that plots of logarithmic number of the variable such as number of viable organisms *versus* a linear axis of dose/concentration would thereby derive a precise definition of additivity: namely, the sum of the mathematical functions of drug responses, $f_a + f_b = 1$.

The concept of synergy was expanded and advanced by the findings of Hitchings [12] that the combination of trimethoprim (TMP) and sulfonamides (SA) produced a broader spectrum of action, more rapid bactericidal activity, and reduced incidence of emergence of bacterial resistance than either drug alone.

The major problem in the pre-1980 era for dissecting the interactions of drug combinations was the apparent lack of a vigorous theoretical basis to define "synergism", "additive effect" or "antagonism". For example, the review article of Berenbaum entitled "What is synergy?" [13] cites 560 references, which demonstrates that more confusion than clarification of the problem exists.

Hypotheses to explain drug synergy

At least four hypotheses have been proposed to explain the mechanisms of synergy of two drugs. First, the agents may interact with one another chemically (or physically) to generate a product with unique effects. Second, one drug may alter the physiology of the target in such a way that facilitates the action of the second drug. Third, one drug may alter the availability of substrate so as to potentiate the effect of the second agent. For example, Seydel et al. [14] published an extensive analysis of the mechanism of synergy of TMP and SA. They proposed that TMP has two modes of action on bacteria, at least one of which depends upon the concomitant presence of SA, rather than the result of two agents acting sequentially on a single pathway. They based their theory on the observation that pre-incubation with SA potentiated the effects of subsequent incubation of the organisms with TMP. Using isobologram analysis, the *in vitro* results were judged to be highly synergistic. Fourth, simultaneous blockade of multiple interacting pathways enhances drug-induced inhibitory effects. This last explanation has been proposed to explain the marked degree of synergism between cyclosporine (CsA) and rapamycin (RAPA).

Rationale for the development of synergistic combinations

The three "ideals" for any immunosuppressive agent are a virtual lack of toxicity, an abrogation of all alloimmune responses, and a satisfactory profile of absorption, distribution, and action in host tissues. The fact that none of the available agents individually meets these criteria has led to greater use of "shotgun" immunosuppressive regimens, i.e., agents administered in arbitrary combinations.

The criteria for rational combination therapy are (a) qualitatively broadened spectrum of therapeutic activity; (b) avoidance of the physiologically harmful effects of a response-equivalent dose of one drug alone; (c) increased response above that predicted from the separate drug action; (d) reduced occurrence or delayed onset of drug resistance due to the lower doses, shorter durations of drug exposure, and/or multiple targets of attack; and (e) economic savings.

The increased pharmacologic efficacy of a synergistic drug combination against the cellular target(s) of action should make it possible to lower the dose(s) of each agent required to produce a given effect, thereby decreasing the toxicity or untoward side-effects against the host and thus increasing the ratio of the toxic dose to the therapeutic dose, which may be defined as the therapeutic index.

This strategy for drug combinations has been widely used in cancer, chemo-, and radio-, as well as in antimicrobial-therapy, particularly for AIDS [9, 15]. However, quantitative assessments of drug interactions *in vitro* and *in vivo* have rarely been applied as rational approaches to design optimal clinical protocols, due to inadequate or even erroneous data analysis [9, 16]. Many studies purporting to demonstrate synergy in fact do not. Faulty experimental design or misguided data analysis often precludes such a demonstration even when synergism exists; in many other cases, claims of synergism are not supported by the available data.

Definition of synergism

When two or more treatment modalities are used for combination therapy, the effect can be "synergistic", "additive", "antagonistic", or mixed (for instance, antagonistic at low-dose levels, and synergistic at high-dose levels). The concept of synergy has only recently been rigorously defined in mathematical terms [9, 17]. A combination is defined as showing "synergism" if it produces a more-than-additive effect; it shows "antagonism" if it produces a less-than-additive effect. Crucial to these concepts, of course, is the determination of what constitutes an "additive effect".

The Webb fractional product

Because of the sigmoidal nature of most dose-effect curves, defining an "additive effect" is not as simple as many investigators believe. This chapter aims to simplify the discussion of synergism by considering the combination of only two drugs, although the general equation for an *n*-drug combination has been recently derived [9, 17].

The additive effect of two drugs cannot be determined by simple arithmetic addition of the effects of the drugs. Under this analysis, if given doses of drug A and drug B each inhibit a system by 70%, the combined additive effect of drugs A and B would be 70% + 70%, or 140%, which is impossible. Some researchers may argue that, based on the fractional product method of Webb [18], if A and B each inhibit a system by 70%, then the combined additive effect is 91%, since $(1-0.7)(1-0.7) = 0.09$ and $1-(0.09) = 0.91$. However, it is well known that Webb's method is valid only when two drugs and their combination have hyperbolic dose-effect curves and when the effects of two drugs are mutually nonexclusive, namely, the drugs display independent modes of action. Unfortunately, this assumption of a hyperbolic dose-effect relation is inaccurate, for biological systems, since the dose-effect curves are most frequently sigmoidal at the cellular or organismic level. To date, only two methods, namely, the isobologram and the combination index (CI) method of Chou-

Talalay, have actually yielded explicit general equations that can be used to define synergism, antagonism, or additive effect [9].

The mass-action law approach and the combination index equation (Chou-Talalay) for drug combinations

By using enzyme-kinetic systems and the pharmacological receptor theory as models, several hundred equations have been systematically derived for a variety of drugs (substrates, products, and inhibitors), mechanism of reactions (ordered, ping-pong, and random-reaction sequences), as well as types and permutations of inhibitory patterns (competitive, noncompetitive, and uncompetitive) [19]. Further mathematical induction and deduction of several hundred specific equations yields only a few general equations. These equations are represented for single drugs by the median-effect equation and the median-effect plot [9], and for multiple drugs by the CI equation and fa-CI plot [17]. The CI method has frequently been used for the analysis of drug interactions in the biomedical literature [16].

The median effect equation and the median effect plot
Regardless of either the shape of the dose-effect curve or the mechanism of inhibition by the agent, its action obeys the median-effect equation [9] as given by:

$$f_a/f_u = (D/D_m)^m \qquad\qquad \text{Eq. (1)}$$

where D is the dose or concentration of a drug and f_a is the fraction of the reaction affected by a dose (D) or concentration of a drug. Thus, f_a can represent the fractional inhibition (i.e., percent inhibition/100), while f_u is the fraction unaffected by a dose (D), such as fractional survival; therefore, $f_a + f_u = 1$ or $f_a = 1 - f_u$. D_m is the median-effect dose (ED_{50}) or concentration (IC_{50}) that affects the system under investigation by 50%, whereas m is the coefficient signifying the shape of dose-effect relationship. Values of $m = 1$, >1, and <1 indicate a hyperbolic, sigmoidal, and flat sigmoidal dose-effect curve, respectively, for an inhibitory drug. Equation (1) is the simplest possible form to express the relationship of dose (right side) to effect (left side).

Rearrangement of Equation (1) gives

$$D = D_m [f_a/(1-f_a)]^{1/m} \qquad\qquad \text{Eq. (2)}$$

$$f_a = 1/[1 + (D_m/D)^m] \qquad\qquad \text{Eq. (3)}$$

Equation (2) allows the determination of the dose (D) for any given degree of effect (f_a) if the parameters D_m and m are known. Conversely, Equation (3) allows the determination of effect at any given dose if f_a and D_m values are known. The D_m and m values are easily determined by the median-effect plot: namely, using the x-axis as log (D) and the y-axis as log (f_a/f_u), as stipulated by the logarithmic form of Equation (1):

$$\log (f_a/f_u) = m \log (D) - m \log (D_m) \qquad \text{Eq. (4)}$$

where m is the slope and log (D_m) is the x-intercept of the median-effect plot. Thus, Equation (4) has the form of the classic straight-line equation, y = mx + b. The conformity of the data to the median-effect principle can be readily manifested by a high linear correlation coefficient (r value) of the median-effect plot, namely, >0.80. The median-effect equation takes account of both "the potency" and "the shape" of the dose-effect response curves, namely, the potency (D_m) of each drug *versus* the potency of the combinations, and the degree of sigmoidicity of the dose-effect curves of each drug alone, as well as their combinations (m-value).

The combination index equation
An equation determines only the additive effect of a drug combination, rather than synergism or antagonism. However, Chou and Talalay define synergism as a more-than-expected, and antagonism as a less-than-expected additive effect. Based on theoretical derivations [17], the additive effect is designated as a CI value equal to unity; thus, for any two-drug combination:

$$CI = \frac{(D)_1}{(D_x)_1} + \frac{(D)_2}{(D_x)_2} \qquad \text{Eq. (5)}$$

where CI values <1, =1, and >1 indicate synergism, additive effect, and antagonism, respectively. Equation (5) dictates that the doses of drug 1, $(D)_1$, and drug 2, $(D)_2$ (in the numerators) in combination inhibit a system by x% in the actual experiment. Thus, the experimentally observed x% inhibition may not be a round number, and more frequently is a decimal fraction. $(D_x)_1$ and $(D_x)_2$ (in the denominators) are the doses of drug 1 and drug 2 alone, respectively, inhibiting x%. D_x can be readily calculated from Equation (2).

By substituting Equation (2) into Equation (5), the algorithms for automated computerized quantitation of synergism and antagonism of two drugs are expressed as follows. For f_a at x% affected by D_1, D_2, or their mixture (i.e., at iso-effective doses) and in the mixture where $(D_x)_{1,2} = (D)_1 + (D)_2$ and $(D)_1/(D)_2 = P/Q$, we get:

$$CI = \frac{(D_x)_{1,2}[P/(P+Q)]}{(D_m)_1\{(f_{ax})_1/[1-(f_{ax})_1]\}^{1/m}{}_1} + \frac{(D_x)_{1,2}[Q/(P+Q)]}{(D_m)_2\{(fa_x)_2/[1-(f_{ax})_2]\}^{1/m}{}_2} \qquad \text{Eq. (6)}$$

where $(D_x)_{1,2} = \{(f_{ax})_{1,2}/[1-(f_{ax})_{1,2}]\}^{1/m}_{1,2}[(D_m)_{1,2}]$ and $(f_{ax})_1 = (f_{ax})_2 = (f_{ax})_{1,2}$ (i.e., iso-effective). Diagnosis: CI = 1, additive; CI < 1, synergistic; and CI > 1, antagonistic.

Equation (6) is used to calculate CI values at different effect levels, or fa (fraction affected; e.g., 5% to 99% inhibition for fa = 0.05 to 0.99). The computer software automatically generates dose-effect curves, the median-effect plot, fa-CI plots, and isobolograms [20–22].

For more drug combinations, the general equation is given by:

$$CI = \sum_{i=1}^{n} \frac{(D)_i}{(Dx)_i}$$
Eq. (7)

Since all terms in Equation (7) are ratios, they are dimensionless quantities. Thus, each component drug may have different units (e.g., μM, μg/ml, IU, etc.) or different modalities of effect (e.g., drug, radiation or hyperthermia).

Thus, the "net result" of the combination n drugs, in terms of synergism or antagonism, can be quantitatively determined regardless of their mechanisms. In these studies the component drugs can have various interactions with each other: all mutually synergistic, all mutually antagonistic, or some synergistic and some antagonistic.

Isobologram analysis

Although Loewe [23] proposed the isobologram more than 45 years ago using empirical approaches, a major advance was proposed by Berenbaum [24], namely the "sham" test, whereby one drug was divided into two aliquots and used in double-blinded fashion by a third party to conduct drug combination studies. This test provided some restricted theoretical bases for defining an additive effect. Indeed an isobologram can be generated directly from the CI equation (Eq. (5), with CI = 1) for each combination data point, as well as for any effect level, by computer simulation [17]. Thus,

$$\frac{(D)_1}{(D_x)_1} + \frac{(D)_2}{(D_x)_2} = 1$$
Eq. (8)

where (D_x) can be obtained from Equation (2). Using $(D)_1/(D_x)_1$ as the x-axis and $(D)_2/(D_x)_2$ as the y-axis in the coordinates for the isobol (i.e., the equi-effective graph), the arrangement of combination points on the hypotenuse (diagonal) indicates an additive effect; on the lower-left of the hypotenuse, synergism; and on the upper-right of the hypotenuse, antagonism (Fig. 1).

The fa-CI plot
The fa-CI plot and the isobologram are inversely related concepts; the former is effect-oriented, while the latter is dose-oriented. Although both methods

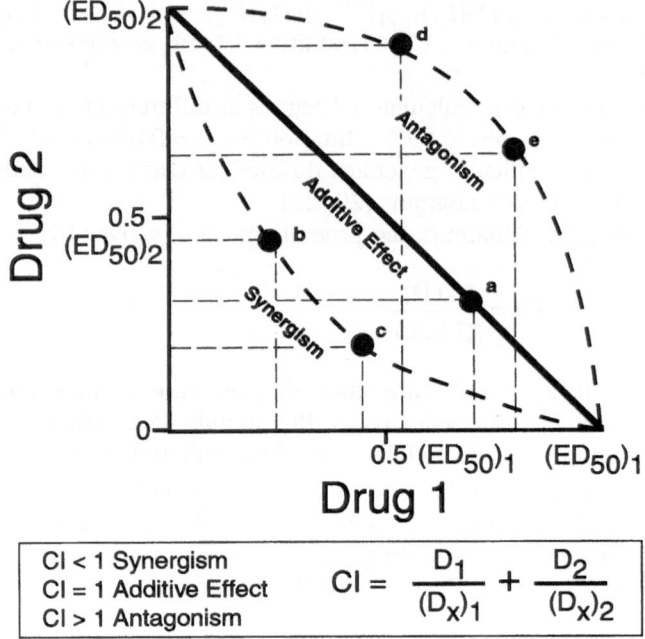

Figure 1. Illustration of ED_{50}-isobologram using the combination index (CI) equation. Combination data points on the diagonal line (e.g., point a) indicate an additive effect, whereas those on the lower-left (e.g., points b and c) indicate synergism, and those on the upper-right (points d and e) indicate antagonism. Isobologram at ED_{50} effect levels or other effect levels (e.g., ED_{70}, ED_{90} and ED_{95}) can also be constructed instantly using the computer software [20–22].

should yield identical conclusions [9, 17], the isobologram suffers serious practical limitations. First, each isobol represents one particular effect level. If isobols are generated for more than three effect levels, the isobologram is messy and hard to read. Second, the x- and y-axes depict individual drugs on two-dimensional graphs. If three or more drugs are used in combination, the construction and interpretation of the graphs becomes difficult. These limitations are overcome by the fa-CI plot (or the fa-CI table; Fig. 2).

The dose-reduction index
The term "dose-reduction index" (DRI) [20, 25] has been widely applied [9, 21, 26]. DRI depicts the number of folds by which a synergistic interaction allows the drug dose(s) to be reduced yet produces a given degree of effect, compared to the concentration required with a single drug alone. Therefore, for drug 1, $(DRI)_1 = (D_x)_1/(D)_1$, and for drug 2, $(DRI)_2 = (D_x)_2/(D)_2$. Substituting these terms into Equation (5), we obtain the relationship between CI and DRI:

$$CI = \frac{(D)_1}{(D_x)_1} + \frac{(D)_2}{(D_x)_2} = \frac{1}{(DRI)_1} + \frac{1}{(DRI)_2} \qquad \text{Eq. (9)}$$

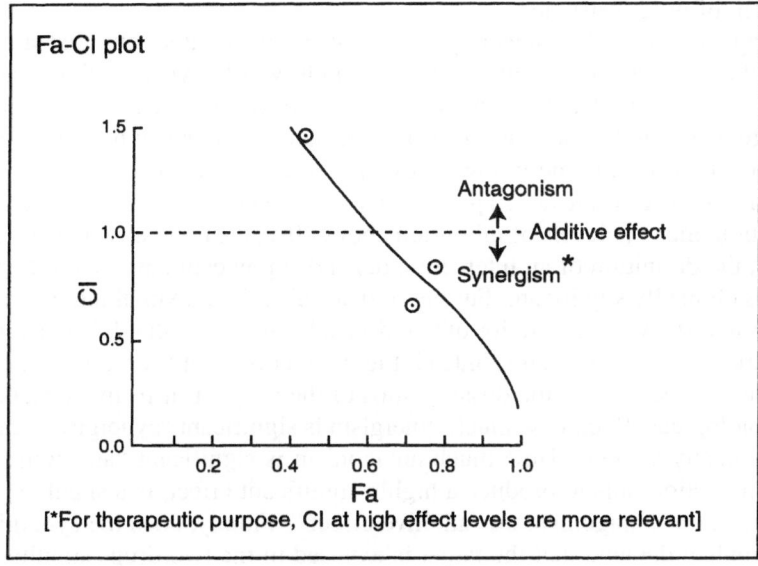

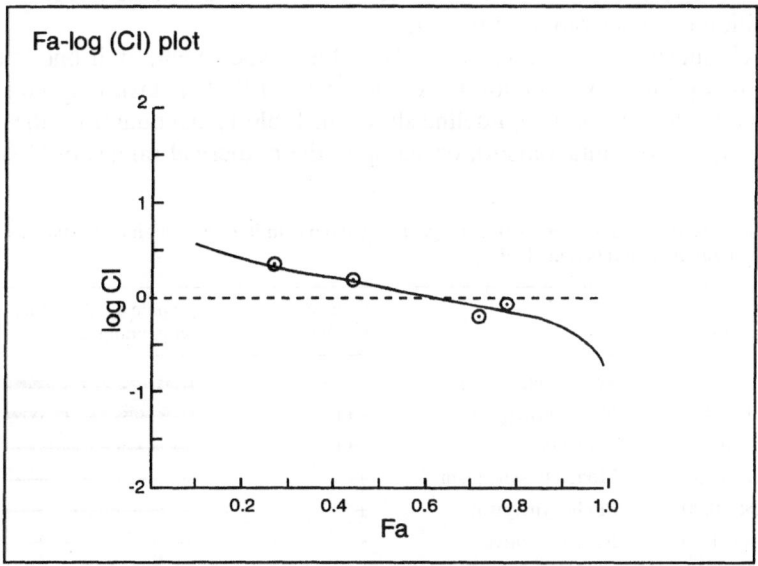

Figure 2. Typical fa-CI plot or fa-log (CI) plot showing synergism, additive effect, and antagonism. Circles represent actuarial combination data points, and the curves are based on computer simulation using the computer software [20–22] in conjunction with Equations (3) and (5).

Equation (9) permits ready calculation of DRI values for each drug used in the combination at different effect levels. While maintaining therapeutic efficacy, dose reduction produces less toxicity and may also reduce or delay the development of drug resistance.

Applications to biological systems may produce situations that are more complicated than those implicit in the single word "synergism" or "antagonism". For example, the combination of two or more drugs may result in antagonism at low dose or low effect levels, and synergism at high dose or high effect levels. Furthermore, our analysis of the interaction between CsA and tacrolimus (FK506) revealed particularly strong synergism at low effect levels, but autogonism at levels of inhibition above 40%, the clinically relevant range. Thus, the definition of an interaction depends upon estimating the effect level that is clinically significant. Further to determine the maximal interaction, one needs to test a variety of ratios of two drugs, beginning with a 1:1 (equal potency) drug combination ratio. Indeed, the interactions between drugs in combination may depend on the dosage ratios of the drugs. But from the standpoint of a biological effect, how much synergism is significant "synergism" that will be clinically evident? How much antagonism is significant "antagonism"? If the interaction fails to produce a highly significant effect, is a small degree of synergism or antagonism an "additive effect"? Finally, does the synergism or antagonism demand that the target is exposed to the two drugs simultaneously *versus* sequentially? And do the synergistic or antagonistic effects relate to inhibition or to activation of the target?

Each question must be individually tackled experimentally if one is to discern the optimal combination for clinical trials [9]. This task may be simplified somewhat by a scale guideline shown in Table 1, that quantifies the degree of synergism (or antagonism), based upon the numerical ranges of CI values.

Table 1. Description and symbols of synergism or antagonism in drug combination studies analyzed with the combination index method

Range of combination	Description	Graded symbols	graphic symbols for polygonograms
<0.1	Very strong synergism	+++++	▬▬▬▬▬▬
0.1–0.3	Strong synergism	++++	▬▬▬▬▬
0.3–0.7	Synergism	+++	————
0.7–0.85	Moderate synergism	++	———
0.85–0.90	Slight synergism	+	——
0.80–1.10	Nearly additive	±	·············
1.10–1.20	Slight antagonism	–	– – – – – –
1.20–1.45	Moderate antagonism	——	–·–·–·–·–·
1.45–3.3	Antagonism	——	– – – – – –
3.3–10	Strong antagonism	———	▬ ▪ ▬ ▪ ▬
>10	Very strong antagonism	————	▬ ▬ ▬ ▬ ▬

Combination index method is based on those described by Chou and Talalay [9, 17] and the computer software of Chou and Chou [20–22]. The ranges of CI and the symbols are refined from those described earlier by Chou [9]. CI values <1, =1, and >1 indicate synergism, additive effect and antagonism, respectively [9, 17].

Indeed, this scale of graphic symbols can be incorporated into polygonogram presentations for combinations of three to *n*-drugs [26, 27] (Figs 3, 4).

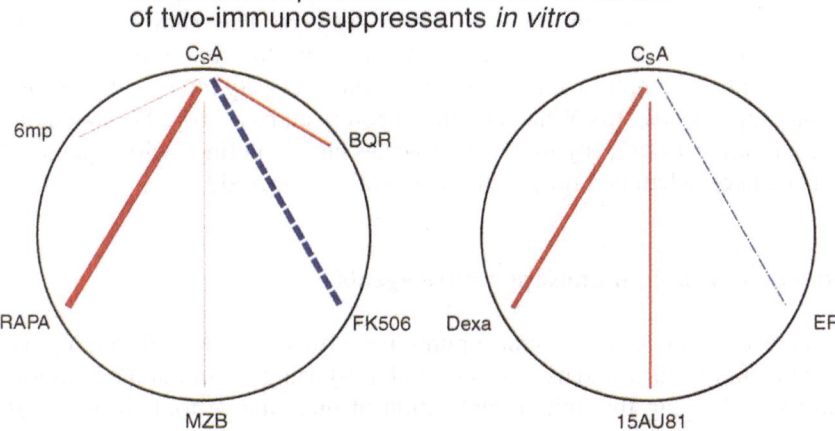

Figure 3. Schematic representation of the immunosuppressive effects of combinations of CsA with other agents *in vitro*. Graphic symbols depicting degrees of synergism and antagonism are given in Table 1.

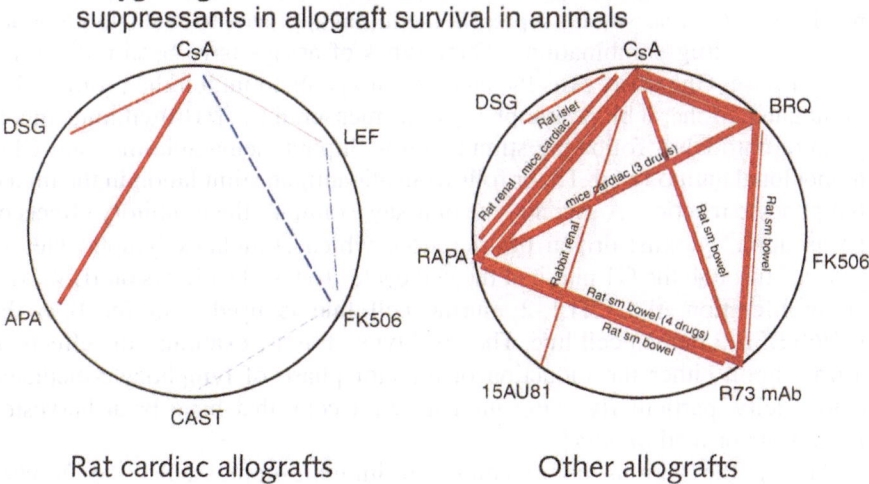

Figure 4. Polygonogram for the effects on allograft survival of combinations including two to four immunosuppressants in mice or rats. Graphic symbols depicting degrees of synergism and antagonism are given in Table 1.

Other approaches to synergy analysis

The terms synergy, synergism and synergistic effect are being used over 4500 times annually in biomedical publications as subject key words [16]. The review article "What is synergy?" indicated above cites over 560 references, but the review raised more questions than answers. This short article is not intended to settle these monumental differences in different aproaches. What we would like to emphasize to the reader is the necessity to critically evaluate various approaches: (a) What are the theoretical basis for the statements, claims, or allegations?; (b) are the approaches clearly defined with equations?; and (c) where, when and how were the equations derived?

Combinations of immunosuppressive agents

To achieve synergistic immunosuppressive effects, a clinical finding was experimentally confirmed by Vathsala et al. [29] using the initial median-effect analysis. Following this initial application of quantitative tools to assess the interactions of immunosuppressants using a computerized method [29], at least 38 papers have been published in this field using the CI method by workers worldwide [28–43].

Combination of immunosuppressants in vitro

Because of the large number of ratios necessary to determine the optimal results, *in vitro* assessments represent the initial approach to evaluate immuno-suppressive drug combinations. Three types of assays have been utilized for this purpose. One assay tests the capacity of agents to inhibit the proliferation of human peripheral blood lymphocytes as measured by ^{3}[H]-thymidine incor-poration into DNA following stimulation with phytohemagglutinin, anti-CD3 monoclonal antibody OKT3, or following alloantigen stimulation in the mixed lymphocyte reaction. A second type of assay examines the inhibitory effects of drugs upon cytokine-driven proliferation, which stimulates lymphocytes to proceed through the G1 phase of the cell cycle. To test the effects on IL-2-driv-en proliferation, the CTLL-2 murine cell line is used, and for IL-6 the MH60.BSF-2 human cell line. The third type of assay examines the effects of a drug upon either the induction or effector phase of lymphocyte-mediated cytotoxicity, particularly using human or rat cells that have been harvested from hosts primed *in vivo*.

Among the various combinations of immunosuppressants, the *in vitro* results summarized in Table 2 document that CsA in combination with RAPA shows very strong synergism, whereas CsA and tacrolimus (FK506) showed marked antagonism.

Table 2. Interactions of various combinations of two immunosuppressants *in vitro*

Immunosuppressants	Combination index (CI)	End results of interaction	Reference
CsA + 6MP	0.48–1.08	Slight synergism	Vathsala et al. [28]
+ Dexa	0.05–0.47	Strong synergism	"
+ EP	1.5–2.6	Modest antagonism	"
+ FK506	1.2–10	Very strong antagonism	"
+ FK506	1.5–10	Very strong antagonism	Vathsala et al. [31]
CsA + RAPA	0.001–0.1	Very strong synergism	Kahan et al. [29]
CsA + RAPA	0.003–0.07	Very strong synergism	Kahan et al. [30]
+ Dexa	0.001–0.66	Strong synergism	"
CsA + RAPA + Dexa	0.001–0.1	Very strong synergism	"
RAPA + Dexa	0.01–0.08	Very strong synergism	"
CsA + RAPA	0.0005–0.005	Very strong synergism	Kahan et al. [27]
+ FK506	4–60	Very strong antagonism	"
+ 6MP	0.8–1.1	Nearly additive	"
+ MZB	0.7–0.95	Slight synergism	"
+ BQR	0.5–0.7	Synergism	"
CsA + 15Au81	0.13–1.07	Synergism	Dumble et al. [32]

The results are based on the lymphocyte stimulation assays of peripheral blood lymphocytes: stimulation induced by phytohemaglutinin, anti-CD3 antibody OKT-3, or by allogeneic cells in mixed lymphocyte reactions.

Drug abbreviations: CsA, cyclosporine; 6MP, 6-mercaptopurine; Dexa, dexamethasone; EP, enisoprost; FK506, tacrolimus; RAPA, rapamycin; MZB, mizorbine; BQR, brequinar; 15Au81, prostacyclin analog.

Combination analysis in vivo

Thereafter *in vitro* observations are tested in organ transplant models in animals (Tab. 3), as illustrated with polygonograms (Figs 3 and 4). These combinations have proved useful for clinical protocol design in neoplastic disease [9], in AIDS [15], and in organ transplantation [28, 43]. For example, the CsA and RAPA combination have proved particularly useful in clinical practice [43]. The safety and efficacy of the CsA and RAPA combination have been reported in an open-label single-center phase I/II dose-escalation trial. The addition of RAPA to a CsA-based regimen reduced the overall incidence of acute rejection episodes to 7.5% from 32% in the immediately precedent CsA/Prednison-treated patients. Although RAPA-treated patients displayed reduced platelet and white blood cell counts, and higher levels of serum cholesterol and triglycerides, RAPA did not augment the nephrotoxic or hypertensive proclivities of CsA [43].

Table 3. Effects of combinations of two to four immunosuppressants upon allograft survival in animals

Allograft donor/recipient	Organ grafted	Combination treatment	Combination index (CI)	End-results of interaction	References
Rat (BuF → WFu)	Heart	CsA + RAPA	0.38 0.01–0.64 0.001–0.2	Synergism Synergism Very strong synergism	Kahan et al. [30] Stepkowski et al. [38] Stepkowski et al. [39]
Rat (PVG → DA)	Heart	CAST + FK506	>1 <1	Low dose → Antagonism High dose → synergism	Grochowicz et al. [40]
Rat (DA → Lewis)	Heart	LEF + CsA LEF + CsA LEF + FK506	0.75–1.97 0.75 1.84–3.37	Additive High dose → synergism Antagonism	Candinas et al. [41] " "
Rat → (BuF → Wfu)	Heart	CsA + FK506	1.32–2.07	Antagonism	Vathsala et al. [31]
Rat (Copenhagen → Lewis)	Heart	CsA + DSG CsA + DSG	0.01–0.30 0.27–0.14	Strong synergism Synergism	Kaji et al. [33] Kaji et al. [34]
Rat (Wistar-Furth → Lewis)	Islet	CsA + DSG	0.48–0.83	Synergism	Gores et al. [35]
Rat (Brown Norway → Lewis)	Small Bowel	CsA + RAPA + BQR + R73mAb	0.006	Very strong synergism	Wang et al. [37]
		CsA + R73mAb RAPA + R73mAb BQR + R73mAb	0.07 0.07 0.80	Strong synergism Srong synergism Moderate synergism	" " "
Rat (BuF CsA → WFu)	Kidney	CsA + RAPA	0.03–0.5	Strong synergism	Stepkowski [39]
Mouse (BALB/c → C3H) (C57BL/10 → C3H)	Heart	CsA + RAPA	0.1–0.6	Synergism	Tu et al. [36]
	Kidney	CsA + RAPA + BQR	0.001–0.02	Very strong synergism	"
Rabbit (New Zealand White → → Anglo lop-ear)	Kidney	CsA + 15Au81	0.15	Synergism	Dumble et al. [32]

Compound abbreviations: CsA, cyclosporine; RAPA, rapamycin; LEF, leflunomide; DSG, 15-deoxyspergualin; BQR, brequinar sodium, 15Au81, asynthetic prostacyclin immunosuppressive analog

Impact of pharmacokinetic interactions on combination index analysis

Due to the dependence of xenobiotics on hepatic metabolizing enzymes, and particularly the cytochrome P450 3A4 system, there are at least theoretical reasons to suspect pharmacokinetic interactions. Thus, before a final determination can be made that a given combination of agents displays immunosuppressive synergy, it must be documented that there is no kinetic interaction by examining drug concentrations in the presence *versus* absence of the second agent. For example, CsA and ketoconazole are both metabolized by cytochrome P450 3A4; thus, combination therapy with the two agents increases the concentration of CsA, thereby enhancing the potency of a given CsA dose. However, this combination would not be defined as synergistic, since ketoconazole has no immunosuppressive effect by itself. Furthermore, when the analysis is performed as a concentration-effect rather than dose-effect plot, there is no difference between the effect of the combination *versus* that of CsA alone. In contrast, although a pharmacokinetic interaction occurs at high drug doses, the synergistic effects of the CsA/RAPA combination are predominantly dynamic in nature, unexplained by their metabolic interactions, either based on their blood [39] or tissue concentrations [44].

Concluding remarks

The evaluation of drug interactions has progressed from an anecdotal pursuit to a rigorous discipline befitting the significance of the findings for the design and conduct of clinical trials. While the occurrence of immunosuppressive drug synergy has not been demonstrated unequivocally, the RAPA/CsA combination is under evaluation for its synergistic capacity, in particular to potentiate rejection prophylaxis yet permit dramatic reduction of the doses of each drug. The process toward development of this drug combination revealed the importance of pharmacokinetic analyses to exclude (or at least account for) the contribution of pharmacokinetic as distinct from pharmacodynamic interactions as a cause for the supra-additive effects. During the coming decade, one can anticipate that concentration-controlled clinical trials will be based upon comprehensive and rigorous *in vitro* analyses, confirmed by *in vivo* animal transplantation experiments, as a basis for clinical trials that recognize and quantitate drug synergy. The availability of mathematical tools, including the median-effect equation and combination index analysis, afford robust parameters for this enterprise.

References

1 Levey M (1973) *Early Arabic pharmacology.* EJ Brill, Leiden
2 Siraisi NG (1990) *Medieval and early renaissance medicine.* University of Chicago Press,

Chicago

3 Thatcher SF (1949) Synergism between antibacterial substances with special reference to streptomycin. *In*: SA Waksman (ed.): *Streptomycin, its nature and practical application.* Williams and Wilkins, Baltimore

4 Lankford CE, Lacy H (1949) *In vitro* responses of staphylococcus to aureomycin, streptomycin and penicillin. *Texas Rep Biol Med* 7: 111

5 Price CW, Randall WA, Welch H, Chandler VL (1949) Studies of the combined action of antibiotics and sulfonamides. *Amer J Public Health* 39

6 Jawetz E, Gunnison JB, Coleman VR (1950) The combined action of penicillin with streptomycin or chloromycetin on enterococci *in vitro*. *Science* 111: 254

7 Jawetz E, Gunnison JB, Speck RS (1951) Antibiotic synergism and antagonism. *N Engl J Med* 245: 966

8 Jawetz E, Gunnison JB, Bruff JB, Coleman VR (1952) Studies on antibiotic synergism and antagonism. *J Bacteriol* 64: 29

9 Chou T-C (1991) The median-effect principle and the combination index for quantitation of synergism and antagonism. *In*: T-C Chou, DC Rideout (eds): *Synergism and antagonism in chemotherapy.* Academic Press, San Diego, 61

10 Jawetz E, Gunnison JB (1952) Studies on antibiotic synergism and antagonism: a scheme of combined antibiotic action. *Antibiot Chemother* 243

11 Garrett ER (1958) Classification and evaluation of combined antibiotic activity. *Antibiot Chemother* VIII, 8

12 Hitchings GH (1973) Biochemical background of trimethoprim-sulphamethoxazole. *Med J Australia* 1 Suppl: 5–9

13 Berenbaum MC (1989) What is synergy? *Pharmacol Rev* 41: 93–141

14 Seydel JK, Wempe E, Miller GH, Miller L (1972) Kinetics and mechanisms of action of trimethoprim and sulfonamides, alone or in combination, upon *Escherichia coli*. *Chemotherapy* 17: 217–258

15 Chou T-C, Rideout D, Chou J, Bertino JR (1991) Chemotherapeutic synergism, potentiation and antagonism. *In*: Dulbecco R (ed.): *Encyclopedia of human biology.* Academic Press, 371

16 Chou T-C (1998) Drug combinations: from laboratory to practice. *J Lab Clin Med* 132: 6–8

17 Chou T-C, Talalay P (1984) Quantitative analysis of dose-effect relationships: the combined effects of multiple drugs or enzyme inhibitors. *Adv Enzyme Regul* 22: 27–55

18 Webb JL (1963) Effect of more than one inhibitor. *Enzyme and metabolic inhibitors.* Academic Press, New York, 66

19 Chou T-C, Talalay P (1981) Generalized equations for the analysis of inhibitors of Michaelis-Menten and higher order kinetic systems with two or more mutually exclusive and nonexclusive inhibitors. *Eur J Biochem* 115: 207–216

20 Chou J, Chou T-C (1987) *Dose-effect analysis with microcomputers: quantitation of ED50, LD50, synergism, antagonism, low-dose risk, receptor-ligand binding and enzyme kinetics.* [Manual and software]. Biosoft, Cambridge, UK

21 Chou J (1991) Quantitation of synergism and antagonism of two or more drugs by computerized analysis. *In*: RD Chou (ed.): *Synergism and antagonism in chemotherapy.* Academic Press, San Diego, 223

22 Chou T-C, Hayball M (1996) *CalcuSyn for Windows: Multiple-drug dose-effect analyzer and manual.* Biosoft, Cambridge, UK

23 Loewe S (1953) The problem of synergism and antagonism of combined drugs. *Arzneim-Forsch-Drug Res* 3: 285

24 Berenbaum MC (1981) Criteria for analyzing interactions between biologically active agents. *Adv Cancer Res* 35: 269–335

25 Chou J, Chou T-C (1988) Computerized simulation of dose reduction index (DRI) in synergistic drug combinations. *Pharmacologist* 30: A231

26 Chou T-C, Motzer RJ, Tong Y, Bosl GJ (1994) Computerized quantitation of synergism and antagonism of taxol, topotecan and cisplatin against teratocarcinoma cell growth: a rational approach to clinical protocol design. *J Natl Cancer Inst* 86: 1517–1524

27 Chou T-C, Chou JH (1998) Computerized indexing of drug combinations: prediction of synergism and anagonism of more that two drugs by polygonogram. *FASEB J* 12: A143

28 Kahan BD, Gibbons-Stubber S, Tejpal N, Chou T-C (1992) Prospects for synergistic immunosuppressive drug therapy in the coming decade. *Transplant Proc* 24: 1263–1265

29 Vathsala A, Chou TC, Kahan BD (1990) Analysis of the interactions of immunosuppressive drugs with cyclosporine in inhibiting DNA proliferation. *Transplantation* 49: 463–472
30 Kahan BD, Gibbons S, Tejpal N, Stepkowski SM, Chou TC (1991) Synergistic interactions of cyclosporine and rapamycin to inhibit immune performances of normal human peripheral blood lymphocytes *in vitro*. *Transplantation* 51: 232–239
31 Kahan BD, Gibbons S, Tejpal N, Chou T-C, Stepkowski S (1991) Synergistic effect of the rapamycin-cyclosporine combination: median-effect analysis of *in vitro* immune performances by human T lymphocytes in PHA, CD3, and MLR proliferative and cytotoxic assays. *Transplant Proc* 23: 1090–1091
32 Vathsala A, Goto S, Yoshimura N, Stepkowski S, Chou TC, Kahan BD (1991) The immunosuppressive antagonism of low doses of FK506 and cyclosporine. *Transplantation* 52: 121–128
33 Dumble LJ, Gibbons S, Tejpal N, Chou TC, Redgrave NG, Boyle MJ, Kahan BD (1993) 15Au81, a prostacyclin analog, potentiates immunosuppression and mitigates renal injury due to cyclosporine. *Transplantation* 55: 1124–1128
34 Kaji H, Chou T-C, Sutherland DER, Stephanian E, Gores PF (1993) 15-deoxyspergualin (DSG) and cyclosporin (CsA) act synergistically to prolong the survival of rat cardiac allografts. *Amer College Surg Surgical Forum* 44: 454
35 Kaji H, Chou T-C, Sutherland DE, Stephanian E, Gores PF (1994) Synergistic effect of 15-deoxyspergualin and cyclosporine in prolonging survival of rat cardiac allografts. *Transplant Proc* 26: 869–970
36 Gores PF, Field JF, Sutherland DE, Chou T-C (1994) Synergistic interaction of 15-deoxyspergualin and cyclosporine to prolong the survival of rat islet allografts. *Transplant Proc* 26: 745
37 Tu Y, Stepkowski SM, Chou TC, Kahan BD (1995) The synergistic effects of cyclosporine, sirolimus, and brequinar on heart allograft survival in mice. *Transplantation* 59: 177–184
38 Wang M, Qu X, Stepkowski SM, Chou T-C, Kahan BD (1996) Beneficial effect of graft perfusion with anti-T cell receptor monoclonal antibodies on survival of small bowel allografts in rat recipients treated with brequinar alone or in combination with cyclosporine and sirolimus. *Transplantation* 61: 458–464
39 Stepkowski SM, Napoli KL, Wang ME, Qu X, Chou T-C, Kahan BD (1996) Effects of the pharmacokinetic interaction between orally administered sirolimus and cyclosporine on the synergistic prolongation of heart allograft survival in rats. *Transplantation* 62: 986–994
40 Stepkowski SM, Tian L, Napoli KL, Ghobrial R, Wang ME, Chou TC, Kahan BD (1997) Synergistic mechanisms by which sirolimus and cyclosporine inhibit rat heart and kidney allograft rejection. *Clin Exp Immunol* 108: 63–68
41 Grochowicz PM, Hibberd AD, Bowen KM, Clark DA, Pang G, Cowden WB, Chou TC, Grochowicz LK, Smart YC (1997) Synergistic interaction between castanospermine and tacrolimus in the rat heart allograft model. *Transplant Proc* 29: 1259–1260
42 Candinas D, Mills C, Lee S et al (1997) Effect of combination schedules of leflunonide. *Cardiovasc Engin* 2: 145
43 Kahan BD, Podbielski J, Napoli KL, Katz SM, Meier-Kriesche H-U, Van Buren CT (1998) Immunosuppressive effects and safety of a sirolimus/cyclosporine combination regimen for renal transplantation. *Transplantation* 66: 1040–1046
44 Napoli KL, Wang ME, Stepkowski SM, Kahan BD (1998) Relative tissue distributions of cyclosporine and sirolimus after concomitant peroral administration to the rat: evidence for pharmacokinetic interactions. *Ther Drug Monit* 20: 123–133

Modern Immunosuppressives
ed. by H.-J Schuurman, G. Feutren and J.-F. Bach
© 2001 Birkhäuser Verlag/Switzerland

Lessons for transplantation of cyclosporine experience in the treatment of autoimmune diseases

Jean-François Bach

INSERM U 25, Hôpital Necker, 161 rue de Sèvres, F-75015 Paris, France

Introduction

The emergence of cyclosporine A (CsA) has opened a new era in the approach of chemically induced immunosuppression. The discovery of its molecular mode of action unraveled a whole yet unknown pathway of receptor-ligand systems controlling cytokine transcription. Multiple *in vitro* studies have extrapolated to human lymphocytes much of the numerous data obtained in murine models either *in vitro* or *in vivo*. Much less direct information is available though on the precise mode of action of the drug in man.

Such a gap is explained by three main orders of facts:

1. The *in vivo* exploration of the human immune system is complex and essentially limited to the study of peripheral blood lymphocytes, after direct *in vitro* stimulation;
2. The drug effect is for the most part reversible. Lymphocytes from CsA-treated patients rapidly recover normal functional reactivity either *in vivo* when the drug levels become unsignificant or *in vitro* when the lymphocytes are cultured in CsA-free medium;
3. CsA is given to allograft organ recipients in combination with many other drugs making it difficult to precisely analyse the direct drug action among the putative effect of other drugs such as steroids, azathioprine or antilymphocyte antibodies.

An interesting way to circumvent these difficulties is to analyse CsA effects in patients with autoimmune diseases where the drug is given alone and where the immune response (to autoantigens) is usually well characterized. It is the aim of this chapter to review the lessons drawn from the usage of CsA in the multitude of autoimmune diseases where it has been administered.

CsA in autoimmune diseases, a summary

The immunosuppressive treatment of autoimmune diseases before CsA introduction mostly relied on a small number of chemicals that essentially included corticosteroids, azathioprine, cyclophosphamide and more recently low-dose methotrexate. These therapies have proven efficacious in a large number of cases. However, two limitations are to be mentioned. First, patient improvement was not regularly seen, and second, drug toxicity and overimmunosuppression precluded long-term treatment, as would have been indicated by the only suspensive effect of these drugs [1].

In this context, CsA represented a real progress in most autoimmune diseases where T-cells play a major role or are suspected to do so. CsA effects are spectacular in psoriasis [2], in the various forms of uveitis [3], in rheumatoid arthritis [4], in atopic dermatitis [5], in nephrotic syndrome [6], in insulin-dependent diabetes mellitus [7] and chronic asthma [8] (Tab. 1). It is interesting that in most of these diseases with the exceptions of rheumatoid arthritis and nephrotic syndrome, other immunosuppressive drugs had not yet currently been used and, in fact, the immune and sometimes more precisely autoimmune origin of the disease had not been established. Some concern was raised about the drug nephrotoxicity which is still considered as a potential CsA limitation in autoimmune diseases [9]. As we shall see below, this is not so much a problem when the dosage is carefully selected and the patient's renal function adequately monitored.

Table 1. Clinical application of cyclosporine A

Approved	Potential	Possible
Nephrotic syndrome	Chronic asthma	Chronic active hepatitis
Psoriasis	Type 1 diabetes mellitus	Epidermolysis bullosa
Rheumatoid arthritis	Myasthenia gravis	Fibrosing alveolitis
Uveitis	Oral erosive lichen planus	Graves' exophtalmopathy
Aplastic anemia	Polymyositis	Polychondritis
Atopic dermatitis	Primary biliary cirrhosis	Reticulosis
	Psoriatic arthritis	Sarcoidosis
	Pyoderma gangrenosum	Scleroderma
	Systemic lupus erythematosus	Wegener's granulomatosis
	Severe Crohn's disease	

With more than 10 years of experience, comparing CsA action with that of other immunosuppressants in the above-mentioned diseases, one can see two major advantages for CsA. First, the clinical improvement has a more rapid onset and is more complete, and second the drug management is by and large easier with lower risk of overimmunosuppression: no infection is observed and, as we shall discuss in the following, the oncogenic risk is minimal and apparently lower than with azathioprine or cyclophosphamide.

The only real limitations are the absence of effect in some cases where the disease process is too advanced (presence of irreversible lesions), or where the hyperimmune nature of the autoimmune pathogenic responses creates resistance to the drug. Additionally, as discussed above for other immunosuppressive drugs, the drug effect is reversible (the clinical symptoms relapse when the treatment is stopped).

CsA predominantly acts on cell-mediated immunity but may also affect primary T-cell dependent antibody responses

The effect of CsA on cell-mediated immunity is well documented in a large number of experimental systems and clinical settings. This is exemplified by the spectacular effect of the drug on allograft rejection.

The CsA effect in autoimmune diseases also argues in the same direction. The diseases in which the drug is most clearly effective are T-cell mediated or strongly suggested to be so. This is particularly the case for rheumatoid arthritis, uveitis and insulin-dependent diabetes mellitus. The evidence lies on a less firm basis for psoriasis and nephrotic syndrome. Concerning psoriasis, the role of T-cells is suggested by the presence of a large number of T-cells in the skin, particularly at the plaque level. The pathogenic role of such T-cells is suggested by the clear clinical improvement observed after administration of anti-CD4 monoclonal antibodies [10, 11]. No role for anti-skin antibodies has been proposed. In fact, it is the spectacular effect of CsA on the disease that represents the best argument in favor of its immune origin and particularly of T-cell implication. Concerning nephrotic syndrome, the situation is more complex since there is no T-cell infiltrate in the glomeruli. The evidence is here more linked to the effect of other immunosuppressive agents such as corticosteroids and cyclophosphamide, the disease association with Hodgkin's lymphoma and perhaps most importantly the disease improvement observed after plasmapheresis and elution of a cytokine-like material from extracted plasma [12]. A current hypothesis is that nephrotic syndrome (minimal changes or focal sclerosis) is due to the systemic release by T-cells of a still unknown cytokine. This hypothesis would explain disease recurrence (manifested by heavy proteinuria) sometimes observed in the minutes following kidney transplantation.

On the other hand, there is evidence that CsA can favorably influence the course of antibody-mediated diseases. This has been particularly well demonstrated for myasthenia gravis [13] and systemic lupus erythematosus [14, 15]. It is interesting to note, however, that in these two diseases clinical improvement was not always correlated with a decrease in antibody level. It remains to be determined whether this discrepancy is due to a lack of discrimination of the antibody assays that do not pick up the pathogenic antibodies, or to the drug effect on antibody-mediated inflammation. Recent data in systemic lupus erythematosus are in favor of the first hypothesis. It has been shown that CsA selectively affects the production of IgG3 antibodies in lupus mice [16], an isotype known to be associated with particular pathogenicity of anti-DNA antibodies in mice. Our recent results of an isotype dependency of antinucleosome antibodies in human systemic lupus erythematosus could suggest an extrapolation of the isotype-selective effect to CsA activity in man. In this scheme, CsA could selectively inhibit the production of a still unknown cytokine involved in the production of the isotype in question.

Interesting data concerning the *in vivo* CsA effect on antibody production were obtained in diabetic patients. The drug had no effect on serum immunoglobulin levels [17] and on the titre of anti-islet antibodies or anti-insulin antibodies whose production had started several years before diabetes onset and CsA treatment [18]. Conversely, CsA significantly inhibited *de novo* antibody production against exogenously administered insulin in the group of patients who did not show anti-insulin antibodies before CsA treatment. These observations suggest that CsA is a good inhibitor of primary antibody responses, but only a weak inhibitor of secondary (already established) antibody responses, whereas it is effective on already established T-cell mediated immunity. This could explain the very low proportion of patients treated with CsA alone who develop infections (against which established antibody-mediated immunity is important).

CsA is primarily a Th1 cell inhibitor, but it can also act on Th2 cells

The distinction between T-helper type 1 (Th1) and Th2 CD4 cells represents a major progress in the understanding of T-cell functions. Th1 cells are characterized by their capacity to produce interleukin-2 (IL-2) and interferon-γ, whereas Th2 cells produce IL-4, IL-5, IL-10 and IL-13. Th1 cells are the main effectors of T-cell mediated immunity (possibly but not necessarily in collaboration with CD8 T-cells). Th2 cells play a major role for the production of some antibody isotypes notably IgE, eosinophil production, cell-mediated hypersensitivity and down-regulation of Th1 cells. There is little doubt that CsA acts primarily on Th1 cells. This is well illustrated by its effects on allograft rejection and on T-cell mediated autoimmune diseases. The problem is to know whether the drug also affects Th2 cells through the inhibition of the production of their specific cytokines. The study of CsA effect on several immune-mediated diseases argues in that direction. CsA has proven to be capable of improving chronic asthma [8] and atopic dermatitis [5] in a spectacular way, two diseases generally thought to be due to the pathogenic effect of Th2 cells.

The CsA effect on Th2 cytokine production is also suggested by a number of experimental studies. The inhibition of IL-4 production by CsA is well established and its precise level of action on the initiation of gene transcription in activated T-cells is well documented, which contrasts with the CsA resistance of ultimate stages of IL-4 synthesis [19]. CsA (1 µg/ml) markedly reduces IL-4-induced IgE and IgG production [20]. One may also mention that CsA has been reported to inhibit IL-4-receptor expression in human peripheral blood mononuclear cells after T-cell activation by anti-CD3 antibody, but not by IL-2 or IL-4. Interestingly, addition of IL-4 whose production is reduced by CsA prevents the effect of CsA on anti-CD3 induced IL-4 receptor expression [21].

The inhibitory effect on IL-5 production has been observed concomitantly with inhibition of allergic airway eosinophilic inflammation [22]. It was further shown that CsA inhibits IL-5-mediated mechanisms in eosinophils which resulted in enhanced survival and release of granule contents [23]. Detailed biochemical studies directly showed that CsA inhibited IL-5 mRNA levels by inhibition of gene transcription. Thus, CsA inhibits the production of IL-4 and IL-5 by a murine Th2-type cell clone at the IC_{50} value of 73 nmol/l for IL-4 and 242 nmol/l for IL-5 [24]. Finally, it it noteworthy to mention the inhibition of anti-CD3-induced IL-10 production by *in vivo* treatment with CsA at the total dose of 50 mg/kg, both at the mRNA and protein levels. Interestingly, in contrast CsA markedly enhances LPS-induced IL-10 release [25].

The question of a CsA effect on non-Th1/non-Th2 cytokines remains unsolved. The intriguing observation that CsA may enhance the production of transforming growth factor-β in some settings both *in vitro* and *in vivo* [26–30] obscures the problem further, since CsA may inhibit the pharmacological effect of transforming growth factor-β on human lung small airway epithelial cell proliferation [26]. This effect of CsA on transforming growth factor-β production could have implications as a contributing factor to its immunosuppressive effect, but also on the drug induced nephrotoxicity [31, 32].

As a further factor of complication, CsA unexpectedly enhances production of IL-12, a Th1 promoter, in murine splenocytes induced by CpG nucleotide sequences in DNA [33]. This effect could be due to a negative effect of IL-10 on IL-2 production as suggested by the absence of effect of CpG DNA on IL-12 production in IL-10$^{-/-}$ mice [33]. Finally, the picture is complicated by isolated reports indicating enhancement of IgE synthesis [34] or of IL-13 production under the combined influence of anti-CD28, phorbol myristate acetate and anti-CD3 antibody [35].

CsA does not induce tolerance

An important debate in clinical transplantation is to determine whether CsA influences the induction of tolerance to allografts. There no doubt that a state of "almost" tolerance as coined by R. Calne develops in most long-term organ allograft recipients. This is strongly suggested by the possibility of decreasing the strength of immunosuppression in such patients and even stopping it in a few cases, particularly liver transplant recipients, without harm to the graft. Some of these patients received CsA for a long period of time but the drug was given in combination with many other immunosuppressive agents. It has been reported that when CsA is given together with OKT3 rather than sequentially (stopping CsA during the first days of OKT3 administration) the long-term transplantation success was decreased [36]. This unfavorable interaction is also illustrated in experimental models by the inhibition by CsA of the tolerance induced by anti-CD154 (CD40 ligand) antibodies combined with CTLA4-Ig [37].

Data obtained in autoimmune diseases provide a relatively clear answer to this question. CsA does not restore tolerance to autoantigens since in all clinical settings discussed above, the clinical effect disappears some weeks after cessation of treatment. In other words, CsA has a major inhibitory effect on the autoimmune response, but this effect is only suspensive.

On the other hand, there has been no report of worsening of autoimmune diseases under CsA therapy excluding so far the risk of an undesirable effect of CsA on Th2 cytokines which might have led to disease exacerbation. Thus, there is no suggestion that CsA may contribute to the loss of tolerance independently of drug combinations which are not used so far in autoimmune diseases.

CsA-induced nephrotoxicity can be controlled and does not tend to progress after cessation of treatment

Alarming reports have indicated that CsA at high dosage could induce severe irreversible nephrotoxicity, notably in heart allograft recipients in whom the largest doses are used [38]. Similarly, significant nephrotoxicity was reported in patients with uveitis given doses of the order of 10 mg/kg/d for periods of time up to 6–12 months [9]. The problem of nephrotoxicity has been attenuated in organ transplantation by the usage of triple or quadruple therapy that allows reducing CsA dosage very significantly while keeping a satisfactory level of immunosuppression. Even in these conditions though nephrotoxicity remains a significant problem with the double question of distinguishing between CsA induced nephrotoxicity and rejection (in the case of renal transplantation) and assessing the long-term outcome (reversibility) of CsA-induced lesions. Autoimmune patients represent in that regard a unique model to approach these questions.

The most extensive studies of CsA-induced nephotoxicity have been performed in psoriasis [39] and type 1 diabetes [40, 41] and to a lesser degree in patients treated by CsA for rheumatoid arthritis, nephrotic syndrome and systemic lupus erythematosus [1]. Several major observations were derived from these studies [39–41]:

1. At doses around 5 mg/kg/d or less, one may observe an initial rise in creatinine values but this renal failure is functional and usually totally reversible. This benign outcome is also observed in patients with previous glomerular involvement associated with their disease (nephrotic syndrome, systemic lupus erythematosus). Hypertension is exceptionally observed.

2. At higher dosage (5–8 mg/kg/d) chronic nephrotoxicity may be observed in a significant number of cases. In a series of 125 biopsies performed in diabetics treated with an average dosage of 7 mg/kg/d for periods of 1–2 years, we have observed renal lesions in 34% of patients, with minimal or slight lesions in 53% and moderate lesions (arteriolopathy, stripes of interstitial fibrosis). Other recent reports have confirmed this risk in a limited number of patients treated with CsA for psoriasis [42–47], rheumatoid arthritis [48–50] or atopic dermatitis [51, 52]. Hypertension was observed in 13% of patients, always controlled by reduction of CsA dosage or administration of anti-hypertensive agents.

3. A systematic study of factors predictive of histologically-proven nephrotoxicity indicated that the best predictor was the initial rise of creatininemia (even though this rise was usually reversible [39]). There was some correlation with average drug dosage and CsA trough levels, but this correlation was less significant than with creatinine rise.

4. The long-term follow-up (6–10 years) after cessation of CsA therapy (which usually occurred 18–24 months after initiating the treatment) provided highly reassuring information (Tabs 2 and 3).

To assess such long-term nephrotoxicity, 285 recently-diagnosed type 1 diabetic patients having received CsA for a mean of 20 months were monitored for 13 years, in parallel with 100 similar patients treated with insulin alone. Inulin and p-aminohippurate (PAH) clearances remained normal throughout follow-up. Neither permanent renal failure, nor progressive deterioration of renal function occurred in either group, or in individual patients. A 10–12% increase in inulin and PAH clearance was observed by intravenous aminoacid infusion at 7–10 years, a finding consistent with a normal renal functional reserve. Patients with moderate kidney lesions on biopsy at 1 year had normal and stable clearance values at 7–13 years. The prevalence of arterial hyper-

Table 2. Correlation between the kidney lesions on biopsy at 12 months following initiation of CsA treatment and the renal function tested at the same time and 5–13 years later

	Kidney lesion Score	Renal function at 12 months (n)	Renal function after 6–13 years (n)
GFR[a] (ml/min)	0	106 ± 5 (19)	122 ± 9 (4)
	1	97 ± 7 (19)	103 ± 3 (8)
	2–3	89 ± 10 (13)	104 ± 3 (11)
RPF[b] (ml/min)	0	607 ± 43 (39)	564 ± 22 (4)
	1	547 ± 42 (19)	497 ± 28 (8)
	2–3	513 ± 39 (13)	459 ± 25 (11)

Histological score: 0, absence of visible tubulo-interstitial lesions; 1, minimal interstitial fibrosis; 2, slight tubulo-interstitial lesions; 3, moderate to severe tubulo-interstitial and/or arteriolar lesions.
[a] Glomerular filtration rate corresponds to the inulin clearance.
[b] Renal plasma flow corresponds to the p-aminohippurate (PAH) clearance.
Data presented are mean values ± SEM

Table 3. Serum creatinine levels over short time in a cohort of adult diabetic patients receiving CsA treatment for a mean duration of 15 months (median)[a]

	Baseline	Follow-up time[b] (years)							
		1	2	3	4	5	6	7	8–10
	(n=174)	(n=129)	(n = 99)	(n = 60)	(n = 42)	(n = 41)	(n = 39)	(n = 27)	(n =12)
Serum creatinine (µmol/l)	77 ± 1	92 ± 2	7 ± 1	86 ± 2	81 ± 4	81 ± 2	86 ± 3	82 ± 5	73 ± 6
Percent change over baseline	–	19 ± 2	14 ± 2	14 ± 3	20 ± 6	10 ± 2	14 ± 3	10 ± 2	0

Data presented are mean values ± SEM.
[a] Started between 1983 and 1989
[b] Taken from the initiation of CsA treatment.

tension and retinopathy was paradoxically lower in the CsA-treated group than in the control group, possibly due to the tighter metabolic control obtained in the CsA group. These results suggest that moderate-dose CsA treatment combined with thorough monitoring does not result in long-term renal dysfunction.

Concerning other diseases, one has to mention that CsA nephrotoxicity was apparently more severe in rheumatoid arthritis [1], probably due to the concomitant usage of nonsteroidal anti-inflammatory agents.

Dose-dependency of the immunosuppressive effect of CsA

It has been well established in autoimmune diseases that the dose dependency of the therapeutic effect of CsA varies according to the disease state, whether one considers the dosage effectively given (expressed in mg/kg/d) or, perhaps in a more relevant fashion, the CsA blood levels (peak level, area under the curve, or most often trough level). Taking drug dosage as a reference, it appears that the minimal effective dosage is 6–7 mg/kg/d in insulin-dependent diabetes mellitus [7], 5–6 mg/kg/d in uveitis [3], 5 mg/kg/d in nephrotic syndrome [6] and rheumatoid arthritis [4], and, intriguingly enough, significantly less (2–5 mg/kg/d) in psoriasis [2]. The reasons for such variations are not known. One may think that the drug has different modes of action in these various diseases. There is indeed some suggestion from *in vitro* studies that CsA could act in psoriasis directly on keratinocyte proliferation (independently of immunosuppression). The recent observation discussed above that anti-CD4 monoclonal antibodies achieve the same effect as CsA [10, 11] and the observation that the CsA induced disease remission is associated with disappearance of CD4[+] T-cells from the skin, do not favor this hypothesis. More likely, the difference in minimal efficacious dosage relates to the intensity of T-cell preactivation which is probably higher in recently diagnosed diabetics than in psoriatic patients. Studies of the drug effect at various phases of the natural history of non-obese diabetic (NOD) mice have indeed shown that CsA was much more efficient early in the disease than in the late stages (independently of the size of beta-cell mass) [53]. Extrapolated to transplantation these data indicate that there is not a unique efficacious CsA dosage (or blood level), but that the useful dosage depends on the individual patient (the intensity of the T-cell response).

It is interesting in this regard to note that CsA is not commonly used to cure hyperacute T-cell mediated pathogenic responses, except perhaps at very high dosage. Similarly, in most severe forms of inflammatory bowel diseases (ulcerative colitis and Crohn's disease), CsA is not efficacious when given orally, but is fully efficacious when given as a continuous infusion at the dosage of 4 mg/kg/d for 14 days. In these conditions, CsA has proven capable of avoiding colectomy in such patients [54, 55]. This observation might suggest that at such intravenous dosage, CsA could be efficacious in treating rejection episodes. This is just a theoretical comment though, at variance with inflammatory bowel disease, one cannot really afford such therapy for allograft rejection episodes inasmuch as transplanted patients are usually already impregnated with CsA at the time of rejection and will receive it ultimately as maintenance therapy: this makes the increased risk of acute nephrotoxicity brought by this short-term intensive CsA therapy hardly acceptable.

The risk of overimmunosuppression (particularly of tumors) is tightly dosage and duration dependent and is not specific to the drug

At variance with understandable fears, CsA therapy in autoimmune diseases has never been reported to be associated with increased risk of opportunistic infections. One does not observe in particular cytomegalovirus or Epstein-Barr virus infections seen in transplant recipients treated with multiple immunosuppressive therapy. Even "benign" infections do not show an increased frequency as demonstrated by a placebo-controlled study [7]. This is a highly satisfactory observation which poses, however, the question of how clinically immunosuppressive doses of CsA are not associated with increased risks of infection. As discussed above, one explanation is that CsA is essentially immunosuppressive on primary immune responses while many if not most severe opportunistic infections are due to widely represented pathogens that have already elicited primary immune responses.

The case of malignancies presents similar features with, however, more uncertainty. Lymphoma, the most commonly observed neoplasia in organ allograft recipients, is exceptionally seen in CsA-treated patients with autoimmune diseases (Tab. 4). The rate of 1 per 1000 should be regarded in relation to the apparently increased incidence of such lymphomas in the autoimmune diseases in question. There is thus a well-known association of lymphoma with

Table 4. Incidences of malignancies in CsA-treated patients

	n	Skin cancers	Solid tumors	Lymphomas
Kidney transplant recipients	4040	5	8	3
Heart transplant recipients	800		1	15
Psoriasis	2520	10	10	1
Rheumatoid arthritis	1000	4	13	1
Type 1 diabetes	480	0	0	0
Nephrotic syndrome	661	0	4	2

Data presented are incidences per 1000
Data from references [57–59]

Table 5. Factors predisposing to cancer in autoimmune diseases

		Nb of reported cases	Relative risk
Psoriasis			
PUVA therapy			23.8
Others			1.7
Rheumatoid arthritis			
Solid tumors	Breast	3	<2.5
	Lung	2	(age 55–65 years)
	Colon	3	
	Others	5	
Nephrotic syndrome			
Hodgkin's lymphoma		2	
Others		3	

Data from references [57–59]

nephrotic syndrome. Malignancies other than lymphomas have been reported in CsA-treated autoimmune patients (Tabs 4 and 5), but again one has to carefully assess the direct causal relationship with CsA. Such a relationship is unlikely for tumors whose frequency is not increased in transplant recipients submitted to heavy T-cell directed multiple immunosuppressive therapy, e.g., breast, colon or lung cancers. It remains open for other tumors even when considering previous potentially oncogenic therapy received by the patients (e.g., psoralen ultraviolet A (PUVA) therapy in psoriasis, alkylating agents in rheumatoid arthritis or systemic lupus erythematosus). It is noteworthy that monitoring a cohort of diabetic patients treated for 1–2 years by CsA at doses of 6–7 mg/kg/d, we did not observe either a single case of malignancy or any restriction of serum immunoglobulin heterogeneity and rise in antibodies to Epstein-Barr virus, two biological manifestations known to accompany (or precede) the Epstein-Barr virus-associated Burkitt's type lymphomas favored by CsA therapy [56].

Taken together, these data do not allow to exclude the infectious or the malignant risks in patients treated with CsA alone, and they urge for caution in long-term treatment, but they also indicate that if it exists the risk is minimal. An important problem is to determine the threshold under which this risk becomes negligible.

References

1 Bach JF, Strom TB (eds) (1985) *The mode of action of immunosuppressive agents. (Research Monographs in Immunology, vol. 9)*. Amsterdam: Elsevier

2 Lebwohl M, Ellis C, Gottlieb A, Koo J, Krueger G, Linden K, Shupack J, Weinstein G (1998) Cyclosporine consensus conference: with emphasis on the treatment of psoriasis. *J Amer Acad Dermatol* 39: 464–475

3 Dick AD, Azim M, Forrester JV (1997) Immunosuppressive therapy for chronic uveitis: optimising therapy with steroids and cyclosporin A. *Brit J Ophtalmol* 81: 1107–1112

4 Yocum DE, Torley H (1995) Cyclosporine in rheumatoid arthritis. *Rheum Dis Clin N Amer* 21: 835–844

5 Stephens RB, Lee ML, Cooper A (1994) Cyclosporin treatment of atopic dermatitis: five case studies and literature review. *Australas J Dermatol* 35: 55–59

6 Meyrier A (1997) Treatment of idiopathic nephrotic syndrome with cyclosporine A. *J Nephrol* 10: 14–24

7 Feutren G, Papoz L, Assan R, Vialettes B, Karsenty G, Vexiau P, Du Rostu H, Rodier M, Sirmai J, Lallemand A et al (1986) Cyclosporin increases the rate and length of remissions in insulin-dependent diabetes of recent onset. Results of a multicentre double-blind trial. *Lancet* 2: 119–124

8 Coren ME, Rosenthal M, Bush A (1997) The use of cyclosporin in corticosteroid dependent asthma. *Arch Dis Child* 77: 522–523

9 Palestine AG, Austin Ha 3D, Balow JE, Antonovych TT, Sabnis SG, Preuss HG, Nussenblatt RB (1986) Renal histopathologic alterations in patients treated with cyclosporine for uveitis. *N Engl J Med* 314: 1293–1298

10 Nicolas JF, Chamchick N, Thivolet J, Wijdenes J, Morel P, Revillard JP (1991) CD4 antibody treatment of severe psoriasis. *Lancet* 338: 321

11 Bachelez H, Flageul B, Dubertret L, Fraitag S, Grossman R, Brousse N, Poisson D, Knowles RW, Wacholtz MC, Haverty TP et al (1998) Treatment of recalcitrant plaque psoriasis with a humanized non-depleting antibody to CD4. *J Autoimmun* 11: 53–62

12 Dantal J, Bigot E, Bogers W, Testa A, Kriaa F, Jacques Y, Hurault de Ligny B, Niaudet P, Charpentier B, Soulillou JP (1994) Effect of plasma protein adsorption on protein excretion in kidney-transplant recipients with recurrent nephrotic syndrome. *N Engl J Med* 330: 7–14

13 Tindall RS, Rollins JA, Phillips JT, Greenlee RG, Wells L, Belendiuk G (1987) Preliminary results of a double-blind, randomized, placebo-controlled trial of cyclosporine in myasthenia gravis. *N Engl J Med* 316: 719–724

14 Feutren G, Querin S, Noel LH, Chatenoud L, Beaurain G, Tron F, Lesavre P, Bach JF (1987) Effects of cyclosporine in severe systemic lupus erythematosus. *J Pediat* 111: 1063–1068

15 Favre H, Miescher PA, Huang YP, Chatelanat F, Mihatsch MJ (1989) Cyclosporin in the treatment of lupus nephritis. *Amer J Nephrol* 9: 57–60

16 Takahashi S, Nose M, Sasaki J, Yamamoto T, Kyogoku M (1991) IgG3 production in MRL/lpr mice is responsible for development of lupus nephritis. *J Immunol* 147: 515–519

17 Muller C, Zielinski CC, Kalinowski W, Wolf H, Mannhalter JW, Aschauer Treiber G, Klosch Kasparek D, Gaube S, Eibl MM, Schernthaner G (1989) Effects of cyclosporin A upon humoral and cellular immune parameters in insulin-dependent diabetes mellitus type I: a long-term follow-up study. *J Endocrinol* 121: 177–183

18 Boitard C, Feutren G, Castano L, Debray-Sachs M, Assan R, Hors J, Bach JF (1987) Effect of cyclosporin A treatment on the production of antibody in insulin-dependent (type I) diabetic patients. *J Clin Invest* 80: 1607–1612

19 Terada N, Or R, Weinberg K, Domenico J, Lucas JJ, Gelfand EW (1992) Transcription of IL-2 and IL-4 genes is not inhibited by cyclosporin A in competent T cells. *J Biol Chem* 267: 21 207–21 210

20 Renz H, Mazer BD, Gelfand EW (1990) Differential inhibition of T- and B-cell function in IL-4-

dependent IgE production by cyclosporin A and methylprednisolone. *J Immunol* 145: 3641–3646

21 Foxwell BM, Woerly G, Ryffel B (1990) Inhibition of interleukin 4 receptor expression on human lymphoid cells by cyclosporin. *Eur J Immunol* 20: 1185–1188

22 Wada K, Kaminuma O, Mori A, Nakata A, Ogawa K, Kikkawa H, Ikezawa K, Suko M, Okudaira H (1998) IL-5-producing T cells that induce airway eosinophilia and hyperresponsiveness are suppressed by dexamethasone and cyclosporin A in mice. *Int Arch Allergy Immunol* 117 Suppl 1: 24–27

23 Meng Q, Ying S, Corrigan CJ, Wakelin M, Assoufi B, Moqbel R, Kay AB (1997) Effects of rapamycin, cyclosporin A, and dexamethasone on interleukin 5-induced eosinophil degranulation and prolonged survival. *Allergy* 52: 1095–1101

24 Schmidt J, Fleissner S, Heimann Weitschat I, Lindstaedt R, Szelenyi I (1994) The effect of different corticosteroids and cyclosporin A on interleukin-4 and interleukin-5 release from murine TH2-type T cells. *Eur J Pharmacol* 260: 247–250

25 Durez P, Abramowicz D, Gerard C, Van Mechelen M, Amraoui Z, Dubois C, Leo O, Velu T, Goldman M (1993) *In vivo* induction of interleukin 10 by anti-CD3 monoclonal antibody or bacterial lipopolysaccharide: differential modulation by cyclosporin A. *J Exp Med* 177: 551–555

26 Zhang JG, Walmsley MW, Moy JV, Cunningham AC, Talbot D, Dark JH, Kirby JA (1998) Differential effects of cyclosporin A and tacrolimus on the production of TGF-beta: implications for the development of obliterative bronchiolitis after lung transplantation. *Transplant Int* 11 Suppl 1: S325-S327

27 Shin GT, Khanna A, Ding R, Sharma VK, Lagman M, Li B, Suthanthiran M (1998) *In vivo* expression of transforming growth factor-beta1 in humans: stimulation by cyclosporine. *Transplantation* 65: 313–318

28 Wolf G, Zahner G, Ziyadeh FN, Stahl RA (1996) Cyclosporin A induces transcription of transforming growth factor beta in a cultured murine proximal tubular cell line. *Exp Nephrol* 4: 304–308

29 Ahuja SS, Shrivastav S, Danielpour D, Balow JE, Boumpas DT (1995) Regulation of transforming growth factor-beta 1 and its receptor by cyclosporine in human T lymphocytes. *Transplantation* 60: 718–723

30 Prashar Y, Khanna A, Sehajpal P, Sharma VK, Suthanthiran M (1995) Stimulation of transforming growth factor-beta 1 transcription by cyclosporine. *FEBS Lett* 358: 109–112

31 Khanna A, Li B, Sharma VK, Suthanthiran M (1996) Immunoregulatory and fibrogenic activities of cyclosporine: a unifying hypothesis based on transforming growth factor-beta expression. *Transplant Proc* 28: 2015–2018

32 Shihab FS, Andoh TF, Tanner AM, Noble NA, Border WA, Franceschini N, Bennett WM (1996) Role of transforming growth factor-beta 1 in experimental chronic cyclosporine nephropathy. *Kidney Int* 49: 1141–1151

33 Redford TW, Yi AK, Ward CT, Krieg AM (1998) Cyclosporin A enhances IL-12 production by CpG motifs in bacterial DNA and synthetic oligodeoxynucleotides. *J Immunol* 161: 3930–3935

34 Chang CC, Aversa G, Punnonen J, Yssel H, de Vries JE (1993) Brequinar sodium, mycophenolic acid, and cyclosporin A inhibit different stages of IL-4- or IL-13-induced human IgG4 and IgE production *in vitro*. *Ann N Y Acad Sci* 696: 108–122

35 Van Der Pouw Kraan TC, Boeije LC, Troon JT, Rutschmann SK, Wijdenes J, Aarden LA (1996) Human IL-13 production is negatively influenced by CD3 engagement. Enhancement of IL-13 production by cyclosporin A. *J Immunol* 156: 1818–1823

36 Opelz G (1995) Efficacy of rejection prophylaxis with OKT3 in renal transplantation. Collaborative Transplant Study. *Transplantation* 60: 1220–1224

37 Larsen CP, Elwood ET, Alexander DZ, Ritchie SC, Hendrix R, Tuckerburden C, Cho HR, Aruffo A, Hollenbaugh D, Linsley PS et al (1996) Long-term acceptance of skin and cardiac allografts after blocking CD40 and CD28 pathways. *Nature* 381: 434–438

38 Myers BD, Ross J, Newton L, Luetscher J, Perlroth M (1984) Cyclosporine-associated chronic nephropathy. *N Engl J Med* 311: 699–705

39 Feutren G, Mihatsch MJ (1992) Risk factors for cyclosporine-induced nephropathy in patients with autoimmune diseases. (International kidney biopsy registry of cyclosporine in autoimmune diseases). *N Engl J Med* 326: 1654–1660

40 Bach JF, Feutren G, Noel LH, Hannedouche T, Landais P, Timsit J, Boitard C, Bougneres P, Grunfeld JP, Assan R (1990) Factors predictive of cyclosporine-induced nephrotoxicity: the role of cyclosporine blood levels. *Transplant Proc* 22: 1296–1298

41 Assan R, Timsit J, Feutren G, Bougneres P, Czernichow P, Hannedouche T, Boitard C, Noel LH, Mihatsch MJ, Bach JF (1994) The kidney in cyclosporin A-treated diabetic patients: a long-term clinicopathological study. *Clin Nephrol* 41: 41–49

42 Young EW, Ellis CN, Messana JM, Johnson KJ, Leichtman AB, Mihatsch MJ, Hamilton TA, Groisser DS, Fradin MS, Voorhees JJ (1994) A prospective study of renal structure and function in psoriasis patients treated with cyclosporin. *Kidney Int* 46: 1216–1222

43 Pei Y, Scholey JW, Katz A, Schachter R, Murphy GF, Cattran D (1994) Chronic nephrotoxicity in psoriatic patients treated with low-dose cyclosporine. *Amer J Kidney Dis* 23: 528–536

44 Lowe NJ, Wieder JM, Rosenbach A, Johnson K, Kunkel R, Bainbridge C, Bourget T, Dimov I, Simpson K, Glass E et al (1996) Long-term low-dose cyclosporine therapy for severe psoriasis: effects on renal function and structure. *J Amer Acad Dermatol* 35: 710–719

45 Grossman RM, Chevret S, Abi Rached J, Blanchet F, Dubertret L (1996) Long-term safety of cyclosporine in the treatment of psoriasis. *Arch Dermatol* 132: 623–629

46 Zachariae H, Kragballe K, Hansen HE, Marcussen N, Olsen S (1997) Renal biopsy findings in long-term cyclosporin treatment of psoriasis. *Brit J Dermatol* 136: 531–535

47 Powles AV, Hardman CM, Porter WM, Cook T, Hulme B, Fry L (1998) Renal function after 10 years' treatment with cyclosporin for psoriasis. *Brit J Dermatol* 138: 443–449

48 Rodriguez F, Krayenbuhl JC, Harrison WB, Forre O, Dijkmans BA, Tugwell P, Miescher PA, Mihatsch MJ (1996) Renal biopsy findings and followup of renal function in rheumatoid arthritis patients treated with cyclosporin A. An update from the International Kidney Biopsy Registry. *Arthritis Rheum* 39: 1491–1498

49 Sund S, Forre O, Berg KJ, Kvien TK, Hovig T (1994) Morphological and functional renal effects of long-term low-dose cyclosporin A treatment in patients with rheumatoid arthritis. *Clin Nephrol* 41: 33–40

50 Landewe RB, Dijkmans BA, Van Der Woude FJ, Breedveld FC, Mihatsch MJ, Bruijn JA (1996) Longterm low dose cyclosporine in patients with rheumatoid arthritis: renal function loss without structural nephropathy. *J Rheum* 23: 61–64

51 Zonneveld IM, de Rie MA, Beljaards RC, Van Der Rhee HJ, Wuite J, Zeegelaar J, Bos JD (1996) The long-term safety and efficacy of cyclosporin in severe refractory atopic dermatitis: a comparison of two dosage regimens. *Brit J Dermatol* 135 Suppl 48: 15–20

52 Berth-Jones J, Graham Brown RA, Marks R, Camp RD, English JS, Freeman K, Holden CA, Rogers SC, Oliwiecki S, Friedmann PS et al (1997) Long-term efficacy and safety of cyclosporin in severe adult atopic dermatitis. *Brit J Dermatol* 136: 76–81

53 Wang Y, McDuffie M, Nomikos IN, Hao L, Lafferty KJ (1988) Effect of cyclosporine on immunologically mediated diabetes in nonobese diabetic mice. *Transplantation* 46: 101S-106S

54 Hanauer SB, Smith MB (1993) Rapid closure of Crohn's disease fistulas with continuous intravenous cyclosporin A. *Amer J Gastroenterol* 88: 646–649

55 Actis GC, Ottobrelli A, Pera A, Barletti C, Ponti V, Pinna Pintor M, Verme G (1993) Continuously infused cyclosporine at low dose is sufficient to avoid emergency colectomy in acute attacks of ulcerative colitis without the need for high-dose steroids. *J Clin Gastroenterol* 17: 10–13

56 Feutren G, de The G, Bach JF (1992) Epstein-Barr virus serology and isoelectrofocusing pattern of serum immunoglobulins in cyclosporin or placebo-treated type I diabetics. *J Autoimmun* 5: 161–172

57 Cockburn IT, Krupp P (1989) The risk of neoplasms in patients treated with cyclosporine A. *J Autoimmun* 2: 723–731

58 Arellano F, Krupp P (1993) Malignancies in rheumatoid arthritis patients treated with cyclosporin A. *Brit J Rheumatol* 32 Suppl 1: 72–75

59 Collaborative Study Group of Sandimmun in Nephrotic Syndrome (1991) Safety and tolerability of cyclosporin A (Sandimmun) in idiopathic nephrotic syndrome. *Clin Nephrol* 35 Suppl 1: S48–S60

Subject index